Management of Complex Cardiovascular Problems

FOURTH EDITION

D1073349

EDITED BY

Thach Nguyen, MD, FACC FSCAI
Director of Cardiovascular Research
Methodist Hospital
Merrillville IN 46410

Dayi Hu, MD FACC FHRS FESC
Director of the Intervention Center at Peking
University People's Hospital,
President, Chinese College of Cardiovascular
Physician (CCCP), Beijing, China

Shao Liang Chen MD
Professor of Cardiology
Professor of Internal Medicine
Deputy President, Nanjing First Hospital,
Nanjing Medical University
Director of Catheterization Laboratories,
Nanjing First Hospital
Chief of Cardiology Nanjing First Hospital
Nanjing, China

Moo-Hyun Kim, MD, FACC
Associate Professor of Medicine
Director, Cardiology Department
Dong A University
Busan, Korea

Cindy Grines, MD
Vice President Academic and Clinical Affairs,
Detroit Medical Center Heart Hospital
Detroit, MI

ASSOCIATE EDITOR

Faisal Latif, MD
Associate Professor of Medicine,
University of Oklahoma, OKC, OK

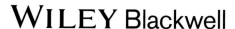

This edition first published 2016 © 2016 by John Wiley & Sons Ltd

Registered office: John Wiley & Sons, Ltd, The Atrium, Southern Gate, Chichester, West Sussex, PO19 8SQ, UK

Editorial offices: 9600 Garsington Road, Oxford, OX4 2DQ, UK
The Atrium, Southern Gate, Chichester, West Sussex, PO19 8SQ, UK
111 River Street, Hoboken, NJ 07030-5774, USA

For details of our global editorial offices, for customer services and for information about how to apply for permission to reuse the copyright material in this book please see our website at www.wiley.com/wiley-blackwell

Library of Congress Cataloging-in-Publication Data:

Names: Nguyen, Thach, editor. | Hu, Dayi, editor. | Chen, Shao Liang, editor.
| Kim, Moo-Hyun (Cardiologist), editor. | Grines, Cindy, editor.
Title: Management of complex cardiovascular problems / edited by Thach Nguyen, Dayi Hu, Shao Liang Chen, Moo-Hyun Kim, Cindy Grines ; associate editor, Faisal Latiff.
Description: Fourth edition. | Chichester, West Sussex, UK ; Hoboken, NJ : John Wiley & Sons Inc., 2016. | Includes bibliographical references and index.
Identifiers: LCCN 2015035763 (print) | LCCN 2015036342 (ebook) | ISBN 9781118965030 (cloth) | ISBN 9781118965047 (Adobe PDF) | ISBN 9781118965054 (ePub)
Subjects: | MESH: Cardiovascular Diseases–therapy. | Evidence-Based Medicine.
Classification: LCC RC671 (print) | LCC RC671 (ebook) | NLM WG 120 | DDC 616.1/2–dc23
LC record available at http://lccn.loc.gov/2015035763

A catalogue record for this book is available from the British Library.

Wiley also publishes its books in a variety of electronic formats. Some content that appears in print may not be available in electronic books.

Cover image: gettyimages.com © Janulla

Set in 8/10pt Frutiger Light by Aptara Inc., New Delhi, India

Printed in Singapore by C.O.S. Printers Pte Ltd

1   2016

Contents

List of Contributors

NABEEL ALI, MD
Xavier University School of Medicine, Aruba

HY TAT AN
MS Class of 2020 Tan Tao University School of Medicine
Tan Duc E-City, Duc Hoa – Long An Vietnam

KHALID NUMAN AL AZZA, MD
Jordan University of Science and Technology
Irbid, Jordan

AMAN M. AMANULLAH, MD, PhD, FACC, FAHA
Clinical Professor of Medicine
Sidney Kimmel Medical College of Thomas Jefferson University
Section Chief, Noninvasive Cardiology, Albert Einstein Medical Center
Philadelphia, PA 19141

AMSA ARSHAD, MD
Xavier University School of Medicine, Aruba

NISA ARSHAD, MD
Xavier University School of Medicine, Aruba

CHRISTOPHER M. BIANCO, MD
Cardiology Fellow
The Brody School of Medicine at East Carolina University
Greenville, NC

THOMAS BUMP, MD
Clinical Associate Professor, University of Chicago
Clinical Assistant Professor, University of Illinois at Chicago
Chicago, IL

PATRICK T. CAMPBELL, MD
Advanced Heart Failure Fellow
Section of Cardiomyopathy & Heart Transplantation
Ochsner Heart and Vascular Center, New Orleans

MIHAIL G. CHELU, MD, PHD, FHRS
Assistant Professor University of Utah School of Medicine
Electrophysiology Division Salt Lake City, UT

SHAO LIANG CHEN, MD, PhD, FACC
Professor of Cardiology
Professor of Internal Medicine
Deputy President, Nanjing First Hospital, Nanjing Medical University
Director of Catheterization Laboratories, Nanjing First Hospital
Chief of Cardiology, Nanjing First Hospital
Nanjing, China

NGUYEN DUC CONG, MD, PhD
Professor of Medicine
Director of Thong Nhat Hospital
Director of Geriatric Department of Pham Ngoc Thach Medical
    University
Vice Director of Geriatric Department, The University of Medicine and
    Pharmacy
Vice Director Department of Internal Medicine, School of Medicine, the
    National University of Hochiminh City, Hochiminh City, Vietnam

VIJAY DAVE, MD
Director of Medical Education
St Mary Medical Center Hobart, IN

HO THUONG DUNG, MD, PhD, FSCAI
Vice Director of Thong Nhat Hospital, HCM City
Vice Chairman of Interventional Cardiology Association of HCM City
Hochiminh City, Vietnam

MARVIN H. ENG, MD
Structural Heart Disease Fellowship Director
Center for Structural Heart Disease, Division of Cardiology
Henry Ford Health System, Detroit, MI

DANIEL FORMAN, MD
Professor of Medicine, University of Pittsburgh
Chair, Geriatric Cardiology Section, University of Pittsburgh Medical
    Center
Director, Cardiac Rehabilitation, VA Pittsburgh Healthcare System
Pittsburgh, PA

RUNLIN GAO, MD, FACC, FESC, FSCAI
Professor of Medicine
Member, Chinese Academy of Medical Sciences
Chief Cardiologist, Fuwai Hospital Beijing, China

C. MICHAEL GIBSON, MD
Director, TIMI Data Coordinating Center; *and* Associate Professor
Harvard Medical School; *and* Chief of Clinical Research, Cardiovascular
Division, Beth Israel Deaconess Medical Center, Boston, MA

CINDY GRINES MD
Vice President Academic and Clinical Affairs, Detroit Medical Center
  Heart Hospital
Professor of Medicine, Wayne State University School of Medicine,
  Detroit MI

RAJIV GOSWAMI DO
Assistant Professor of Medicine, Baylor College of Medicine
Ben Taub Hospital, Houston, Texas

NGUYEN LAN HIEU, MD, PhD
Vice director, Heart Center
Hanoi Medical University Hospital
Hanoi, Vietnam

BAO V. HO, MD, MSC
New York Institute of Technology, College of Osteopathic Medicine
Old Westbury, NY

DAYI HU, MD, FACC, FESC
Director of the Heart Center at Peking University People's Hospital,
  Beijing China
President of the China Heart Federation Beijing China

PHAM MANH HUNG, PHD, MD, FACC, FESC
Associate Professor, Hanoi Medical University
Secretary General, Vietnam National Heart Association
Director, Cardiac Catheterization Laboratories Vietnam National
  Heart Institute
Hanoi, Vietnam

PHAM NHU HUNG, MD, PhD, FACC, FASCC
Consultant of Cardiology and Electrophysiology
Director of Electrophysiology Laboratories, Hanoi Heart Hospital
Hanoi, Vietnam

PHAN NAM HUNG, MD
General Secretary, the Internal Medicine Society of Vietnam
Vice Chief, Cardiovascular Medicine Department, Binh Dinh
  General Hospital
Qui Nhon, Vietnam

AN HUYNH
MS Class of 2019, Tan Tao University School of Medicine
Tan Duc E-City, Duc Hoa – Long An Vietnam

HUNG D. HUYNH
Senior Research Associate, Community Healthcare System, St Mary
Medical Center, Hobart, IN; *and* Webmaster, Riverside, CA

KIM N. HUYNH
Honor Student, Miss Hall's School
Vice President, International Student Alliance
Pittsfield, MA

KAHROBA JAHAN MD
Division of Cardiology, Sarver Heart Center
Banner University Medical Center South Campus
University of Arizona, Tucson, AZ

DEEPAK JOSHI, MD
Cardiology Fellow
The Brody School of Medicine at East Carolina University
Greenville, NC

MOO-HYUN KIM, MD, FACC, FSCAI
Director, Global Clinical Trial Center
Professor, Dept. of Cardiology, Dong-A University Hospital
Busan, Korea

NEAL KLEIMAN MD
Professor, Department of Medicine
Weill Cornell Medical College of Cornell University
Director, Applied Platelet Physiology Lab
Director, Cardiac Catheterization Laboratories
Houston Methodist DeBakey Heart & Vascular Center
Houston, TX

SELIM R. KRIM, MD
Staff, Section of Cardiomyopathy & Heart Transplantation
Ochsner Heart and Vascular Center, New Orleans LA

FAISAL LATIF, MD, FACC, FSCAI
Associate Professor of Medicine
Associate Program Director, Cardiology Fellowship Program
University of Oklahoma Health Sciences Center
Director, Cardiac Catheterization Laboratories
VA Medical Center, Oklahoma City, OK

SORIN LAZAR, MD
Electrophysiologist
Methodist Hospital, Merrillville, IN

DAN D. LE, MD
Cardiology Fellow
The Brody School of Medicine at East Carolina University
Greenville, NC

TRONG HA LE
MS Class of 2019 Tan Tao University School of Medicine
Tan Duc E-City, Duc Hoa – Long An Vietnam

KWAN S. LEE, MD FACC FSCAI
Medical Director of Cardiology
Director Cardiac Catheterization Laboratory
Banner University Medical Center South Campus
Sarver Heart Center, Banner University Medical Center South Campus
University of Arizona Tucson, AZ

XIAN KAI LI, MD, PhD
Cardiology Department
Shanghai Tenth People's Hospital of Tongji University
Shanghai, China

TUNG DINH MAI, DO
Resident, Department of Internal Medicine
Detroit Medical Center – Sinai Grace Hospital
Wayne State University – School of Medicine, Detroit, Michigan
Clinical faculty, Department of Medicine
Michigan State University – College of Osteopathic Medicine
East Lansing, Michigan

ARAVINDA NANJUNDAPPA, FACC, FSCAI, RVT
Professor of Medicine and Surgery
Director of TAVR Program
West Virginia University, Charleston, WV

CHISALU NCHEKWUBE, MD
Internal Medicine Residency Program
Department of Internal Medicine
University of Illinois Hospital and Health Sciences System
Chicago, IL

RAJASEKHAR NEKKANTI, MD FACC FASE CCDS
Associate Professor of Medicine
Program Director, Cardiology Fellowship Program
Director, Continuing Medical Education-Cardiovascular Series
East Carolina Heart Institute
The Brody School of Medicine at East Carolina University
Director, Echocardiography Laboratories
East Carolina Heart Institute at Vidant Medical Center
Greenville, NC

TAM NGO, MD
Resident in ophthalmology
University of Medicine and Pharmacy, Ho Chi Minh City, Viet Nam

LAN NGUYEN, MD
Universidad Autonóma de Guadalajara
Guadalajara, MX

NGUYEN PHUC NGUYEN, MD
Cardiology Department
St Mary Medical Center, Hobart, IN

NGOC-QUANG NGUYEN, MD, PhD, FASCC, FSCAI
Department of Cardiology, Hanoi Medical University
Head of Coronary Care Unit (C7), Vietnam National
    Heart Institute
Bach Mai Hospital, Hanoi, Vietnam

QUANG TUAN NGUYEN, MD, PHD, FACC, FSCAI
CEO, Hanoi Heart Hospital
Medical Director, Hanoi Heart Hospital
Associate professor, Hanoi Medical University
President, Vietnam Interventional Cardiology Society
President, Hanoi Heart Association, Hanoi, Vietnam

THACH NGUYEN, MD, FACC, FSCAI
Deputy Editor-in-chief, Interventional Cardiology Grand Rounds, NYC,
    NY, *and* Associate-editor-in-chief, Journal of Geriatric Cardiology,
    Beijing, China; *and* Editorial Consultant, Journal of Interventional
    Cardiology; Hoboken, NJ, *and* Chinese Medical Journal, Beijing,
    China, *and* Honorary Professor of Medicine, Hanoi Medical University,
    and Vietnam Heart Institute, Hanoi, Vietnam, *and* Capital University
    of Medical Sciences, Beijing, China; *and* The Institute of Geriatric
    Cardiology, 301 Hospital of the Chinese People's Liberation Army,
    Beijing, China; *and* Friendship Hospital, Beijing, *and* the Tenth

People's Hospital, Shanghai, China, *and* Visiting Professor, Nanjing First Hospital, Nanjing Medical University, Nanjing, China; *and* Clinical Assistant Professor of Medicine, Indiana University Northwest, IN, USA, Director of cardiovascular research Methodist hospital, Merrillville, IN; *and* Director of Cardiology, Community Healthcare System, St Mary Medical Center, Hobart, IN, USA

TUAN D. NGUYEN, DO
Candidate, Class of 2017
New York Institute of Technology, College of Osteopathic
  Medicine
Old Westbury, NY

ALI OTO, MD, FESC, FACC, FHRS
Professor of Cardiology
Chairman, Department of Cardiology,
MHG, Memorial Ankara Hospital
Ankara, Turkey

PHAN DINH PHONG, MD, PhD
Head of Training Center
Vietnam National Heart Institute
Bach Mai Hospital, Hanoi, Vietnam

DUANE PINTO, MD FACC FSCAI
Associate Professor of Medicine, Harvard Medical School
Director, General Cardiology Fellowship Program
Director, Cardiac Intensive Care Unit, Beth Israel Deaconess
  Medical Center
Boston MA

GIANLUCA RIGATELLI, MD, PhD, EBIR, FACP, FACC, FESC, FSCAI
Cardiovascular Diagnosis and Endoluminal Interventions Unit
Rovigo, General Hospital, Rovigo, Italy

MICHAEL RINALDI, MD
Interventional Cardiology and Vascular Medicine
Director, Clinical Research, Sanger Heart and Vascular Institute
Professor of Medicine, Carolinas HealthCare System
Charlotte, NC

MADHUR ROBERTS, MD
Cardiovascular Fellow, PGY 6
University of Tennessee Medical Center
Knoxville, TN

AINOL SHAREHA SAHAR, MD FACC FSCAI FNHAM SCIM
Senior Consultant Cardiologist
Deputy Head, Department of Cardiology
Penang General Hospital
Penang Malaysia

SARA SHAH
Honor Student, Munster High School
National Society of High School Scholar
Delegate, the Congress of Future Medical Leaders
2015 Nominee, National Youth Leadership Forum in Medicine

EVGENY SHLYAKHTO, MD, PhD, FESC, FACC
President, Russian Society of Cardiology
Director, Federal Almazov Heart Blood Endocrinology Centre
St Petersburg, Russian Federation

UDHO THADANI, MD, MRCP, FRCPC, FACC, FAHA
Professor Emeritus of Medicine University of Oklahoma Health Sciences
    Center
Consultant Cardiologist Oklahoma University Medical Center and VA
    Medical Center
Oklahoma City, OK

LÊ HOÀNG ĐỨC TOÀN
MS Class of 2019 Tan Tao University School of Medicine
Tan Duc E-City, Duc Hoa – Long An Vietnam

LÊ THỊ NGỌC TRÂM
MS Class of 2019, Tan Tao University School of Medicine
Tan Duc E-City, Duc Hoa – Long An Vietnam

HAU TRAN, MD, DO
New York Institute of Technology, College of Osteopathic Medicine
Old Westbury, NY

PHILLIP TRAN, DO
Cardiology fellow
Mercy Medical Center – North IA

HUÝNH THỊ THU TRÚC
MS Class of 2019 Tan Tao University School of Medicine
Tan Duc E-City, Duc Hoa – Long An Vietnam

VIEN THANH TRUONG, MD
Resident in Internal Medicine
Junior Lecturer, Internal Medicine Department
Pham Ngoc Thach University of Medicine, Ho Chi Minh City, Vietnam

M. HARIS U. USMAN, MD, MS
Interventional Cardiology Fellow
Detroit Medical Center, Wayne State University
Detroit MI

HECTOR O. VENTURA, MD, FACC, FACP
Director, Section of Cardiomyopathy & Heart Transplantation
Ochsner Heart and Vascular Center, New Orleans
New Orleans, LA

VÕ MINH VIỆT
MS Class of 2019 Tan Tao University School of Medicine
Tan Duc E-City, Duc Hoa – Long An Vietnam

YIDONG WEI, MD, FACC
Professor, Chief, Department of Cardiology
Shanghai Tenth People's Hospital of Tongji University
Shanghai, China

NANETTE K. WENGER, MD, MACC, MACP, FAHA
Professor of Medicine (Cardiology) Emeritus
Emory University School of Medicine
Consultant, Emory Heart and Vascular Center
Atlanta, GA

BO XU, MBBS
Director, Catheterization Laboratory
Fu Wai Hospital, National Center for Cardiovascular Diseases
Beijing, China

HAN YALING, MD, FACC, FESC
Academician of Chinese Academy of Engineering
President, Institute of Cardiovascular Medicine of PLA
Director, Department of Cardiology
General Hospital of Shenyang Military Region
Shenyang, Liaoning China

Foreword to the Third Edition

The modern cardiologist is confronted with a bewildering amount of new information. At last count there were more than one hundred cardiology journals. Many cardiology textbooks, covering every aspect of the field and dozens of symposia are published each year. The major cardiovascular centers all have their 'in house' publications, which emphasize their local accomplishments. In addition, industry bombards cardiologists with many reviews, each placing the sponsor's project and trial in the best light.

What the practicing cardiologist really needs is a text that emphasizes unbiased, up to date information and that places this information into an appropriate context. The third edition of *Management of Complex Cardiovascular Problems*, carefully edited by Dr. Nguyen, does precisely this.

Particularly new, reader friendly, features are the boxes of 'Take Home Messages' [Action Points in the Fourth Edition] which give succinct summaries of each chapter, together with *Critical Thinking* (new concepts); *Evidence-Based Medicine* (the key results of important clinical trials); and *Clinical Pearls* (advice from master clinicians).

This unique format provides busy cardiologists with an approach to deal with information overload and will thereby enhance the quality of care delivered to the cardiac patient. Thus, Dr. Thach Nguyen and his talented authors have again provided us with important ammunition for the war against heart disease. This fine book describes clearly some of the most difficult problems that cardiovascular specialists face, and it provides enormously helpful directions in dealing with them. This eminently readable book should be equally valuable to practicing cardiologists in the front lines of the battle against the global scourge of cardiovascular disease and to trainees in the field.

Eugene Braunwald, M.D.
Boston, Massachusetts

Preface

PRACTICING CARDIOLOGY IS LIKE CAR RACING AT THE INDY 500

When driving to work, do you drive in the fast lane? When using the internet, do you use a shortcut to open a new window? For short and quick communication, do you text or pick up the phone? In 2016, do cardiologists still work with 20th century mentality or do they see and work through a 21st century lens or Google Glass? In this fourth edition of *Management of Complex Cardiovascular Problems*, the authors and editors offer new strategic views and tactical maps similar to the ones used in car racing; they are presented, however, with the wit of a young broker in the middle of the New York Stock Exchange pit.

When confronting a cardiac problem, the first strategy is to identify the challenges. How long is the race? Where are there dangerous turns? Which slippery slope could dump the best and most promising rider? If this vital information is available ahead of the game, the practicing cardiologists could program their brain, rewire the shortcuts, and reserve enough adrenaline needed for the run.

The second strategy when examining a patient is to risk profile the patient thereby discriminating the sickest from the less sick. By doing so, more resources, time, and manpower could be allocated for the small number of patients who need it the most without compromising quality of care for the entire group.

Then the authors and editors would offer a strategic map which prioritizes the process of investigation and management. Which is the straight line to the target (direct tests to confirm a clinical diagnosis)? How does one rule out the most important differential diagnoses? Which option offers the best cost and time effective (most fuel efficient) treatment? At the same time, signposts warning of imminent risks or end of danger zones are positioned in strategic locations dotting the horizons. Signs predicting the near future (or prognostic factors) are also prominently posted. Metrics which monitor the progress (follow-up) and evaluate the performance of the operators (practicing cardiologists) are positioned on large billboards or LED screens along the track. All of these signs are transparently posted for the practicing cardiologists without a paternalistic overtone.

Instead of arguing for a preferred solution to a particular problem, the authors and editors provide raw data in the form of abstracts detailing important randomized clinical trials; this enables the practicing cardiologist readers to scrutinize the main results and understand their differences. By so doing, they are able to intelligently select the best between multiple options. There is no need to spoonfeed readers with digested and regurgitated data. The numbers speak for themselves. However, the editors and authors do give practical pearls (which are shortcuts in real life) in order to cut time and cost.

Information is provided by the writers and editors utilizing short paragraphs so that readers will be able to store them in their short-term memory and analyze them before storing them in different compartments of their long-term memories. The strategy is to tailor these messages for today's cardiologists who may be overbooked, impatient, and/or hyperactive.

To all of our readers: The authors and editors of this book have shared many of your trials and tribulations. We have experienced the many sleepless nights. We labor every day in the hospital, at the patient's bedside, like yourself. We too have felt the need for the practical advices found in this book; indeed, that is why we have written them. We are, like all of you, our colleagues, both experienced and beginners, young and old, men and women; there are no divisions of class, age, sex, or race here. This book is not written from an ivory tower perspective – we aim to practice what we preach. Although much practical information and suggestions are given, we have also written from our subjective experience and from our hearts. After all, there is much drama and many ups and downs occurring daily on every cardiac floor in every healthcare facility across the globe. Hopefully, the outcome of our care and treatment will always be a happy and beneficial one for the patients. The bottom line is that we practice cardiology to the best of our ability in a responsible manner that is both cost-effective and time-effective and provides excellent patient-centered care. We are all equal in our quest of striving for the best management and clinical success.

That is the goal of this handbook. To give you, the cardiologist (racing car driver), the tools, the data, and the resources that you need to successfully navigate the race to the finishing line.

Acknowledgements

For the completion of this book, we owe much to our teachers, friends, colleagues, families, staff and patients. I (TNN) am indebted to Dr Eugene Braunwald, who wrote the foreword of the first to the third editions, for his invaluable encouragement, very kind words and advices. My deepest appreciation goes to my fellow editors and contributors and to my family, with the dedicated support of Huang Weitao, NNG CN; my parents Sau N. Nguyen (+ 2012) and Hanh T.H. Tran, and my family in Irvine CA and La Porte IN, especially Robert Luscomb Jr, Le Cong Dinh JD, Lê Gia Long and Lê Trung Hưng, SGN, VN; Dr Huynh Duong Hung, Webmaster Riverside CA; Professor Bui Duy Tam, SFO, Lê Hoàng Đức Toàn, Võ Minh Việt, Huỳnh Trọng Ân, Lê Trọng Hà, Huỳnh Thị Thu Trúc, Lê Thị Ngọc Trâm, Hy Tat An, *Hoàng Quốc Bảo*, Truyện Thiện Tấn Trí Tài of Tan Tao University School of Medicine, Long An, Vietnam; special assistance was given by Cindy Macko at the Library of St Mary Medical Center, Hobart, IN and Yin Rong-Xiu at the Institute of Cardiovascular Disease, Capital University of Medical Sciences, Beijing, China. Above all, we are indebted to our patients – the purpose of our care, the source of our quests, the inspiration of our daily work. To them we give our heartfelt thanks.

CHAPTER 1

Hyperlipidemia

Vien T. Truong, Kim N. Huynh, Tam Ngo, Sara Shah, Hau Van Tran, Chisalu Nchekwube, Nabeel Ali and Faisal Latif

Management of Complex Cardiovascular Problems, Fourth Edition. Edited by Thach N. Nguyen, Dayi Hu, Shao Liang Chen, Moo Hyun Kim and Cindy L. Grines.
© 2016 John Wiley & Sons, Ltd. Published 2016 by John Wiley & Sons, Ltd.

BACKGROUND

Hyperlipidemia – in particular, elevated low-density lipoprotein cholesterol (LDL-C) – is a major risk factor for various forms of cardiovascular (CV) diseases (CVDs). Hyperlipidemia occurs secondary to diet, genetic factors, and/or the presence of other diseases.

CHALLENGES

In the treatment of hyperlipidemia, there are four groups of patients who benefit from statin therapy [1], as listed in Table 1.1. Clinical atherosclerotic CVD (ASCVD) includes acute coronary syndromes (ACS) or a history of myocardial infarction (MI), stable or unstable angina, coronary or other arterial revascularization, stroke, transient ischemic attack (TIA), or peripheral arterial disease (PAD) presumed to be of atherosclerotic origin [1]. The **first challenge** is for all patients who need to be treated to be identified and treated accordingly. No patient should be left behind without treatment.

The second issue is that up to 20% of patients are intolerant to statin therapy due to side-effects [2]. In addition, 5% of patients are resistant to statins [3]. How to treat these patients optimally is the **second challenge.** The **third challenge** is to optimize the treatment for the patients not addressed in the American College of Cardiology/American Heart Association (ACC/AHA) guidelines. The **fourth challenge** is to select the effective management for high triglyceride (TG) or low high-density lipoprotein cholesterol (HDL-C) levels.

Table 1.1 Four statin benefit groups

1. Patients with clinical atherosclerotic cardiovascular disease.
2. Patients with an LDL-C level of 190 mg/dL or higher without secondary cause.
3. Primary prevention: patients with diabetes, aged 40 to 75 years, or with an LDL-C level of 70 to 189 mg/dL.
4. Primary prevention: patients aged 40 to 75 years with an LDL-C level of 70 to 189 mg/dL and atherosclerotic cardiovascular disease risk estimate of 7.5% or higher.

STRATEGIC MAPPING

The 2013 ACC/AHA guidelines heralded a radical change in the management of hyperlipidemia, which was a shift in focus from achieving certain numerical targets (LDL-C in particular) to ensuring application of evidence-based dosage of statins shown to improve CV outcomes. The strategy is to identify the patients with hyperlipidemia through a comprehensive history and physical examination. For any adults aged 20 years or older, questions concerning a high-cholesterol diet, obesity in the family, and dietary habits should be asked. Then, a history of atherosclerosis of any major vascular bed should be documented, because this information is very important in classifying patients into a high- or low-risk group. Other medical conditions or the use of drugs causing high cholesterol levels should also be investigated. After these investigations, blood tests are ordered to confirm the diagnosis of hyperlipidemia and its possible etiologies. Once the diagnosis is confirmed, education and treatment may be started, and follow-up results monitored. In the new management strategy, the patients should be involved deeply in the discussion of risks and the decision to start statin therapy. This strategy is to keep treatment not only 'evidence-based' but also 'patient-centered'.

HIGH-RISK MARKERS

According the 2013 ACC/AHA guidelines, ASCVD risks can be calculated using the new Pooled Cohort Equations for ASCVD risk prediction, developed by the Risk Assessment Work Group [1]. It is a tool to help formulate clinical judgment when there is uncertainty about a patient's risk.

EVIDENCE-BASED MEDICINE
The ASCVD risk estimator This new risk calculator was derived from four community-based population studies that directly measured risk factors in black and white people free of known CVD at entry, and then recorded heart attack and stroke rates over at least 10 years. Being based on actual observations from contemporary US community cohorts, this new risk estimator reflects the high long-term risk of CVD among black and white Americans [4]. This risk calculator may overestimate the score in Hispanics and East Asians. On the other hand, it does not estimate the risk of angioplasty or hospitalization for unstable

angina or TIA, so it underestimates global CV risks. The major components in the risk calculator are listed in Table 1.2 (link for app: www.cardiosource.org/Science-And-Quality/Practice-Guidelines-and-Quality-Standards/2013-Prevention-Guideline-Tools.aspx).

Table 1.2 High-risk markers in the new ACC/AHA ASCVD risk estimator

1. Age (range from 20 to 59 years)
2. Race/ethnicity (white or other or African American)
3. Total cholesterol (mg/dL)
4. HDL-C (mg/dL)
5. LDL-C (mg/dL)
6. Systolic blood pressure (mmHg)
7. Blood pressure treated (yes or no)
8. Smoker (yes or no)
9. Diabetes (yes or no)
10. Has ASCVD (yes or no)

CRITICAL THINKING
Why treat patients with a risk of 7.5%? According to the 2013 ACC/AHA guidelines, a risk of 7.5% or higher is the threshold to be considered for lifestyle and statin therapy because meta-analyses of clinical trials showed statins reduced CV events and strokes in individuals with a risk as low as 5% to less than 10%. While a 7.5% or greater chance of a heart attack or stroke in 10 years does not seem high enough to warrant drug treatment, it is important to recognize that this translates into a cumulative risk of fatal or non-fatal heart attack or stroke of about 22% over 30 years (7.5% for each of three decades) [1].

Additional high-risk markers

For patients who are not included in the four statin benefit groups given earlier, if the patients and their physicians believe that their lifetime risk may be higher than the 10-year calculator estimates, a positive family history or abnormal results of the tests listed in Table 1.3 could guide the patient to the decision to start statin therapy [1].

Table 1.3 High-risk markers for decision to start statin therapy

1. Family history of premature atherosclerotic cardiovascular disease.
2. Elevated lifetime risk of atherosclerotic cardiovascular disease.
3. LDL-C of 160 mg/dL or greater.
4. High-sensitivity C-reactive protein (hs-CRP) of 2.0 mg/L or greater.
5. Subclinical atherosclerosis: coronary artery calcium (CAC) score of 300 or greater or ankle brachial index (ABI) of less than 0.9.

INTRIGUING OBSERVATIONS: VALIDATION OF THE NEW RISK CALCULATOR FOR US PATIENTS – THE REGARDS STUDY [5]

Among other changes, the 2013 ACC/AHA lipid guidelines focus on risk prediction of individuals for experiencing adverse CV events over a 10-year period and using them to identify who will benefit from statins. In the Reasons for the Geographic And Racial Differences in Stroke (REGARDS) study, 10,997 patients aged 45 to 79 years (2003 to 2007 and followed until 2010) were studied with a follow-up of 5 years for atherosclerotic CV events (non-fatal MI, cardiac death, stroke) [5]. In total, there were 338 CV events (192 coronary artery disease [CAD] events, 146 strokes). The observed and predicted 5-year CVD incidence per 1000 person-years for participants with a 10-year predicted ASCVD risk of less than 5% was 1.9 and 1.9; risk of 5% to 7.5% was 4.8 and 4.8; risk of 7.5% to 10% was 6.1 and 6.9; and risk of 10% or greater was 12.0 and 15.1, respectively (Hosmer–Lemeshow $\chi^2 = 19.9$, $P = .01$) [5].

According to this study, among adults for whom statin therapy was initiated based on the ACC/AHA Cohort risk equations, the observed and predicted 5-year ASCVD (non-fatal MI, cardiac death, stroke) risks were similar, indicating that these risk equations were well-calibrated in the US population for whom they were designed to be used and demonstrated moderate to good discrimination [5].

High-risk predictors

The clinical entities that mark high-risk category resulting in early clinical events are listed in Table 1.4 [1]. Elderly patients, who were excluded in the randomized clinical trials (RCTs), may have more side-effects from treatment. Patients with liver disease are also at high risk, because they may encounter problems taking statins due to side-effects from impaired

---

Table 1.4 Predictors determining the poor prognosis

1. Older than 75 years.
2. Multiple major risk factors (especially diabetes).
3. Severe and poorly controlled risk factors (especially continued cigarette smoking).
4. Chronic kidney disease (CKD) based on proteinuria or reduced glomerular filtration rate (GFR).
5. Statin intolerance or muscle disorders.
6. Hepatic or renal impairment.
7. Frailty or small body size.
8. South Asian ancestry.
9. History of hemorrhagic stroke.

---

liver metabolism. South Asian patients originating from the Indian subcontinent had higher CV risk.

INVESTIGATIONS

Symptoms to look for
Hyperlipidemia does not cause symptoms by itself. The symptoms exhibited are the symptoms of the organ or system affected by atherosclerosis.

Signs to look for
Long-standing hyperlipidemia can lead to corneal arcus, corneal opacification, xanthelasma, or tendon xanthomas. A clinician should look for clinical manifestations of atherosclerosis, such as decreased peripheral pulses, ischemic ulcers, vascular bruits, and abdominal aortic aneurysm, as well as sequelae of a previous cerebrovascular or CV event.

Smart testing
The selection of a diagnostic test depends on the level of certainty of evidence regarding risks and benefits, how these risks and benefits compare with potential alternatives, and what the comparative cost or cost-effectiveness of the diagnostic test would be. An informed patient should ask his or her physician this question: Could you tell me the purpose and the diagnostic accuracy of this test?

Laboratory Fasting lipid profile, fasting glucose, liver enzyme, and thyroid function tests should be ordered if indicated. Calculation of LDL-C level using the Friedewald equation is highly robust and reproducible with respect to accuracy in laboratories that participate in standardization programs. It is useful only when TG levels are lower than 400 mg/dL and when the calculated LDL level is greater than 70 mg/dL. Baseline measurement of creatine kinase is reasonable for individuals believed to be at increased risk for adverse muscle events because of a personal or family history of statin intolerance or muscle disease, clinical presentation, or concomitant drug therapy that might increase the risk of myopathy [1].

INTRIGUING OBSERVATIONS: LIPID LEVEL CHANGES WITH SEASON

In a study of 2.8 million adults that evaluated seasonal lipid trends, it was found that lipid profiles were unfavorable in the colder months compared with the warmer months, closely following the trends known about patterns in acute MI and related mortality. Total cholesterol, LDL-C, and non–HDL-C levels were higher in the winter than in the summer months. During the winter months, LDL-C and non–HDL-C levels were 3.5% and 1.7% higher among women, while TG levels were 2.5% higher in men [6].

Looking forward: A new biomarker – HDL-C efflux capacity in the Dallas Heart Study

It is unclear whether HDL-C concentration plays a causal role in atherosclerosis. A more important factor may be the HDL-C efflux capacity, the ability of HDL to accept cholesterol from macrophages, which is a key step in reverse cholesterol transport. In a large, multi-ethnic population cohort, the HDL-C level, HDL particle concentration, and cholesterol efflux capacity were measured at baseline in 2924 adults free from CVD. The primary endpoint was ASCVD, defined as a first non-fatal MI, non-fatal stroke, or coronary revascularization or death from CV causes. The results showed that baseline HDL-C level was not associated with CV events in an adjusted analysis (hazard ratio [HR] 1.08, 95% confidence interval [CI] 0.59 to 1.99). On the other hand, there was a 67% reduction in CV risk in the highest quartile of cholesterol efflux capacity versus the lowest quartile (HR 0.33, 95% CI 0.19 to 0.55). Therefore, cholesterol efflux capacity may become a better biomarker identifying a high-risk patient with CVD [7].

MANAGEMENT

The treatment goal of hyperlipidemia is to achieve the maximum reduction of the long-term total risk of CV events from atherosclerotic diseases. The patients who were found to benefit most from statin are listed in Table 1.1 [5]. Once the patients are risk stratified, they will be assigned to receive high- or moderate-intensity statin therapy. The high-intensity statin therapy is expected to decrease the LDL-C level 50% from baseline, while the moderate-intensity statin therapy is expected to decrease the LDL-C level 30% to 50% from baseline. The schema for selection of patient and indication for statin therapy is shown in Figure 1.1 [1].

Strategic mapping for therapy

Drug therapy with statins is often considered simultaneously with the decision to initiate therapeutic lifestyle changes (TLC) including diet and exercise. After initiation of statin therapy, a follow-up lipid profile should be obtained every 3 to 12 months to assess response and medication compliance. The AHA/ACC guideline provides a weak recommendation that the statin dose may be decreased if there are two consecutive LDL levels below 40 mg/dL. Once the patient has achieved these treatment goal(s), follow-up intervals may be reduced to every 4 to 6 months. The primary focus of these visits is encouragement of long-term compliance with therapy and check for side-effects [1].

When discussing the strategy for treatment, a well-informed patient should ask about treatment options and question the success and complications of the proposed treatment. The detailed investigative questions from a patient's perspective are listed below.

1 What are the level of certainty of evidence regarding risk and benefits?
2 How do these risks and benefits compare with potential alternatives?
3 What are the treatment options available?
4 What are the rates of success or failure of these treatment options?
5 What kind of side-effects or complications are to be expected with these treatment options?
6 What would be the comparative cost or cost-effectiveness of the treatment?
7 What happens if this treatment approach does not work for me?
8 How will you help me balance my treatment with the demand of active life?

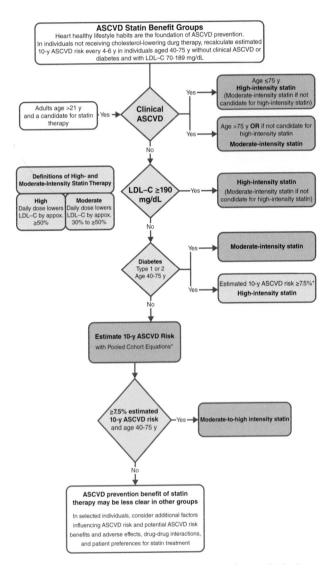

Figure 1.1 Schema for selection of patients to be treated for hyperlipidemia (adapted from Stone et al [1]).

Lifestyle modification   Lifestyle changes are the first requisites of the treatment plan, including adherence to a Heart Healthy Diet, regular exercise habits, avoidance of tobacco products, and maintenance of a healthy weight.

The AHA/ACC guideline is promoting a Heart Healthy Diet based on their evidence review of different diet/lifestyle-focused studies. The Heart Healthy Diet is defined as a diet rich in vegetables, fruits, low-fat dairy products, whole grains, poultry, fish, legumes, nuts, and vegetable oil. It limits intake of red meat, sweets, sugar-containing beverages, *trans*-fat, and sodium, and it restricts intake of saturated fat to 5% to 6% of total daily calories. The Heart Healthy Diet emphasizes caloric intake levels consistent with achieving and maintaining a healthy weight and has shown a benefit with respect to lipid profiles and blood [1]. Weight reduction by at least 5% to 10% and weight maintenance are best achieved by a combination of caloric reduction and increased physical activity. Lifestyle changes are the most cost-effective means to reduce risk for CAD. One of common questions is about the benefits and risks of diet drinks (DDs) to reduce weight.

INTRIGUING OBSERVATIONS: DIET DRINKS
Researchers analyzed 59,614 women from the Women's Health Initiative study who had available DD intake data without pre-existing CVD. A composite of incident CAD, congestive heart failure (CHF), MI, coronary revascularization, ischemic stroke, PAD, and CV death was used as the primary outcome. It was found that 8.5% of the women consuming 2 DDs/day or more experienced the primary endpoint compared with 6.9% who consumed 5 to 7 DDs/week and 7.2% who consumed 0 to 3 DDs/month. After adjustment for CV risk factors, women who consumed 2 DDs/day or more had a higher risk of CV events (HR 1.3, 95% CI 1.1 to 1.5), CVD mortality (HR 1.5, 95% CI 1.03 to 2.3), and overall mortality (HR 1.3, 95% CI 1.04 to 1.5) compared with the 0 to 3 DDs/month group [8].

Statin therapy
Once the patient is risk stratified, the patient is assigned to receive high- or intermediate-intensity statin therapy. Table 1.5 shows the priority ranks comparing one statin with another and their dosages. In a meta-analysis including five randomized controlled trials comparing rosuvastatin with atorvastatin for the treatment of coronary atherosclerotic plaques, rosuvastatin was shown to reduce total atheroma volume further and

Table 1.5 Priority ranks comparing high-, intermediate-, and low-intensity statins

High-intensity statin
Atorvastatin 40 to 80 mg
Rosuvastatin 20 to 40 mg
Moderate-intensity statin
Atorvastatin 10 (20) mg
Rosuvastatin (5) 10 mg
Simvastatin 20 to 40 mg
Pravastatin 40 (80) mg
Lovastatin 40 mg
Fluvastatin XL 80 mg
Fluvastatin 40 mg bid
Pitavastatin 2 to 4 mg
Low-intensity statin
Simvastatin 10 mg
Pravastatin 10 to 20 mg
Lovastatin 20 mg
Fluvastatin 20 to 40 mg
Pitavastatin 1 mg

improve the lumen volume significantly more compared with atorvastatin [9].

Combination therapy

When the patient receives statin and the level of LDL is not satisfactory or when the patient has side-effects from statin use, then combination therapy (statins with non-statins) should be considered. Non-statins include fibrates, ezetimibe, bile acid sequestrants, etc. Among all current agents, ezetimibe is the latest medication with strongest evidence-based effectiveness as seen in the IMPROVEd Reduction of Outcomes: Vytorin Efficacy International (IMPROVE-IT) trial [10]. The considerations for combined therapy are listed in Table 1.6.

Table 1.6 Considerations for combination therapy

1. Failure of statin monotherapy to achieve treatment goals.
2. Intolerance, adverse drug interactions with higher-dose statin monotherapy.
3. Complementary benefits toward further reduction in CAD risk.

EVIDENCE-BASED MEDICINE
Statin and ezetimibe combination – The IMPROVE-IT Trial [10] The study included more than 18,000 patients who were stable after ACS (10 days or less) who had a mean age of 64 years; 25% were female, 36% were receiving prior lipid treatment, and the median LDL-C at ACS event was 95 mg/dL. Patients were randomized to simvastatin 40 mg alone or simvastatin 40 mg plus ezetimibe 10 mg. Over a period of 7 years, the addition of ezetimibe to simvastatin 40 mg reduced the primary endpoint – a composite of CV death, MI, unstable angina requiring rehospitalization, coronary revascularization, or stroke. The absolute reduction in risk over 7 years was 2.0%, with 32.7% in the ezetimibe/simvastatin arm experiencing a primary endpoint compared with 34.7% in the simvastatin arm ($P < .016$). The detailed results of IMPROVE-IT are listed in Table 1.7 [10].

Table 1.7 Primary endpoint and individual components

Clinical Outcomes	Simvastatin, n = 9077 (%)	Ezetimibe/ Simvastatin, n = 9067 (%)	P
Primary end point (Cardiovascular death. MI, unstable angina, coronary revascularization, or stroke)	34.7	32.7	0.016
All-cause death	15.3	15.4	0.782
MI	14.8	13.1	0.002
Stroke	4.8	4.2	0.052
Ischemic stroke	4.1	3.4	0.008
Unstable angina	1.9	2.1	0.618
Coronary revascularization	23.4	21.8	0.107

CRITICAL THINKING
Lower is better The IMROVE-IT trial supported the 'lower is better' cholesterol hypothesis. In this study, the mean LDL-C level among the ACS patients was 95 mg/dL in both treatment arms at baseline. LDL-C levels were reduced to 69.9 mg/dL at 1 year with simvastatin 40 mg. The

addition of ezetimibe 10 mg to simvastatin further lowered LDL-C levels to 53.2 mg/dL at 1 year. Over 7 years, there remained a significant difference between the two treatments in the achieved LDL-C levels. The incremental benefit was achieved in patients treated well below the previously recommended threshold of 70 mg/dL. These great benefits were driven mainly by a significant reduction in MI ($P < .002$) and ischemic stroke ($P < .008$) in the simvastatin/ezetimibe group [11].

The results of the IMPROVE-IT trial give room to use other non-statins to lower LDL-C if a patient is unable to tolerate a statin or unable to achieve the recommended 50% reduction by the ACC/AHA guidelines [1].

Patients intolerant of statins

From 10% to 25% of patients in clinical practice report statin intolerance. How to treat these patients is very difficult, as large, well-controlled RCTs of cholesterol-lowering drugs in statin-intolerant patients are lacking. The results of the ODYSSEY ALTERNATIVE trial for patients intolerant to statin using a proprotein convertase subtilisin/kexin type 9 (PCSK9) inhibitor were presented at the 2014 annual scientific meeting of the AHA, and are shown next.

EVIDENCE-BASED MEDICINE
The PCSK9 ODYSSEY ALTERNATIVE Trial [12] The ODYSSEY ALTERNATIVE trial enrolled 361 patients with statin intolerance and an LDL-C level of 70 mg/dL or higher at very high CV risk or LDL-C level of 100 mg/dL or higher and at high or moderate CV risk. Mean baseline LDL was 190 mg/dL. The primary endpoint was the percentage change from baseline in LDL-C at week 24. After a placebo run-in phase for 4 weeks, the patients were randomized to alirocumab 75 or 150 mg subcutaneously every 2 weeks ($n = 126$), ezetimibe 10 mg once daily ($n = 125$), or atorvastatin 20 mg once daily ($n = 63$). At week 24, the alirocumab group had shown a much greater reduction in LDL than the ezetimibe group. Mean LDL level was reduced to 154 mg/dL with ezetimibe vs. 96 mg/dL in the alirocumab group. The results of LDL reduction of the patients based on intention to treat or based on treatment received are listed in Table 1.8.

Table 1.8 Percentage of LDL-C decrease in the ODYSSEY ALTERNATIVE Trial

Analysis	Alirocumab (%)	Ezetimibe (%)	P
Intention to treat	−45.0	−14.6	<0.0001
On treatment	−52.2	−17.1	<0.0001

Adverse effects of statins

In clinical practice, because the statins are very effective in lowering LDL-C, the main focus of clinicians in the first few months of follow-up is to check the side-effects of statin. They are rare, but they are real and they can be controlled or reversed if detected early. In the approach to the patient with possible statin intolerance, readers can follow the algorithm suggested by the American College of Cardiology and download the free apps (https://itunes.apple.com/en/app/statin-intolerance/id985805274).

Data from both primary and secondary prevention RCTs indicate that no clinically significant liver problems are associated with statin therapy. Elevated hepatic transaminase levels (aspartate aminotransferase [AST] and/or alanine aminotransferase [ALT]) associated with high-intensity statin therapy occurred in fewer than 1.5% of individuals over 5 years, and elevations associated with low- or moderate-intensity statin therapy occurred at rates similar to those seen with placebo or no statin treatment controls [3]. Therefore, the US Food and Drug Administration (FDA) no longer requires routine monitoring of liver function tests. However, it is reasonable to measure hepatic function if symptoms suggesting hepatotoxicity arise (e.g., unusual fatigue or weakness, loss of appetite, abdominal pain, dark-colored urine, or yellowing of the skin or sclera) [1].

The risk of a statin causing a life-threatening effect on muscles is less than 2:100,000. It is reasonable to measure creatine kinase (CK) levels in individuals with muscle symptoms, including pain, tenderness, stiffness, cramping, weakness, or generalized fatigue [1].

Finally, the risk of cognitive impairment from statins is based primarily on individual reports to the FDA [1]. A recently published meta-analysis showed no short-term effects of statins on cognition and a possible long-term protective effect against dementia [1].

CLINICAL PEARLS
Tactics when encountering possible side-effects with statins [1] The AHA/ACC expert opinion suggests as follows:

1 Obtain a history of prior or current muscle symptoms to establish a baseline before initiating statin therapy.

2 If the ALT or AST level increases above three times the upper limit of normal, in case of a normal baseline, statin should be discontinued and a repeat value in 2 weeks to 1 month obtained to ascertain if it was due to the statin.

3 If mild to moderate muscle symptoms develop during statin therapy: Discontinue the statin therapy until the problem can be evaluated. Evaluate the patient for other conditions that might increase the risk for muscle symptoms (e.g., hypothyroidism, reduced renal or hepatic function, rheumatic disorders such as polymyalgia rheumatica, steroid myopathy, vitamin D deficiency, or primary muscle diseases, many medications which can interfere with the metabolism of statin).

4 If muscle symptoms resolve, and if no contraindication exists, give the patient the original or a lower dose of the same statin to establish a causal relationship between the muscle symptoms and statin therapy. If a causal relationship exists, discontinue the original statin. Once muscle symptoms resolve, use a low dose of a different statin. Once a low dose of a statin is tolerated, gradually increase the dose as tolerated.

5 If unexplained severe muscle symptoms or fatigue develop, promptly discontinue the statin and address the possibility of rhabdomyolysis by evaluating CK and creatinine and a urinalysis for myoglobinuria.

6 If, after 2 months without statin treatment, muscle symptoms or elevated CK levels do not resolve completely, consider other causes of muscle symptoms. If persistent muscle symptoms are determined to arise from a condition unrelated to statin therapy or if the predisposing condition has been treated, resume statin therapy at the original dose [1].

Risk of development of diabetes with statin There is moderate evidence that statin therapy is associated with an excess risk for incident diabetes (number needed to harm = 100 in primary prevention and 500 to 1000 in secondary prevention). The risk of diabetes occurs almost exclusively in those with 'prediabetes' and appears to be proportional to the intensity of statin therapy. However, the adverse outcome of incident (or earlier diagnosis of) diabetes must be weighed in the context of the potentially fatal or debilitating occurrence of MI or stroke that could be prevented by statin therapy [1]. Individuals receiving statin therapy should be evaluated for new-onset diabetes according to the current diabetes-screening guidelines [13]. Those who develop diabetes during statin therapy should be encouraged to adhere to a heart-healthy dietary pattern, engage in physical activity, achieve and maintain a healthy body weight, cease tobacco use, and continue statin therapy to reduce their risk of ASCVD events. The early signs of patients who may develop DM with statin therapy are evidenced in the Multi-Ethnic Study of Atherosclerosis (MESA) study [14].

EVIDENCE-BASED MEDICINE

The MESA Study In the MESA study of patients without CVD, T2D/impaired fasting glucose, or baseline statin therapy, high liver fat and statin therapy were associated with DM (HR 2.06 [95%CI 1.52–2.79, $P < 0.0001$] and 2.01 [95%CI 1.46–2.77, $P < 0.0001$], respectively). With low liver fat and CAC = 0, the number needed to treat (NNT) for statin to prevent one CVD event (NNT 218) was higher than the number needed to harm (NNH) with an incident case of T2D (NNH 68). Conversely, those with CAC >100 and low liver fat were more likely to benefit from statins for CVD reduction (NNT 29) relative to T2D risk (NNH 67). Among those with CAC >100 and fatty liver, incremental reduction in CVD with statins (NNT 40) was less than incremental risk increase for T2D (NNH 24) [14].

So, liver fat is associated with incident T2D and stratifies competing metabolic/CVD risks with statin therapy. The presence of hepatic fat may suggest further T2D surveillance and lipid therapeutic strategies [14].

STRONG WARNING: INTERACTIONS BETWEEN CLARITHROMYCIN AND STATINS

Most macrolides inhibit the cytochrome P450 isoenzyme CYP3A4, by which some statins such as simvastatin and atorvastatin are metabolized. Concurrent use of macrolide antibiotics may increase statin toxicity [15].

Table 1.9 Patients not on the recommendation list of the ACC/AHA Guidelines [1]

1. Patients with CKD without ASCVD, not on hemodialysis.
2. Patients with end-stage renal disease not on hemodialysis.
3. Patients with diabetes mellitus without ASCVD.
4. Patients with heart failure.

EVIDENCE-BASED MEDICINE
Statin toxicity from macrolide antibiotics
Antibiotic coprescription in a population-based cohort study was conducted at Canada, from 2003 to 2010, to examine the frequency of statin toxicity after coprescription of a statin with clarithromycin or erythromycin in older adults. Compared with azithromycin, coprescription of a statin with clarithromycin or erythromycin was associated with a higher risk for hospitalization with rhabdomyolysis (absolute risk increase, 0.02% [95% CI 0.01% to 0.03%]; relative risk [RR], 2.17 [CI, 1.04 to 4.53]) or with acute kidney injury (absolute risk increase, 1.26% [CI, 0.58% to 1.95%]; RR, 1.78 [CI, 1.49 to 2.14]) and for all-cause mortality (absolute risk increase, 0.25% [CI, 0.17% to 0.33%]; RR, 1.56 [CI, 1.36 to 1.80]). The message from this study was that coprescription of clarithromycin or erythromycin with a statin that is metabolized by cytochrome P450 isoenzyme 3A4 (CYP3A4) increases the risk for statin toxicity in older adults. Then, in this situation, we should use a statin not metabolized by the P450 isoenzyme CYP3A4, such as rosuvastatin, pravastatin, or fluvastatin [15].

MANAGEMENT OF PATIENTS NOT ON THE RECOMMENDATION LIST OF THE ACC/AHA GUIDELINES

The authors of the 2013 AHA/ACC guidelines found insufficient evidence for or against the use of statin therapy for the purpose of ASCVD risk reduction in some population groups, as listed in Table 1.9 [1].

Patients with CKDs
Secondary prevention for CKD patients not requiring hemodialysis The ACC/AHA guidelines suggest intensive statin for moderate CKD and clinical ASCVD (excluding patients receiving

hemodialysis) (secondary prevention) through the evidence from the subanalysis from the Treating to New Targets (TNT) study [16].

Primary prevention for CKD patients not requiring hemodialysis   Even the ACC/AHA guidelines did not make recommendation for CKD patients without ASCVD (primary prevention); the benefits with a statin were evidenced in the results of the *Study* of Heart and Renal Protection (SHARP) trial [17]. The readers can read and assess the results of the study (as did the authors of the guidelines) and make their own judgment about the validity and clinical applications of the results.

EVIDENCE-BASED MEDICINE
The SHARP Trial [17] In this double-blind RCT, 9720 patients with CKD without history of CAD or MI were randomized to either simvastatin 20 mg plus ezetimibe 10 mg daily or placebo. The primary endpoint was first major atherosclerotic event (non-fatal MI or coronary death, non-hemorrhagic stroke, or any arterial revascularization procedure) [17]. Patients in the simvastatin/ezetimibe group experienced a lower level of LDL during a median follow-up of 4.9 years. Patients in the simvastatin/ezetimibe group also experienced a 17% risk reduction in major atherosclerotic events (11.3% for simvastatin plus ezetimibe vs. 13.4% for placebo; 95% CI 0.74 to 0.94; log-rank $P = .0021$). Overall, patients in the simvastatin/ezetimbibe group demonstrated a trend toward a reduced incidence of non-fatal MI and CV death (4.6% vs. 5.0%; RR 0.92, 95% CI 0.76 to 1.11; $P = .37$), and there was a significant reduction in non-hemorrhagic stroke (2.8% vs. 3.8%; RR 0.75, 95% CI 0.60 to 0.94; $P = .01$) and arterial revascularization procedures (6.1% vs. 7.6%; RR 0.79, 95% CI 0.68 to 0.93; $P = .0036$) [17].

Based on the same data assessed by the ACC/AHA guideline writers, the 2013 Kidney Disease: Improving Global Outcomes (KDIGO) Clinical Practice Guideline for Lipid Management in Chronic Kidney Disease suggested lipid therapy by the absolute risk of coronary events based on patient age and stage of CKD or estimated GFR (eGFR) [18]. The KDIGO guidelines recommend that patients already receiving statins or statin/ezetimibe combination at the time of dialysis initiation continue therapy. In adults with new dialysis-dependent CKD, the KDIGO guidelines [18] suggest that statin or statin/ezetimibe combination not be initiated (as per the results of the AURORA study [A study to Evaluate the Use of

Table 1.10 Suggestions for therapy for non-hemodialysis CKD patients

Adults aged 50 years or older with eGFR less than 60 mL/min/ 1.73 m [2] but no chronic dialysis or kidney transplantation:
Statin or statin/ezetimibe

Adults aged 50 years or older with CKD and eGFR60 mL/min/1.73 m [2] or higher:
Statin

Adults aged 18 to 49 years with CKD and no chronic dialysis:
Statin

Or kidney transplantation, if one of the following is present:
1. Known coronary heart disease (MI or coronary revascularization)
2. Diabetes mellitus
3. Prior ischemic stroke, or
4. Estimated 10-year incidence of coronary death or non-fatal MI greater than10% on the Framingham risk score.

Adult kidney transplant recipients:
Statin

Rosuvastin in Subjects on Regulat Hemodialysis]) [19]. They are listed in Table 1.10.

 CLINICAL PEARLS
Why did CKD patients respond less with statins? One reason why these studies in dialysis and post-transplant patients have shown only mixed results and not clear benefits may be because these patients have had such long-standing CKD and diabetes, so their CVD becomes too advanced and less responsive to statins. Second, these patients develop heavy calcification of atherosclerotic plaques, which is likely a barrier to potential regression in plaque volume.

As GFR falls, the dosages of many of the drugs that are used for the treatment of hypercholesterolemia need to be modified. However, atorvastatin and fluvastatin dosages do not have to be modified [20]. Combinations of statins and fibrates should be avoided, and fenofibrate should be avoided in patients with GFR levels of less than 50 mL/min [21].

Patients who were receiving dialysis treatment for up to 4 years could have produced greater calcification of the coronary arteries, which is a known side-effect of hemodialysis. Even though the results of the AURORA study were negative, dialysis patients should still receive a statin if they have other risk factors associated with the coronary arteries or other parts of their vascular tree. These patients may not die from a heart attack or stroke; they may die of kidney failure from their end-stage renal disease [19].

Patients with diabetes

The ACC/AHA guidelines state that there is insufficient evidence to make recommendations for statin therapy in diabetics younger than 40 or older than 75 years with clinical evidence of ASCVD (primary prevention). However, for diabetics under the age of 40 years, the American Diabetes Association (ADA) and the American Association of Clinical Endocrinology (AACE) suggest that statin therapy be considered in those with multiple CVD risk factors or with an LDL-C level of greater than 100 mg/dL after therapeutic lifestyle change. They agreed with the ACC/AHA that there was very little clinical trial evidence in this patient population (Level of Evidence: C) [13].

Patients with heart failure

The authors of the 2013 AHA/ACC guidelines found insufficient evidence for or against the use of statin therapy for the purpose of ASCVD risk reduction in patient with heart failure per se [1]. In the two large RCTs in patients with heart failure, the Controlled Rosuvastatin in Multinational Trial in Heart Failure (CORONA) and the Gruppo Italiano per lo Studio della Sopravvivenza nell'Infarto Miocardio (GISSIHF), there was no statistically significant difference between groups in the primary composite outcome of death from CV causes, non-fatal MI, or non-fatal stroke [22,23]. Patient ASCVD risk factors and risk/benefit of statins should be considered on an individual basis.

Patients younger than 40 years

The ACC/AHA recommendations for the benefits of statin therapy in patients with LDL-C of 190 mg/dL or higher and/or familial hypercholesterolemia extend to all adults aged 21 years or older, many of whom will have initiated therapy during childhood or adolescence due to the high lifetime risk for ASCVD events [1]. Because the hypercholesterolemia in these high-risk individuals is often genetically determined, family screening is especially important to identify additional family members who would benefit from assessment and early treatment [1]. Secondary causes of severe elevations of LDL-C of 190 mg/dL or higher and TG levels of

500 mg/dL or higher often contribute to the magnitude of the hyperlipidemia and should be evaluated and treated appropriately [1].

Pregnant women
Cholesterol and TG levels rise progressively throughout pregnancy, while treatments with statins, niacin, and ezetimibe are contraindicated during pregnancy and lactation [1]. If the pregnant woman is young, it is hoped that she can wait a few years before embarking on a medical journey for the prevention of ASCVD.

Patients with an ASCVD risk of less than 7.5%
Available RCT evidence indicates that when baseline ASCVD risk is 5.0% to less than 7.5%, there is still net absolute benefit with moderate-intensity statin therapy. However, the trade-offs between the ASCVD risk-reduction benefit and adverse effects are less clear. Thus, a clinician–patient discussion is even more important for individuals with this range of ASCVD risk. The net benefit of high-intensity statin therapy may be marginal in such individuals [1].

Race/Ethnicity
The current recommendations modify statin therapy intensity only in individuals of East Asian ancestry, who have been reported to have genetically based differences in the metabolism of statins at the level of hepatic enzymes and drug transporters. Lower statin doses have been demonstrated to achieve lipid improvements in Asian patients comparable with those observed with higher doses in white people [1].

HYPERTRYGLYCERIDEMIA

Rationale for the treatment of high TG levels
Elevated TG levels, especially in individuals with additional lipoprotein abnormalities, predict higher CVD risk. However, there is a lack of data regarding the benefits of strategies directly targeting elevated TG levels [1]. The factors contributing to elevated TG levels are listed in Table 1.11.

Management
The ACC/AHA guidelines advocate use of medications to lower TG levels only when the TG level is above 500 mg/dL. They recommend evaluating and addressing secondary causes of elevated TG levels and implementing diet and lifestyle modifications first for these patients [1].

Table 1.11 Factors contributing to elevated TG levels

1. Obesity
2. Physical inactivity
3. Cigarette smoking
4. Excess alcohol intake
5. High-carbohydrate diets (60% of energy intake)

Diseases:
6. Type 2 diabetes
7. Chronic renal failure
8. Nephrotic syndrome
9. Genetic disorders (familial combined hyperlipidemia, familial hypertriglyceridemia, and familial dysbetalipoproteinemia)

Drugs:
10. Corticosteroids, estrogens, retinoids, higher doses of beta-adrenergic blocking agents

For many patients with mild increase in TG, a lifestyle change program alone will normalize the TG levels. The limitation of the intake of complex carbohydrates can be very beneficial in lowering TG levels [1]. When lifestyle change cannot achieve the desired TG goal, pharmacological therapy is to be considered. According to the 2013 guidelines, for elevated TG, there are three choices: fibrates, niacin, or omega-3 formulas [1]. The most commonly used drug for isolated hypertriglyceridemia is the fibrates.

Fibrates and statin   The Action to Control Cardiovascular Risk in Diabetes (ACCORD) Lipid Trial [24] compared combination therapy of statin plus a fibrate with statin monotherapy on CVD event rate in patients with type 2 diabetes. The study consisted of 5518 patients with type 2 diabetes who were being treated to receive either masked fenofibrate or placebo. The mean follow-up was 4.7 years. The primary outcome was the first occurrence of a major CV event that included non-fatal MI, non-fatal stroke, or death from CV causes. The study showed no significant decrease in major CV events, with an annual event rate of 2.2% in the fenofibrate group and 2.4% in the placebo group (HR in the fenofibrate group 0.92; 95% CI 0.79 to 1.08; $P = .32$). To date, no trial has provided statistically or clinically compelling evidence to routinely recommend the addition of a fibrate to statin therapy [24].

Statin and niacin   In the Atherothrombosis Intervention in Metabolic Syndrome with Low HDL/High Triglycerides: Impact on Global Health

Outcomes (AIM-HIGH) trial [25], niacin therapy had significantly increased the median HDL-C level, lowered the TG level, but showed no overall significant difference in the primary endpoint (16.4% in patients randomly assigned to niacin vs. 16.2% in patients assigned to placebo). Overall, niacin-laropiprant was associated with an increased incidence of disturbances in diabetes control, diabetes diagnoses, gastrointestinal disturbances, infections, and bleeding. These data confirm that the use of niacin in statin-treated patients is not associated with a reduction in CV events but may be associated with a significant increase in serious adverse events.

Treatment of low HDL-C   HDL-C levels are inversely correlated with CAD risk. Low HDL-C levels (less than 40 mg/dL) may be due to a genetic disorder or to secondary causes. Strategies to raise HDL-C levels have also been studied. Non-pharmacologic therapy, such as exercise, weight loss, and smoking cessation, should be stressed. Exercise increases HDL-C about 3% to 9%, but the increase is related to the frequency and intensity of the exercise. Smoking cessation will increase HDL by about 4 mg/dL. Weight loss is another effective way to increase HDL, but the increase in level is related to the number of pounds lost and kept off [1].

Treatment of hypercholesterolemia in patients with liver disease   Biliary obstruction can lead to severe hypercholesterolemia that is resistant to conventional cholesterol-lowering drugs. The only effective therapy is treatment of the underlying liver or biliary tract disease [26]. Patients with borderline elevation of liver enzymes should undergo frequent laboratory testing. If there is persistent or substantial elevation of liver enzymes, the statin should be discontinued [26]. Different tactics of how to use statins in patients with baseline elevation of liver enzymes are listed in Table 1.12.

Treatment of hypercholesterolemia in HIV patients taking protease inhibitor   Dyslipidemia associated with the treatment of HIV infection, particularly with the use of protease inhibitors (PIs), can raise cholesterol and TG levels to the thresholds indicated for therapy. Diet modification and exercise should be tried first. If results are unsatisfactory, alternative retrovirals can be tried if appropriate, and lipid-lowering drugs started. Selection of drug therapy for lipid lowering depends on the type of predominating dyslipidemia and the potential for drug interactions. The use of the statins is recommended for the treatment of patients with elevated LDL-C levels and gemfibrozil or fenofibrate for patients with

---

Table 1.12 Tactics for treatment of hypercholesterolemia in patients with liver disease

---

1. Measure baseline electrolyte, liver function, renal function, and thyroid-stimulating hormone levels.
2. Evaluate for nondrug causes of elevation of ALT or AST such as alcohol use, non-immune hepatitis, infectious hepatitis, or non-alcoholic fatty liver disease.
3. Statin can be started if the ALT and AST levels are not more than three times the upper limit of normal.
4. After starting the statin, monitor ALT and AST levels every 6 and 12 weeks and after dose increase.
5. If the levels of AST and ALT are elevated more than three times normal during monitoring:
   Repeat measurement in 1 week.
   If the level is still high, decrease the dose or stop the medication if the patient has chronic liver disease or chronic alcohol abuse.
   If decreasing the dose, repeat measurement in 2 to 4 weeks.
   If level returns to baseline, continue lower dose and monitor.
6. If statin is discontinued, consider rechallenge with the same statin at lower dose or another statin [26].

---

elevated TG concentrations. Because atorvastatin and some antiretroviral drugs are metabolized by the same cytochrome C-450 isoenzyme CYP3A4, inhibition of the isoenzyme may result in an excessive high level of statin (raising the risk of rhabdomyolysis). Therefore, simvastatin and lovastatin should be avoided, and atorvastatin should be used instead at a lower dose. Pravastatin can be used, but its efficacy is questionable. Rosuvastatin is a better choice for the patients receiving antiretroviral drugs, because it may have slightly more CYP3A4 activity [27]. Ezetimibe alone reduces LDL-C in HIV-infected patients receiving combination antiretroviral therapy [27]. Its high tolerability and the lack of interactions with the cytochrome CYP3A4 indicate that ezetimibe will not increase the risk of toxicity or pharmacokinetic interactions with antiretrovirals.

Treatment of children and young adults in a family of patients with hypercholesterolemia   The process of ASCVD begins early in life and is progressive throughout the lifespan. Clinical evidence suggests that serum cholesterol measured at 22 years of age is predictive of risk of

CAD over the next 30 to 40 years [28]. The National Cholesterol Education Program (NCEP) recommends screening children over 2 years of age with parental hypercholesterolemia or a first-degree family history of premature CVD [29]. Pharmacologic intervention should be considered for patients 8 years and older with an LDL-C of 190 mg/dL or higher. The AHA has recommended that TG concentrations of greater than 150 mg/dL and HDL-C concentrations of less than 35 mg/dL be considered abnormal for children and adolescents [29]. Treatment of hypercholesterolemia during childhood and adolescence is based on dietary treatment and lifestyle modification. Drug therapy should be limited to children with levels above the 99th percentile who fail to reduce their levels after 6 to 12 months. A treatment is considered successful if any reduction of LDL-C is accomplished by appropriately changing lifestyle and incorporating healthy eating habits [29].

CLINICAL PEARLS
Statins for hypercholesterolemia in children
Lovastatin is the only statin currently approved for children, but simvastatin, pravastatin, and atorvastatin have also been used. LDL-C decreased by 17% on 10 mg/day and by 27% on 40 mg/day lovastatin in boys aged 10 to 14 years [30] without an adverse effect on growth and development. LDL-C was reduced by 41% and apolipoprotein B by 34% with 40 mg/day simvastatin [31] in 173 boys and girls with heterozygous hypercholesterolemia.

Hypercholesterolemia in Asians The pattern of lipid abnormalities and their relative impact on CVD risk may vary among ethnic groups. Asians include several distinct ethnic subpopulations (South Asians, Chinese, etc.), who may differ in their lipid profiles [32]. These differences may be the result of both genetic and environmental factors (high-carbohydrate diets, reduced physical activity, and so on). In a case-control study, 65 centers in Asia recruited 5731 cases of a first acute MI and 6459 control subjects. Among both cases and controls, mean LDL-C levels were about 10 mg/dL lower in Asians compared with non-Asians. A greater proportion of Asian cases and controls had LDL-C 100 mg/dL or less (25.5% and 32.3% in Asians vs. 19.4% and 25.3% in non-Asians, respectively). HDL-C levels were slightly lower among Asians compared with non-Asians. There was a preponderance of people with low HDL-C among South Asians (South Asia vs. rest of Asia: cases 82.3% vs. 57.4%;

controls 81% vs. 51.6%; $P < .0001$ for both comparisons). However, despite these differences in absolute levels, the risk of acute MI associated with increases in LDL-C and decreases in HDL-C was similar for Asians and non-Asians [33]. In the treatment, a lower dose of statin may reduce the risk of CAD similarly among Asians, as higher doses have in populations of Europe and the United States.

ACTION POINTS

1 Collect all the data about the patient's history (history of smoking, high sodium, high-cholesterol diet, alcohol abuse, lack of exercise, hypertension, diabetes, high cholesterol level, etc.), family history (of early sudden death due to heart disease, history of early CAD, etc.), and social history (work and behaviors) and perform a complete physical examination (signs of prior stroke, CAD, PAD, carotid murmur, weak peripheral pulses, etc.), all of which weigh in the clinical decision-making.

2 Recommend appropriate and efficacious investigation (including fasting lipid profile, fasting blood glucose, blood urea nitrogen and creatinine levels, weight, body mass index, waist circumference, AST, ALT, CK).

3 Recommend safe, appropriate, and efficacious therapy to maintain the stable health status of the patient over time (low sodium, low-cholesterol diet, stop smoking, losing weight, prevent alcohol abuse, regular aerobic exercise, etc.). Therapeutic lifestyle change should precede or occur with pharmacological therapy, depending on the clinical urgency.

4 Manage to reduce LDL-C and non-HDL-C in accordance with the latest lipid guidelines with focus on moderate- versus high-intensity statins depending on the patient. Treatment of low HDL and hypertriglyceridemia has strong justification as well.

5 Provide patient-centered care. To provide continual care, patients should be encouraged and empowered with the TLC, and their office visits should be scheduled for lipid and liver function testing to ascertain compliance and response to therapy.

REFERENCES

1. Stone NJ, Robinson J, Lichtenstein AH, et al. 2013 ACC/AHA Guideline on the Treatment of Blood Cholesterol to Reduce Atherosclerotic Cardiovascular.

https://circ.ahajournals.org/content/early/2013/11/11/01.cir.0000437738
.63853.7a (figure 2).

2. Ganga HV, Slim HB, Thompson PD. A systematic review of statin-induced muscle problems in clinical trials. *Am Heart J*. 2014;168:6–15.

3. Mampuya WM, Frid D, Rocco M, et al. Treatment strategies in patients with statin intolerance: the Cleveland Clinic experience. *Am Heart J*. 2013;166:597–603. doi:10.1016/j.ahj.2013.06.004. Epub 2013 Aug 5.

4. www.cardiosource.org/Science-And-Quality/Practice-Guidelines-and-Quality-Standards/2013-Prevention-Guideline-Tools.aspx

5. Muntner P, Colantonio LD, Cushman M, et al. Validation of the pooled cohort 10-year atherosclerotic cardiovascular disease risk equations. *JAMA*. 2014;311:1406–1415. doi:10.1001/jama.2014.2630

6. Moura FA, Dutra-Rodrigues MS, Cassol AS, et al. Impact of seasonality on the prevalence of dyslipidemia: a large population study. *Chronobiol Int*. 2013 Oct;30(8):1011–1015. doi: 10.3109/07420528.2013.793698. Epub 2013 Jul 9.

7. Rohatgi A, Khera A, Berry JD, et al. HDL cholesterol efflux capacity and incident cardiovascular events. *N Engl J Med*. doi:10.1056/NEJMoa1409065

8. Vyas A, Rubenstein L, Robinson J, et al. Diet drink consumption and the risk of cardiovascular events: a report from the Women's Health Initiative. *J Am Coll Cardiol*. 2014;63. doi:10.1016/S0735-1097(14)61290-0.

9. Qian, Cheng, et al. Meta-analysis comparing the effects of rosuvastatin versus atorvastatin on regression of coronary atherosclerotic plaques. *Am J Cardiol*. 2015;116:1521–1526.

10. Cannon CP, Blazing MA, Giugliano RP, et al. for the IMPROVE-IT Investigators. Ezetimibe added to statin therapy after acute coronary syndromes. *N Engl J Med* 2015; 372:2387–2397, DOI: 10.1056/NEJMoa1410489.

11. Jarcho JA, Keaney JF Jr. Proof that lower is better – LDL cholesterol and IMPROVE-IT. *N Engl J Med*. 2015;372:2448–2450.

12. Moriarty PM, et al. Efficacy and safety of alirocumab vs ezetimibe in statin-intolerant patients, with a statin rechallenge arm: The ODYSSEY ALTERNATIVE randomized trial. *J Clin Lipidol*. DOI: http://dx.doi.org/10.1016/j.jacl.2015.08.006

13. American Diabetes Association. Standards of medical care in diabetes 2014. *Diabetes Care*. 2014;37:S14–S80.

14. Shah RV, Allison MA, Lima JA Liver fat, statin use, and incident diabetes: The Multi-Ethnic Study of Atherosclerosis. *Atherosclerosis*. 2015;242:211–217. doi: 10.1016/j.atherosclerosis.2015.07.018. Epub 2015 Jul 15.

15. Li D, Kim R, McArthur E, et al. Risk of adverse events among older adults following co-prescription of clarithromycin and statins not metabolized by cytochrome P450 3A4. *CMAJ*. 2014. doi:10.1503/cmaj.140950

16. Shepherd J, Kastelein JJP, Vera B, et al; for the Treating to New Targets Investigators. Intensive lipid lowering with atorvastatin in patients with coronary heart disease and chronic kidney disease: the TNT (Treating to New Targets) Study. *J Am Coll Cardiol*. 2008;51:1448–1454.

17. Baigent C, Landray MJ, Reith C.The effects of lowering LDL cholesterol with simvastatin plus ezetimibe in patients with chronic kidney disease (Study of

Heart and Renal Protection): a randomised placebo-controlled trial. *Lancet.* 2011;377:2181–2192.

18. Kidney Disease: Improving Global Outcomes (KDIGO) Lipid Work Group. KDIGO clinical practice guideline for lipid management in chronic kidney disease. *Kidney Int Suppl.* 2013;3:259–305.

19. Fellstroem BC, Jardine AG, Schmieder RE, et al. Rosuvastatin and cardiovascular events in patients undergoing emodialysis. *N Engl J Med.* 2009;360:1395–1407.

20. Molitch ME. Management of dyslipidemias in patients with diabetes and chronic kidney disease. *Clin J Am Soc Nephrol.* 2006;1:1090–1099.

21. Ritz E, Wanner C. Lipid abnormalities and cardiovascular risk in renal disease. *J Am Soc Nephrol.* 2008;19:1065–1070.

22. Kjekshus J, Apetrei E, Barrios V, et al. Rosuvastatin in older patients with systolic heart failure. *N Engl J Med.* 2007;357:2248–2261.

23. GISSI-HF Investigators, Tavazzi L, Maggioni AP, et al. Effect of rosuvastatin in patients with chronic heart failure (the GISSI-HF trial): a randomised, double-blind, placebo-controlled trial. *Lancet.* 2008;372:1231–1239.

24. The ACCORD Study Group. Effects of combination lipid therapy in type 2 diabetes mellitus. *N Engl J Med.* 2010;362:1563–1574.

25. The AIM-HIGH Investigators. Niacin in patients with low HDL cholesterol levels receiving intensive statin therapy. *N Engl J Med* 2011;365:2255–2267.

26. Vasudevan A, Hamirani Y, Jones P. Safety of statin: effects on the muscle and liver. *CCJM.* 2005;72:990–1000.

27. Calza L, Colangeli V, Manfredi R, et al. Rosuvastatin for the treatment of hyperlipidaemia in HIV-infected patients receiving protease inhibitors: a pilot study. *AIDS.* 2005;19:1103–1105.

28. Klag MJ, Ford DE, Mead LA, et al. Serum cholesterol in young men and subsequent cardiovascular disease. *N Engl J Med.* 1993;328:313–318.

29. Daniels SR, Greer FR and the Committee on Nutrition. Lipid Screening and Cardiovascular Health in Childhood. *Pediatrics* 2008;122;198–208.

30. Kavey RE, Daniels SR, Lauer RM, et al. American Heart Association guidelines for primary prevention of atherosclerotic cardiovascular disease beginning in childhood. *Circulation.* 2003;107:1562–1566; copublished in *J Pediatr.* 2003;142:368–372.

31. McCrindle BW, Helden E, Cullen-Dean G, Conner WT. A randomized crossover trial of combination pharmacogenic therapy in children with familial hyperlipidemia. *Pediatr Res.* 2002; 51:715–721.

32. Karthikeyan G, Teo KK, et al. Lipid profile, plasma apolipoproteins, and risk of a first myocardial infarction among Asians: an analysis from the INTERHEART study. *J Am Coll Cardiol.* 2009;53:244–253.

33. Heng DM, Lee J, Chew SK, Tan BY, Hughes K, Chia KS. Incidence of ischaemic heart disease and stroke in Chinese, Malays and Indians in Singapore: Singapore Cardiovascular Cohort Study. *Ann Acad Med Singapore.* 2000;29:231–236.

CHAPTER 2

Hypertension
Implications of Current JNC 8 Guidelines on Treatment

Udho Thadani and Nguyen Duc Cong

Management of Complex Cardiovascular Problems, Fourth Edition. Edited by Thach N. Nguyen, Dayi Hu, Shao Liang Chen, Moo Hyun Kim and Cindy L. Grines.
© 2016 John Wiley & Sons, Ltd. Published 2016 by John Wiley & Sons, Ltd.

BACKGROUND

Slowly but surely, blood pressure (BP) increases with age [1–4]. Consistent BP readings above 140/90 mmHg indicate high BP (hypertension [HTN]) and are associated with increased risk of death, stroke, heart failure (HF), cardiovascular (CV) morbidity, aortic dissection, renal failure, peripheral arterial disease and memory impairment [5–20]. In the majority of patients (>90% to 95%), no obvious cause for high BP can be found and these patients are considered to have essential HTN [3, 4, 21]. Nearly 67 million Americans have HTN, defined as BP reading >140/90 mmHg [1, 22]; this represents about one of every three US adults [22]. Higher BP is much more prevalent in black people (42.1%) than in white people (28%), Latinos (26%), or Asian Americans (24.7%) [22]. Many others have BP readings between 120–139/80–89 mmHg and are considered to have pre-HTN [1–4, 23]. Men have a higher incidence of HTN before the age of 45, but women catch up, and after the age of 65, more women have HTN than men [1, 2, 4, 21].

CHALLENGES

Treating HTN to desirable BP levels reduces adverse clinical outcomes [2–4, 6]. The first challenge for clinicians is that many patients with HTN are unaware that they have high BP. Early recognition and treatment are essential to prevent the consequences of HTN-related end-organ damage and subsequent complications.

The second challenge is that secondary causes of HTN, especially in younger patients, although less common, need to be excluded at the initial evaluation.

STRATEGIC PLANNING

A detailed history and physical examination at initial encounter are needed to confirm the diagnosis of HTN or the presence of long-standing uncontrolled HTN and for evidence of any end-organ damage related to HTN. Then, secondary causes, if suspected clinically, should be sought. Once the diagnosis of HTN is established, strategies for better control of HTN need to be formulated.

HIGH-RISK MARKERS

Advancing age, genetic factors (family history), race (African Americans), increased body weight, physical inactivity, tobacco use, obstructive sleep apnea, excessive alcohol use, and inadequate adaptation to stress are known risk factors of HTN [1, 2, 24–32].

Sodium and potassium intake may play a role in increasing BP in some patients, but remains controversial at present [21, 33–35].

HIGH-RISK PREDICTORS

The presence of kidney disease, diabetes mellitus (DM), high low-density lipoprotein cholesterol, and left ventricular hypertrophy is a predictor of high risk because these factors all worsen the outcomes of patients with HTN [3, 12, 13, 26, 38–44].

INVESTIGATIONS

In the history, the patient should be checked for possible underlying causes of HTN. These include renal disease, adrenal gland tumor, thyroid problems, coarctation of the aorta, sleep apnea, the use of birth control medications, cold remedies (decongestants), non-steroidal pain-relieving medications, illegal drugs (amphetamines, cocaine), and alcohol in an excessive amount [3, 4, 21]. The patient's social tendency to be compliant or non-compliant with medication, laboratory testing, and follow-up should be documented. It is also important to document any family history of HTN, as this often is suggestive of the presence of primary HTN [21].

Symptoms to look for

HTN does not cause any symptoms per se. The symptoms are usually due to end-organ damage or secondary causes of HTN [75]. In the case of hypertensive crisis, patients may present with severe headache, nausea and vomiting, confusion, acute left HF, or visual changes [21].

Signs to look for

A detailed physical examination should be performed to confirm the presence of HTN, any end-organ damage, or any secondary causes of HTN. If the BP measured by staff is high at the first visit or if it is high at follow-up visit, usually the physician would recheck it herself or himself to confirm the presence of uncontrolled HTN. Ophthalmic examination at the initial visit is important to assess and document any changes in the retinal vessels due to HTN or DM.

Blood pressure readings

BP readings, taken 5 minutes apart after a 5-minute rest in the sitting position, are recommended. It is important that the BP is taken with an adequate sized arm cuff and preferably with a sphygmomanometer [3, 45]. Any US Food and Drug Administration (US)-approved BP measuring device may be used, but it is important that it is accurate and well-calibrated [21]. BP should be measured in both arms. There is often a 5- to 10 mmHg differential in readings between the two arms, and the arm with the higher reading should be used for all subsequent measurements. Consistent high BP readings on two or three separate occasions, over a 2- to 3-week period, are necessary to establish the diagnosis of HTN [21]. Exceptions are when the patient is already taking medications for high BP or if the BP is markedly elevated (>160/110 mmHg), when repeated BP readings over time are not needed to establish a diagnosis of HTN.

CLINICAL PEARLS
How often to measure BP In subjects who have pre-HTN, it is recommended that the BP be measured at least every 2 years by a health care provider. In a recent publication by the prevention panel of health authorities, it is

estimated that 67 million people in the United States have high BP and those with upper-normal BP readings should have their BP checked every year [22]. In those who have HTN, frequency of measurement will vary with response to treatment. A repeat measurement within 1 month is necessary to evaluate response to medication and following a dose adjustment or the addition of a new medication. Once the BP is adequately controlled, measurements may be less frequent, but it is preferable that patients see their health care providers at least once every 6 months or earlier if necessary.

Self-measurement of BP

Many BP devices are currently available, but it is important that these devices are calibrated frequently, as erroneous readings often lead to unnecessary patient anxiety. Occasional measurements, once a week or more often if necessary, are useful in assessing the appropriateness of therapy. Self-monitoring is also important if there are any adverse effects experienced by the patient. However, we discourage measurement of BP many times a day, as fluctuations are common and variable readings often lead to unnecessary patient anxiety and visits to the clinician's office.

Routine ambulatory BP

Diurnal variations in BP are common and may have treatment implications [46]. However, routine monitoring of ambulatory BP is not indicated as evidence-based treatment guidelines [3] are based on office-based BP readings rather than on ambulatory BP readings. Ambulatory BP monitoring may help in identifying patients with white collar HTN and patients who truly have refractory HTN despite multiple antihypertensive medications [46, 47].

Smart testing

A 12-lead electrocardiogram and preferably an echocardiogram should be obtained at baseline to assess for left ventricular hypertrophy, due to its adverse effects on outcomes [21, 38–40]. Blood lipid and glycated hemoglobin (HbA$_{1c}$) levels should be measured, as elevated LDL levels and DM worsen outcomes in patients with HTN [16, 43, 48]. Examination of the urine for proteinuria and the blood for electrolytes and measurement of renal function based on calculated estimated glomerular filtration rate (eGFR) are important, as the presence of kidney disease adversely affects outcomes [37–40]. If clinically suspected, other tests to confirm the secondary causes can be ordered accordingly.

MANAGEMENT

Lifestyle modifications

Although there are no outcome studies showing that lifestyle modifications in patients with HTN decrease mortality or stroke rates, there is substantial evidence that lifestyle changes do lower BP [32, 49]. Restricting sodium intake to 1500–2300 mg/day, achieving an ideal body weight (body mass index [BMI] of 18.5–24.9 kg/m [2]), waist circumference of <102 cm for men and 88 cm for women, and 30 minutes of aerobic exercise daily are recommended in all patients with HTN, as well those with a diagnosis of pre-HTN [32].

Tobacco smoking increases BP and heart rate acutely and is deleterious to CV health [31]. Even second-hand smoking has deleterious health consequences and should be avoided. Excessive use of alcohol increases BP and encourages unhealthy lifestyles and must be avoided by all patients with HTN [28]. Drinking coffee in moderation raises BP acutely, but when drinking on a daily basis, these effects are blunted and have not been shown to exert detrimental health effects [32].

There are no randomized controlled trials documenting that limiting alcohol to two drinks per day for males and one drink per day for females has any beneficial effects on outcome. Observational studies are, however, suggestive of CV health benefits of moderate alcohol consumption and thus are recommended (restricting alcohol to 14 units per week in men and 9 units per week in women) [32].

In addition to lifestyle modifications, the majority of patients will also need pharmacologic treatment to control their HTN more effectively.

Pharmacologic treatment

With the exception of very low BP values [49, 50], observational data showed that both lower diastolic (<90 mmHg) and systolic BP (especially in the elderly) are associated with lower rates of stroke [4]. Until recently, optimal BP was considered to be <140/90 mmHg in all patients with uncomplicated HTN and to values <130/80 mmHg for those who, in addition to HTN, also had either DM or CV or renal disease [4]. These recommendations were based more on expert opinion than on randomized outcome trial results [3]. The new Eighth Joint National Committee on the Prevention, Detection, Evaluation, and Treatment of High Blood Pressure (known as JNC-8) treatment guidelines made recommendations primarily based on randomized clinical trial results that were recently published [51–55]. Age and race of the patient are important considerations in making treatment decisions in these guidelines [20, 52, 55–61]. Many have raised objections to these guideline recommendations for fear that many older patients will be inadequately treated. However, in our opinion, it appears that these objections are not justified in the absence of published randomized trials showing results that are contrary to the JNC 8 published guidelines. Recently, at the AHA meeting in Orlando November 2015, the investigators of the Systolic Blood Pressure Intervention Trial (SPRINT) trial presented their long awaited results and showed the best CV outcomes with a systolic BP less than 120 mmHg [62]. This target BP may become the standard BP in future guidelines.

EVIDENCE BASED MEDICINE
New target of optimal blood pressure in the SPRINT Trial In the SPRINT study, 9361 persons aged 50 years or greater with a systolic BP of 130 mmHg or higher and an increased CV risk, but without DM, were randomized to receive treatment in order to achieve a systolic BP target of less than 120 mmHg (intensive treatment) or a target of less than 140 mmHg (standard treatment). The primary composite outcome was myocardial infarction, other acute coronary syndromes, stroke, heart failure, or death from CV causes.

At 1 year, the results showed that the mean systolic BP was 121.4 mmHg in the intensive-treatment group and 136.2 mmHg in the standard-treatment group. The intervention was stopped early after a median follow-up of 3.26 years owing to a significantly lower rate of the primary composite outcome in the intensive-treatment group than in the standard-treatment group (1.65% per year vs. 2.19% per year; hazard ratio with intensive treatment, 0.75; 95% confidence interval [CI], 0.64 to 0.89; $P < 0.001$). All-cause mortality was also significantly lower in the intensive-treatment group (hazard ratio, 0.73; 95% CI, 0.60 to 0.90; $P = 0.003$). Rates of serious adverse events of HTN, syncope, electrolyte abnormalities, and acute kidney injury or failure, but not of injurious falls, were higher in the intensive-treatment group than in the standard-treatment group.

In conclusion, the SPRINT investigators suggest that among patients at high risk for CV events but without diabetes, targeting a systolic BP of less than 120 mmHg, as compared with less than 140 mmHg, resulted in lower rates of fatal and non-fatal major CV events and death from any cause, although significantly higher rates of some adverse events were observed in the intensive-treatment group [62].

Non-African Americans

Non-African American patients aged 60 years and older with uncomplicated HTN and BP >150/90 mmHg need initial pharmacologic treatment with either an angiotensin-converting enzyme inhibitor (ACEI), an angiotensin type I receptor blocker (ARB), a calcium channel blocker (CCB), or a thiazide-type diuretic. The goal is for a BP of <150/90 mmHg, rather than previous recommendation of ≤140/90 mmHg [3]. Invariably, more than one agent from a different class of drug is needed to achieve the goal (a combination of a CCB and ACEI or an ARB or a thiazide-type diuretic and either an ACEI or ARB or a CCB). More than two classes of drugs may be required to achieve the ideal BP. A combination of an ACEI and an ARB is not recommended due to increased adverse effects from combination treatment [3, 55, 64].

If these patients also have DM or renal disease, the target BP goal is still <150/90 mmHg [3] rather than values lower than 130–140/80–90 mmHg, with the exception that one should incorporate an ACEI in the treatment regimen [47, 65–69].

African Americans

African Americans aged ≥60 years with uncomplicated HTN and BP >150/90 mmHg should be initially treated with a thiazide-type diuretic, preferably chlorthalidone, as was used in the Antihypertensive and Lipid Lowering Treatment to Prevent Heart Attack (ALLHAT) trial [55, 61, 62, 72] and or a CCB (amlodipine). These patients respond less to an ACEI or a β-blocker [3]. If these patients also have DM, recommendations are to incorporate an ACEI to prevent further renal injury. These treatment recommendations are based on trial results that show that both systolic and diastolic BPs are targets for therapy and BP <140/90 mmHg does not reduce adverse clinical outcomes compared with values <150/90 mmHg. In patients aged <60 years (30–59 years), the treatment target is diastolic BP rather than systolic BP [75]. Those with a diastolic BP >90 mmHg should receive pharmacologic treatment aimed at lowering diastolic BP to <90 mmHg. Initial treatment with a CCB, an ACEI, or a thiazide diuretic is recommended. Often, more than one class of agent is needed to achieve the BP goal.

As in patients older than 60 years, African Americans respond better to a thiazide-type diuretic (chlorthalidone) or a CCB or combination of the two than they do to an ACEI or a β-blocker [61, 73].

CLINICAL PEARLS

Systolic BP in patients aged 60 years or less Control of systolic BP in patients aged ≤60 years is relevant, but in randomized trials, the treatment target has been diastolic BP and not systolic BP; systolic BP usually also decreases along with diastolic BP.

What should one do if the BP on treatment is lower than recommended pressures? If the patient is tolerating the medications without any side-effects, one should continue therapy without any change. There is no evidence to the contrary that in the absence of adverse effects from therapy that the patient comes to harm.

Beta-blockers

β-Blockers are proven antihypertensive agents but outcome studies are lacking [3]. A recent study reported that the rates of stroke were higher with atenolol-based treatment compared to an ARB-based treatment [64]. Therefore, these drugs are reserved for patients who also have established coronary artery disease (CAD) or for control of angina or arrhythmias. When using a β-blocker in hypertensive patients, one should avoid a dihyropyridine CCB (diltiazem or verapamil) and clonidine, as combining these drugs is associated with increased side-effects due to bradycardia or heart block. Randomized trials that recommend one β-blocker over another are lacking, regardless of whether they have additional α-blocking or vasodilatory properties.

CLINICAL PEARLS

Medications that should not be used with

HTN α-Blockers are not recommended for the treatment of HTN due to the increased incidence of HF observed in the ALLHAT trial [62]. Non-steroidal anti-inflammatory drugs (NSAIDs) increase BP by decreasing renal sodium excretion and by interfering with the effects of CCBs and ACEIs. Patients should be advised against excessive use of these agents [3]. Regarding birth control pills, some women are especially prone to elevation of BP secondary to hormonal therapy. Individual discussion with the patient and their gynecologist is indicated to modify hormonal therapy and the institution of antihypertensive therapy if indicated [3, 4].

Aldosterone blockers

Aldosterone blockers lower BP [3] but are not used routinely as these agents can cause hyperkalemia when used with an ACEI or an ARB to treat HTN [3]. However, in some patients who have aldosterone escape or evidence of hyperaldosteronism, these agents may be useful if used appropriately [74]. No outcome trials are available to make definite recommendations for their use with other antihypertensive agents.

CLINICAL PEARLS
Hypertension in aortic stenosis There is some evidence (not based on randomized trials) that a careful trial of ACEIs is worth a trial as these agents improve forward output even in the presence of fixed aortic stenosis. When the patient has associated CAD, we often use a β-blocker rather than clonidine for patient with aortic stenosis and HTN.

INFLUENCE OF COMORBID CONDITIONS

Diabetes mellitus

Patients with HTN who also have DM are at increased risk of CV complications. If they also have albuminuria, an ACEI and a statin need to be incorporated in the treatment regimen [3, 43, 48, 75]. The goal of BP control is influenced by age and not by DM alone per se.

INTRIGUING OBSERVATIONS: WHAT IS THE OPTIMAL BLOOD PRESSURE IN DIABETIC PATIENTS ACCORDING TO SPRINT AND ACCORD?
With the substantial reductions of CV events in the SPRINT trial, the question for clinicians who take care of diabetic patients is: Why did the SPRINT trial succeed with a systolic BP target under 120 mmHg

when the ACCORD trial failed with intensive treatment to the same target in diabetes? [62, 76].

In a detailed review of inclusion and exclusion criteria, the results showed that the PRINT trial enrolled 9361 hypertensive patients with additional risk equivalent of a Framingham 10-year cardiovascular disease risk score of 20% while excluding patients with DM, prior stroke, and polycystic kidney disease. The ACCORD trial enrolled 4733 HTN patients with anatomical evidence of a substantial amount of atherosclerosis, albuminuria, left ventricular hypertrophy, or at least two additional risk factors for cardiovascular disease (dyslipidemia, hypertension, smoking, or obesity). By these inclusion and exclusion criteria, the patients with confirmed CAD or CKD were not included. In the review of results, some investigators noted that the ACCORD primary outcomes included a higher proportion of events less sensitive to blood-pressure reduction [77]. So with the strong results of SPRINT, the guideline committees and the cardiovascular community will have to decide whether the SPRINT results should be generalized to patients with HTN and DM.

Chronic kidney disease

Uncontrolled HTN often leads to kidney injury and ultimately to renal failure. Adequate BP control prevents or minimizes renal damage. In addition, one should add a low-dose statin and an ACEI or an ARB to the treatment regimen to slow the progress of renal impairment over time [3, 64, 68, 70, 71].

CLINICAL PEARLS
Diuretics in chronic renal insufficiency We use diuretics in the majority of patients with chronic kidney disease (CKD) who have HTN. When serum creatinine is <3 mg%, the thiazide group of diuretics are indicated. When creatinine is >3 mg% or eGFR is <30 mL/min/1.73 m [2], loop diuretics are indicated. In that situation, one often requires higher doses of furosemide. The only time the use of a diuretic is restricted is when a patient is dehydrated.

Hypertensive urgency

Some patients with HTN present with severe headache, nausea and vomiting, confusion, acute left HF, or visual changes due to high BP with values >180/110 mmHg. Urgent treatment with a vasodilator (nitroprusside or nitroglycerin) and/or labetolol, a β-blocker with α/β-blocking effect, or a CCB (nicardipine) is usually effective in controlling the BP. Subsequently, these patients need long-term oral treatment with oral antihypertensive agents as discussed earlier.

Compliance with antihypertensive medications

HTN is a life-long illness, and it is important that patients take their medications without interruptions throughout their life. Regular visits with a health care provider are important to emphasize the importance of compliance with the medications to prevent a hypertensive emergency and minimize end-organ damage due to high BP.

Resistant hypertension   When the BP remains elevated despite the use of three different classes of antihypertensive drugs including a diuretic, patients are considered to have resistant HTN [3, 78–80]. Often, this is due to poor compliance with the medications or use of inadequate doses of the medications [80].

CLINICAL PEARLS
Medications for resistant HTN There are no randomized clinical trials for the medical treatment of patients with resistant HTN. In the SIMPLICITY 3 trial, doxazosin was used in 12% of patients as the fourth drug with some positive response. Often, one uses hydralazine, before considering an α-blocker, but there is no science behind it in this group of patients. Because doxazosin and other α-blockers increase the incidence of HF in patients with HTN, they are best avoided.

Renal denervation for resistant HTN   Open-label trials showed that renal denervation was very effective in controlling BP in patients with resistant HTN [78]. A subsequent sham-controlled trial failed to confirm these findings [80]. In this large trial of 535 patients, at 6 months after renal denervation, mean systolic BP and mean 24-hour ambulatory pressures were no different from the sham plus medically treated patients [78]. At present, this procedure remains unapproved by the FDA for use in the United States, although it is still used widely in Europe [76]. We do not recommend this procedure in patients with resistant HTN. These patients need close follow-up and adjustment of treatment to achieve BP goals.

Stenting for renal artery stenosis   Many older patients have renal artery stenosis, which accounts for HTN. Stenting of renal artery, however, was not superior to pharmacologic treatment in a recent trial and is not routinely recommended at the present [81].

Hypertension during pregnancy   HTN is not uncommon during pregnancy, and pre-eclampsia and eclampsia carry an increased risk to the fetus as well as to the mother. ACEIs and ARBs are contraindicated due to their known teratogenic effects. Currently, methyldopa and labetalol are the drugs of choice to control BP during pregnancy [21].

SECONDARY CAUSES OF HYPERTENSION

There are many common but potentially reversible causes of secondary HTN. Secondary causes of HTN other than NSAIDs and illicit drugs are uncommon and do not warrant routine work-up for their exclusion in all patients presenting with HTN. Diagnostic yield is low, but when presentations are suggestive of possible underlying causes, a detailed evaluation including specialized tests is indicated as individualized treatment is indicated for each disorder. Some rare but potentially treatable causes of HTN are listed in Table 2.1.

Medications
Many over-the-counter and prescription medications can lead to HTN or cause problems with BP control. The most common offending agents

---

Table 2.1 Rare causes of hypertension

1. Endocrine disorders:
   a Hypothyroidism and hyperthyroidism
   b Parathyroidism
   c Acromegaly
   d Cushing's syndrome
   e Pheochromocytoma
   f Primary aldosteronism
2. Coarctation of aorta
3. Renovascular HTN
4. Genetic disorders with gene mutations

are NSAIDs, decongestants (containing pseudoephedrine), antidepressants (tricyclics and selective serotonin uptake inhibitors), and glucocorticoids. Illicit drugs, especially cocaine and amphetamines, are not uncommon causes of acute presentation with HTN emergency. Avoidance of these medications or judicious use is important to manage HTN better. Cyclosporine, often used following solid organ transplantation, leads to HTN due to decreased renal flow. Treatment with antihypertensive is usually needed to control HTN.

Obstructive sleep apnea

This is not an uncommon cause of HTN. Obese patients who are prone to HTN also have a higher incidence of obstructive sleep apnea. Treatment of obstructive sleep apnea is important and may eliminate the need for medications or reduce their use for controlling BP.

ACTION POINTS

1 BP increases with age, and elevated BP to values >140/90 mmHg is associated with adverse clinical outcomes. The majority of patients do not know that they have HTN, and in nearly 95% of patients one cannot find an underlying cause. These patients are considered to have primary (essential) HTN.

2 Primary HTN is usually an asymptomatic disease, but over time causes arteriosclerosis and end-organ damage, resulting in increased rates of stroke, death from CV causes, HF, renal damage, peripheral arterial disease, impaired vision, and memory problems. It requires treatment for life.

3 Lifestyle modifications with daily exercise, weight control, restriction of daily sodium intake to 1500–2300 mg, and restriction of alcohol use lowers BP, and is recommended in all patients. Smoking tobacco is associated with a rapid increase in BP and smoking cessation, and avoidance of second-hand smoke is important as it lowers CV morbidity and mortality.

4 Treatment of primary HTN with medications reduces stroke rates, HF, renal injury, and CV morbidity and mortality. Current treatment recommendations are based on the results of randomized clinical trials, and age plays an important role in instituting pharmacologic treatment. Patients aged ≥60 years who have BP >150/90 mmHg need pharmacologic treatment to lower BP to values <150/90 mmHg rather than the older recommendations of ≤140/90 mmHg. Often, more than one class of drugs (a thiazide

diuretic, ACEI or an ARB, or CCB) is needed to adequately control BP. A target of treatment in patients younger than 60 years (30–59 years), is diastolic BP rather than systolic BP. When the diastolic BP is >90 mmHg, lowering of diastolic BP to values <90 mmHg is recommended. This often requires treatment with more than one class of antihypertensive agents as discussed earlier.

5 In patients 50 years or older who are at high CV risk, but have no DM, previous stroke nor polycystic kidney diseases, the target of systolic BP to <120 mmHg may be desirable based on the results of the SPRINT trial.

6 β-Blockers are often used in patients with HTN who also have CAD or cardiac arrhythmias. African American patients with essential HTN respond better to a thiazide-type diuretic and/or a CCB rather than an ACEI or a β-blocker. Patients with HTN who also have diabetes and/or CKD should also receive an ACEI and a statin to improve clinical outcomes. At present, the role of renal denervation to treat resistant HTN remains unproved.

REFERENCES

1. Burt VL, Cutler JA, Higgins M, et al. Trends in the prevalence, awareness, treatment, and control of hypertension in the adult US population. Data from the Health Examination Surveys, 1960 to 1991. *Hypertension.* 1995;26:60–69.
2. Joint National Commission on Prevention, Detection, Evaluation, and Treatment of High Blood Pressure. The sixth report of the Joint National Commission on Prevention, Detection, Evaluation, and Treatment of High Blood Pressure. *Arch Intern Med.* 1997;157:2413–2445.
3. James PA, Oparil S, Carter BL, et al. 2014 Evidence-based guideline for the management of high blood pressure in adults: Report from the panel members appointed to the Eighth Joint National Committee (JNC 8). *JAMA.* 2014;311:507–520.
4. Chobanian AV, Bakris GL, Black HR, et al. The Seventh Report of the Joint National Committee on Prevention, Detection, Evaluation, and Treatment of High Blood Pressure: the JNC 7 report. *JAMA.* 2003;289:2560–2572.
5. MacMahon S, Peto R, Cutler J, et al. Blood pressure, stroke, and coronary heart disease. Part 1, Prolonged differences in blood pressure: Prospective observational studies corrected for the regression dilution bias. *Lancet.* 1990;335:765–774.
6. Collins R, Peto R, MacMahon S, et al. Blood pressure, stroke, and coronary heart disease. Part 2, Short-term reductions in blood pressure: Overview of randomised drug trials in their epidemiological context. *Lancet.* 1990;335:827–838.

7. Kannel WB, Gordon T, Schwartz MJ. Systolic versus diastolic blood pressure and risk of coronary heart disease. *The Framingham Study. Am J Cardiol.* 1971;27:335–346.

8. Kannel WB. Blood pressure as a cardiovascular risk factor: Prevention and treatment. *JAMA.* 1996;275:1571–1576.

9. van den Hoogen PC1, Feskens EJ, Nagelkerke NJ, et al. The relation between blood pressure and mortality due to coronary heart disease among men in different parts of the world. *N Engl J Med.* 2000;342:1–8.

10. Levy D, Larson MG, Vasan RS, et al. The progression from hypertension to congestive heart failure. *JAMA.* 1996;275:1557–1562.

11. Novo S, Barbagallo M, Abrignani MG, et al. Increased prevalence of cardiac arrhythmias and transient episodes of myocardial ischemia in hypertensives with left ventricular hypertrophy but without clinical history of coronary heart disease. *Am J Hypertens.* 1997;10:843–851.

12. Freedman BI, Iskandar SS, Appel RG. The link between hypertension and nephrosclerosis. *Am J Kidney Dis.* 1995;25:207–221.

13. Walker WG. Hypertension-related renal injury: A major contributor to end-stage renal disease. *Am J Kidney Dis.* 1993;22:164–173.

14. Kannel WB, Dawber TR, Sorlie P, Wolf PA. Components of blood pressure and risk of atherothrombotic brain infarction: The Framingham Study. *Stroke.* 1976;7:327–331.

15. Shaper AG, Phillips AN, Pocock SJ, et al. Risk factors for stroke in middle aged British men. *BMJ* 1991;302:1111–1115.

16. Prospective Studies Collaboration. Cholesterol, diastolic blood pressure, and stroke: 13,000 strokes in 450,000 people in 45 prospective cohorts. *Lancet.* 1995;346:1647–1653.

17. MacMahon S. Blood pressure and the prevention of stroke. *J Hypertens Suppl.* 1996;14:S39–S46.

18. Nielsen WB, Vestbo J, Jensen GB. Isolated systolic hypertension as a major risk factor for stroke and myocardial infarction and an unexploited source of cardiovascular prevention: A prospective population based study. *J Hum Hypertens.* 1995;9:175–180.

19. Glynn RJ, Field TS, Rosner B, et al. Evidence for a positive linear relation between blood pressure and mortality in elderly people. *Lancet.* 1995;345:825–829.

20. MRC Working Party. Medical Research Council trial of treatment of hypertension in older adults: Principal results. *BMJ.* 1992;304:405–412.

21. Kaplan NM. *Kaplan's Clinical Hypertension*, 9th edn. Philadelphia: Lippincott Williams and Wilkins; 2006.

22. Final Recommendation Statement: High Blood Pressure in Adults: Screening. U.S. Preventive Services Task Force. October 2015. www.uspreventiveservices gtaskforce.org/Page/Document/RecommendationStatementFinal/high-blood-pressure-in-adults-screening

23. Valderrama AL, Gillespie C, King SC, George MG, Hong Y, Gregg E. Vital signs: awareness and treatment of uncontrolled hypertension among adults – United States, 2003–2010. *MMWR Morb Mortal Wkly Rep.* 2012;61:703–709 [Correction added after online publication 26–Dec-2012: The authors in this reference have been updated.]

24. Ebrahim S, Smith GD. Lowering blood pressure: A systematic review of sustained effects of non-pharmacological interventions. *J Public Health Med.* 1998;20:441–448.

25. Marmot MG, Elliott P, Shipley MJ, et al. Alcohol and blood pressure: The INTERSALT study. *BMJ.* 1994;308:1263–1267.

26. Puddey IB, Beilin LJ, Vandongen R, et al. Evidence for a direct effect of alcohol consumption on blood pressure in normotensive men. A randomized controlled trial. *Hypertension.* 1985;7:707–713.

27. Puddey IB, Beilin LJ, Vandongen R. Regular alcohol use raises blood pressure in treated hypertensive subjects. A randomised controlled trial. *Lancet.* 1987;1:647–651.

28. Maheswaran R1, Gill JS, Davies P, Beevers DG. High blood pressure due to alcohol. A rapidly reversible effect. *Hypertension.* 1991;17:787–792.

29. Sacks FM1, Kass EH. Low blood pressure in vegetarians: Effects of specific foods and nutrients. *Am J Clin Nutr.* 1988;48(Suppl):795–800.

30. Jonas BS, Franks P, Ingram DD. Are symptoms of anxiety and depression risk factors for hypertension? Longitudinal evidence from the National Health and Nutrition Examination Survey I Epidemiologic Follow-up Study. *Arch Fam Med.* 1997;6:43–49.

31. Shinton R, Beevers G. Meta-analysis of relation between cigarette smoking and stroke. *BMJ.* 1989;298:789–794.

32. Khan NA, Hemmelgarn B, Herman RJ, et al. The 2009 Canadian Hypertension Education Program recommendations for the management of hypertension: Part 2 – therapy. *Can J Cardiol.* 2009;25:287–298.

33. Law MR, Frost CD, Wald NJ. By how much does dietary salt reduction lower blood pressure? I: Analysis of observational data among populations. *BMJ.* 1991;302:811–815.

34. Cappuccio FP, Markandu ND, Carney C, et al. Double-blind randomised trial of modest salt restriction in older people. *Lancet.* 1997;350:850–854.

35. Whelton PK, He J, Cutler JA, et al. Effects of oral potassium on blood pressure. Meta-analysis of randomized controlled clinical trials. *JAMA.* 1997;277:1624–1632.

36. Koren MJ, Devereux RB, Casale PN, et al. Relation of left ventricular mass and geometry to morbidity and mortality in uncomplicated essential hypertension. *Ann Intern Med.* 1991;114:345–352.

37. Kaplan NM. The deadly quartet. Upper-body obesity, glucose intolerance, hypertriglyceridemia and hypertension. *Arch Intern Med.* 1989;149:1514–1520.

38. Levy D, Garrison RJ, Savage DD, et al. Prognostic implications of echocardiographically determined left ventricular mass in the Framingham Heart Study. *N Engl J Med.* 1990;322:1561–1566.

39. Koren MJ, Devereux RB, Casale PN, et al. Relation of left ventricular mass and geometry to morbidity and mortality in uncomplicated essential hypertension. *Ann Intern Med.* 1991;114:345–352.

40. Schmieder RE, Martus P, Klingbeil A. Reversal of left ventricular hypertrophy in essential hypertension. A meta-analysis of randomized double-blind studies. *JAMA.* 1996;275:1507–1513.

41. Perneger TV, Nieto FJ, Whelton PK, et al. A prospective study of blood pressure and serum creatinine. Results from the 'Clue' Study and the ARIC Study. *JAMA*. 1993; 269:488–493.

42. Klag MJ, Whelton PK, Randall BL, et al. End-stage renal disease in African-American and white men. 16-year MRFIT findings. *JAMA*. 1997;277:1293–1298.

43. Tight blood pressure control and risk of macrovascular and microvascular complications in type 2 diabetes: UKPDS 38. UK Prospective Diabetes Study Group. *BMJ*. 1998;317:703–713.

44. Wright JT Jr, Bakris G, Greene T, et al. Effect of blood pressure lowering and antihypertensive drug class on progression of hypertensive kidney disease: Results from the AASK trial. *JAMA*. 2002;288:2421–2431.

45. Pickering JG, et al. Recommendations for blood pressure measurement in humans and experimental animals: Part 1: Blood pressure measurement in humans. A statement for professionals from the Subcommittee of Professional and Public Education of the American Heart Association Council on High Blood Pressure Research. *Circulation*. 2005;111:697–716.

46. Pickering T. Recommendations for the use of home (self) and ambulatory blood pressure monitoring. American Society of Hypertension Ad Hoc Panel. *Am J Hypertens*. 1996;9:1–11.

47. Redon J, Campos C, Narciso ML, et al. Prognostic value of ambulatory blood pressure monitoring in refractory hypertension: A prospective study. *Hypertension*. 1998;31:712–718.

48. American Diabetes Association. Standards of medical care in diabetes, 2013. *Diabetes Care*. 2013;36(Suppl 1):S11–S66.

49. Oparil S, Calhoun DA. Managing the patient with hard-to-control hypertension. *Am Fam Physician*. 1998;57:1007–1014.

50. The J-curve phenomenon and the treatment of hypertension: Is there a point beyond which pressure reduction is dangerous? *JAMA*. 1991;265:489–495.

51. Tight blood pressure control and risk of macrovascular and microvascular complications in type 2 diabetes: UKPDS 38. UK Prospective Diabetes Study Group. *BMJ*. 1998;317:703–713.

52. Beckett NS, Peters R, Fletcher AE, et al. Treatment of hypertension in patients 80 years of age or older. *N Engl J Med*. 2008; 358:1887–1898.

53. Verdecchia P, Staessen JA, Angeli F, et al. Usual versus tight control of systolic blood pressure in non-diabetic patients with hypertension (Cardio-Sis): An open-label randomised trial. *Lancet*. 2009;374:525–533.

54. Ruggenenti P, et al. Blood-pressure control for renoprotection in patients with non-diabetic chronic renal disease (REIN-2): Multicentre, randomised controlled trial. *Lancet*. 2005;365:939–946.

55. Wright JT Jr[1], Harris-Haywood S, Pressel S, et al. Clinical outcomes by race in hypertensive patients with and without the metabolic syndrome: Antihypertensive and Lipid-Lowering Treatment to Prevent Heart Attack Trial (ALLHAT). *Arch Intern Med*. 2008 Jan 28;168(2):207–217. doi: 10.1001/archinternmed.2007.66.

56. Staessen JA, Fagard R, Thijs L, et al. Randomised double-blind comparison of placebo and active treatment for older patients with isolated systolic

hypertension. The Systolic Hypertension in Europe (Syst-Eur) Trial Investigators. *Lancet.* 1997;350:757–764.

57. Prevention of stroke by antihypertensive drug treatment in older persons with isolated systolic hypertension. Final results of the Systolic Hypertension in the Elderly Program (SHEP). SHEP Cooperative Research Group. *JAMA.* 1991;265:3255–3264.

58. JATOS Study Group. Principal results of the Japanese trial to assess optimal systolic blood pressure in elderly hypertensive patients (JATOS). *Hypertens Res.* 2008;31:2115–2127.

59. Ogihara T, Saruta T, Rakugi H, et al. Target blood pressure for treatment of isolated systolic hypertension in the elderly: Valsartan in Elderly Isolated Systolic Hypertension Study. *Hypertension.* 2010;56:196–202.

60. Curb JD, Pressel SL, Cutler JA, et al. Effect of diuretic-based antihypertensive treatment on cardiovascular disease risk in older diabetic patients with isolated systolic hypertension. Systolic Hypertension in the Elderly Program Cooperative Research Group. *JAMA.* 1996;276(23):1886–1892.

61. ALLHAT Officers and Coordinators for the ALLHAT Collaborative Research Group. Major outcomes in high-risk hypertensive patients randomized to angiotensin-converting enzyme inhibitor or calcium channel blocker vs diuretic: The Antihypertensive and Lipid-Lowering Treatment to Prevent Heart Attack Trial (ALLHAT). *JAMA.* 2002;288:2981–2997.

62. The SPRINT Research Group A Randomized Trial of Intensive versus Standard Blood-Pressure Control November 9, 2015DOI: 10.1056/NEJMoa1511939.

63. Krakoff LR, et al. 2014 HTN recommendations from the Eighth Joint National Committee panel members raise concern for elderly black and female patients. *JACC.* 2014;64:394–402.

64. Dahlöf B, Devereux RB, Kjeldsen SE, et al.; for the LIFE Study Group. Cardiovascular morbidity and mortality in the Losartan Intervention for Endpoint reduction in hypertension study (LIFE): A randomised trial against atenolol. *Lancet.* 2002;359:995–1003.

65. The SOLVD Investigators. Effect of enalapril on mortality and the development of heart failure in asymptomatic patients with reduced left ventricular ejection fractions. *N Engl J Med.* 1992; 327:685–691.

66. Grossman E, Messerli FH. Calcium antagonists in cardiovascular disease: A necessary controversy but an unnecessary panic. *Am J Med.* 1997;102:147–149.

67. Gansevoort RT, de Zeeuw D, de Jong PE. Additive antiproteinuric effect of ACE inhibition and a low-protein diet in human renal disease. *Nephrol Dial Transplant.* 1995;10:497–504.

68. Giatras I, Lau J, Levey AS. Effect of angiotensin-converting enzyme inhibitors on the progression of nondiabetic renal disease: A meta-analysis of randomized trials. Angiotensin-Converting-Enzyme Inhibition and Progressive Renal Disease Study Group. *Ann Intern Med.* 1997;127:337–345.

69. Bauer JH, Reams GP, Lal SM. Renal protective effect of strict blood pressure control with enalapril therapy. *Arch Intern Med.* 1987;147:1397–1400.

70. Maschio G, Alberti D, Janin G, et al. Effect of the angiotensin-converting-enzyme inhibitor benazepril on the progression of chronic renal insufficiency. *N Engl J Med.* 1996;334:939–945.

71. Hall WD, Kusek JW, Kirk KA, et al. Short-term effects of blood pressure control and antihypertensive drug on glomerular filtration rate: The African-American Study of Kidney Disease and Hypertension Pilot Study. *Am J Kidnev Dis.* 1997;29:720–728.

72. Flack JM, Sica DA, Bakris G, et al. Management of high blood pressure in blacks: An update of the International Society on Hypertension in Blacks consensus statement. *Hypertension.* 2010;56:780–800.

73. Leenen FHH, Nwachuku CE, Black HR, et al. Clinical events in high-risk hypertensive patients randomly assigned to calcium-channel blocker versus angiotensin-converting enzyme inhibitor in the Antihypertensive and Lipid-Lowering Treatment to prevent Heart Attack Trial. *Hypertension.* 2006;48:374–384.

74. Vaclavik J, et al. Spironolactone in resistant hypertension. *Hypertension.* 2011;57:1069–1075.

75. Patel A, MacMahon S, et al.; ADVANCE Collaborative Group. Effects of a fixed combination of perindopril and indapamide on macrovascular and microvascular outcomes in patients with type 2 diabetes mellitus (the ADVANCE trial): A randomised controlled trial. *Lancet.* 2007;370:829–840.

76. The ACCORD Study Group. Effects of intensive blood-pressure control in type 2 diabetes mellitus. *N Engl J Med.* 2010; 362:1575–1585.

77. Perkovic V, Rodgers A. Redefining blood-pressure targets – SPRINT starts the marathon November 9. 2015DOI: 10.1056/NEJMe1513301.

78. Krum H, Schlaich M, Whitbourn R, et al. Catheter-based renal sympathetic denervation for resistant hypertension: A multicentre safety and proof-of-principle cohort study. *Lancet.* 2009;373:1275–1281.

79. Esler MD, Krum H, Sobotka PA, et al. Renal sympathetic denervation in patients with treatment-resistant hypertension (the Simplicity HTN-2 trial): A randomised controlled trial. *Lancet.* 2010;376:1903–1909.

80. Bhatt DL, et al. A controlled trial of renal denervation for resistant hypertension. *N Engl J Med.* 2014;370:1393–1401.

81. Cooper CJ, et al. Stenting and medical therapy for atherosclerotic renal artery stenosis. *N Engl J Med.* 2014;370:13–22.

CHAPTER 3

Stable Coronary Artery Disease

Mohammed Haris Umer Usman, Lê Hoàng Đức Toàn, Lê Thị Ngọc Trâm, Huỳnh Thị Thu Trúc, An Huynh and Aman Amanullah

Management of Complex Cardiovascular Problems, Fourth Edition. Edited by Thach N. Nguyen, Dayi Hu, Shao Liang Chen, Moo Hyun Kim and Cindy L. Grines. © 2016 John Wiley & Sons, Ltd. Published 2016 by John Wiley & Sons, Ltd.

BACKGROUND

Stable coronary artery disease (CAD) is defined as a state of myocardial demand/supply mismatch related to coronary blood flow disruption. It is usually related to reversible ischemia induced by exercise, emotion or other stresses with resultant transient chest discomfort (angina pectoris).

CHALLENGES

In the diagnosis and management of stable CAD, the **first challenge** is to confirm the diagnosis of stable CAD. This is a challenge because this is a clinical diagnosis. Not every patient has a significant fixed lesion in the epicardial coronary arteries. The **second challenge** is that there are many medical conditions which increase myocardial O_2 demand or reduce O_2 delivery, triggering chest pain and exacerbating previously stable angina. They are listed in Table 3.1. The **third challenge** is that in many patients with CAD, heart failure (HF) by causing cardiac dilation, mitral regurgitation, or tachyarrhythmias (including sinus tachycardia), could increase myocardial O_2 need and so frequency and severity of angina. These patients may present to the emergency room as acute coronary syndrome (ACS) or acute decompensated HF. So did ACS trigger HF or did HF trigger ACS? (Please see detailed explanations in Chapter 6.)

Although the greatest success of modern day therapeutic intervention has been reduction in mortality, today's challenges in the care of patients with stable CAD are the search for a perfect formula for a cost-effective diagnostic process, patient friendly medical therapy and patient-centered options for surgical and percutaneous interventions.

Table 3.1 Non-cardiac problems of increased oxygen demand

1. Anemia
2. Severe obesity
3. Uncontrolled hyperthyroidism
4. Cigarette smoking
5. Cocaine abuse
6. Fever (infections)
7. Tachycardia
8. Heart failure

Table 3.2 Pretest probability for coronary artery disease

Age	Non-anginal chest pain		Atypical wangina		Typical angina	
	Men	Women	Men	Women	Men	Women
30–39	4	2	34	12	76	26
40–49	13	3	51	22	87	55
50–59	20	7	65	31	93	73
60–69	27	14	72	51	94	86
70–79	54	24	69	37	89	68
>80	65	32	78	47	93	76

Pretest probability <10% = extremely low; 15% = low; 15% to 85% = Intermediate; >85% = very high.

STRATEGIC MAPPING

In the investigation of a patient with possible CAD, the first step is to perform a comprehensive history, physical examination and to order a basic work-up (blood tests, electrocardiogram (ECG), chest X-ray (CXR) or echocardiography). This is the first step in risk profiling the patients and in searching for their predicting factors.

The next step is to calculate the pretest probability (PTP) according to age, gender and the characteristics of symptoms. The results of the PTP are listed in Table 3.2 [1]. Then the patient is scheduled to have non-invasive or invasive testing based on the results of PTP and the sensitivity and specificity of the selected test.[1] As there are many options in the non-invasive approach, an optimal strategy for sequential multimodality imaging is needed in order to give excellent outcomes at the most competitive cost. Once a diagnosis of stable CAD is made, the last step is to give patient-centered medical, percutaneous or surgical treatment in order to prevent mortality and to return the patient to their age-appropriate level of activities.

RISK PROFILING

Based on the atherosclerotic cardiovascular disease (ASCVD) risks prediction calculated by the new Pooled Cohort Equations, the global

Table 3.3 Classification of global coronary artery disease risk

1. **Low risk:** Defined by an age-specific risk level that is below average. In general, low risk will correlate with a 10-year absolute CAD risk <10%. However, in women and younger men, low risk may correlate with 10-year absolute CAD risk <6%.
2. **Intermediate risk:** Intermediate risk is defined as a 10-year CAD risk from 10% to 20%. Among women and younger men can expanded intermediate-risk range of 6% to 20% may be appropriate.
3. **High risk:** High risk is defined as a 10-year CAD risk of >20%. CAD equivalents (e.g., diabetes mellitus, peripheral arterial disease) can also define high risk.

coronary artery disease risks are listed in Table 3.3 [2]. To download the app for the ASCVD risks, here is the link: www.cardiosource.org/ Science-And-Quality/Practice-Guidelines-and-Quality-Standards/2013- Prevention-Guideline-Tools.aspx. The results of the PTP may classify patients into low, intermediate and high global CAD risk (Table 3.3).

HIGH-RISK PREDICTORS

Clinical predictors: There are five clinical predictors (male gender, typical angina, history and EKG evidence of myocardial infarction (MI), diabetes mellitus (DM) and use of insulin). These predictors confer additive value in predicting the extent of CAD or the presence of severe left main or 3-vessel CAD [3,4].

Non-invasive predictors: Between all non-invasive predictors, the functional capacity is most important. Patients with stable CAD who achieved <5 MET of activity were shown to have a >4-fold higher risk of death when compared to patients who exercised to >10.7 metabolic equivalent (MET) [5,6]. Low left ventricular ejection fraction (LVEF) is also a strong negative prognostic factor.

Biomarkers: Because atherosclerosis is an inflammatory process, high-sensitivity C-reactive protein (hs-CRP) which is a marker of inflammation, has been associated with a higher risk of subsequent clinical CV events [7]. The brain natriuretic peptide (BNP) is also a strong negative prognostic predictor for patients with stable CAD [8].

Table 3.4 Definition of angina

Typical angina (definite): (1) Substernal chest discomfort with a characteristic quality and duration that is (2) provoked by exertion or emotional stress and (3) relieved by rest or nitroglycerin.
Atypical angina (probable): Meets 2 of the above characteristics.
Non-cardiac chest pain: Meets ≤1 of the typical angina characteristics.

INVESTIGATIONS

Symptoms to look for
There are three kinds of chest pain: Typical chest pain, atypical chest pain and non-typical chest pain [9]. The definitions are listed in Table 3.4.

CLINICAL PEARLS
Symptoms suggestive of left main disease or chronic total occlusion A patient who has typical angina at rest after a heavy meal may have significant left main artery disease. A patient with prior evidence of CAD has angina in the morning with regular activities (e.g., walking inside the house). The chest pain slowly disappears as the patient continues these regular activities. As the day goes on, even with higher levels of activity, the pain never comes back. This phenomenon is suggestive of chronic total occlusion (CTO). The mechanism is such that the collaterals collapse during the night. In the morning, the patient develops angina because of regular activities due to the mismatch between supply and demand. With chest pain as a trigger, the collaterals open up so that even at a higher level of activity as the day goes by, the pain never comes back. The same phenomenon repeats itself every day. These details in a patient's history help the physician to guess the patency of a recently stented artery without the need for coronary angiography [10].

Signs to look for
There are no specific physical findings for CAD, so often the goal of the physical examination is to detect possible precipitating factors or identify clues of alternative diagnoses. However, several related physical

findings could rank the patients in a higher risk category, especially when patients present with acute coronary syndrome (ACS): pulmonary edema, a worsening mitral regurgitation murmur, a third or fourth heart sound, hypotension, bradycardia, or tachycardia.

Smart testing

The selection of a diagnostic test depends on the level of certainty of evidence regarding risks and benefits, how these risks and benefits compare with potential alternatives, and what the comparative cost or cost-effectiveness of the diagnostic test would be. An informed patient should ask his or her doctor this question: Could you tell me the purpose and the diagnostic accuracy of this test?

Blood tests   The initial investigation includes blood tests to rule out non-cardiac causes of chest pain such as anemia, hyperthyroidism, electrolyte abnormalities, and renal, liver or pancreatic disease. Lipid panel and hemoglobin A1c levels are for assessment of risk factors. The benefits of brain natriuretic peptide (BNP or pro-BNP) levels are for prognostication and assessment of associated asymptomatic and possibly significant LV dysfunction [11]. Very low levels of troponin can be detected in many patients with stable CAD when high-sensitive assays are used. These levels are usually below those for true ACS definition but add to prognostic value [11]. However, troponin elevation does not have independent prognostic significance for recommending systematic measurement for out-of-hospital patients with stable CAD.

Electrocardiogram and chest X-ray   A baseline ECG is carried out to assess the severity and extent of ST depression on the 12 leads. The deeper the ST depression and the higher the number of leads involved, the higher is the likelihood of significant CAD. In addition, the underlying arrhythmias could also manifest as chest pain so the ECG may help, although rarely. Chest X-ray does not provide specific diagnostic information in patients with chest pain, but may be helpful in assessing patients with suspected heart failure (HF) or associated pulmonary pathologies.

Echocardiography   Resting two-dimensional and Doppler transthoracic echocardiography provides information on cardiac structure and function. Aortic stenosis, hypertrophic cardiomyopathy and pulmonary HTN can be ruled out as causes of chest pain. Regional wall motion abnormalities of the LV (e.g., hypokinesis, akinesia, dyskinesia) may be detected, and increase the likelihood of CAD [12].

Abnormalities of LV relaxation, tissue Doppler imaging and strain rate measurements may point towards diastolic dysfunction as an explanation for physical activity-associated symptoms. In addition, when impaired diastolic filling is the first sign of active ischemia, it may indicate the presence of microvascular causes in patients with atypical angina [13].

FUNCTIONAL ASSESSMENT OF ISCHEMIC RISK

Strategic mapping for sequential multi-modalities imaging

At the start of investigating the extent of ischemic burden, based on age, gender and symptoms, a pretest probability is calculated. If the patients have extremely low PTP (<10%), they do not require further testing unless it will modify risk prevention. Patients with very high PTP should go directly to invasive coronary angiography.

Patients with an intermediate risk between 15–85% (and especially those ~40–50%), should undergo functional or stress testing with or without imaging [14]. These patients have many options, from a very affordable exercise stress test to a very expensive (but more accurate) imaging modality. Which test should be the first test? Which would be the next if the prior test is inconclusive? If the patient can adequately exercise on the treadmill and the EKG is interpretable (no severe STT changes and no left bundle branch block) then an exercise ECG testing would be the first step.

If the patient cannot exercise on the treadmill, then the next step will be a choice between pharmacological stress echocardiography, or myocardial perfusion imaging, according to the availability and expertise of the local interpreting cardiologists or radiologists.

CLINICAL PEARLS
When not to do stress tests
1 Don't perform stress cardiac imaging or advanced non-invasive imaging in the initial evaluation of patients without cardiac symptoms unless high-risk markers are present. Testing should be performed only when the following findings are present: DM in patients older than 40-years-old; PAD; or greater than 2% yearly risk for CAD events.
2 Don't perform annual stress cardiac imaging or advanced non-invasive imaging as part of routine follow-up in asymptomatic

patients. An exception to this rule would be for patients who had gone for more than five years after coronary bypass surgery.

3 Don't perform stress cardiac imaging or advanced non-invasive imaging as a preoperative assessment in patients scheduled to undergo low-risk non-cardiac surgery. Non-invasive testing is not useful for patients undergoing low-risk non-cardiac surgery (e.g., cataract removal). These types of test do not change the patient's clinical management or outcomes and will result in increased costs [15].

Exercise ECG testing   As the exercise ECG without imaging has a specificity of 90%, its limited sensitivity (~60%) leads to high false-positive (25%) rates, especially in women [16]. Therefore, in patients with a PTP >65%, exercise ECG testing should be supplemented with imaging [17].

The diagnostic endpoint for an ischemic stress ECG is development of ≥1 mm horizontal or down-sloping ST segment depression at peak exercise 80 ms after the J point. A normal exercise ECG and a lower clinical PTP (<30%) indicate excellent prognosis with the probability of left main disease or risk of CV events being <1% [18].

Other important markers in addition to ECG changes include exercise capacity (~8 minutes), blood pressure (BP) response and exercise-induced ischemic symptoms. Maximum exercise capacity (usually measured as a maximum *Metabolic Equivalent* of Task (MET) level achieved) is a prognostic marker and a surrogate of resting and exercise induced LV dysfunction. However, exercise capacity is also affected by age and physical conditioning. These combined factors constitute the Duke Treadmill Score, which has been validated as an excellent marker of ischemia or risk of CV outcomes [19]. Markers of increased mortality or CV outcome include low exercise capacity (less than stage II of the Bruce protocol or <20% of age- and gender-predicted), failure to increase systolic BP (<120 mmHg or sustained 10 mmHg decrease from baseline), complex ventricular arrhythmias, and delayed heart rate recovery (<10 beats in first minute) [20, 21].

Exercise echocardiography   Stress echocardiography classifies patients according to the presence and extent of wall motion abnormalities [22]. It provides the risk of subsequent CV events and has excellent negative predictive value (predicted risk of death or CV events <0.5% annually) [23]. Any wall motion abnormality extending beyond two segments and one coronary territory is suggestive of higher risk (>3%

annually) and warrants coronary angiography [24]. Exercise echocardiography also provides post-exercise LVEF which is an independent marker of worse prognosis [25].

Exercise stress testing with myocardial perfusion imaging

Myocardial perfusion imaging (MPI) using single photon emission computed tomography (SPECT) is a useful method of risk stratification for subsequent death or CV events. [26] Myocardial perfusion SPECT is generally performed with rest and with stress technetium (Tc-99m) radioisotopes, because thallium (Tl-201) isotope has limited applications (e.g., viability) due to its higher radiation exposure [27]. Reversible perfusion defect involving ≥10% of the myocardium are considered moderately abnormal and warrants invasive coronary angiography [28]. In addition, ventricular volume changes with transient post-stress ischemic LV dilatation and increased tracer lung uptake indicate adverse prognosis [29]. In contrast, normal SPECT imaging is associated with a low risk of CV events or death (<1% annually).

Pharmacologic stress echocardiography   Pharmacologic testing is preferred when there is a significant resting wall motion abnormality (for viability assessment) or if the patient is unable to exercise adequately. For stress echocardiography, the agent of choice is dobutamine, with an endpoint of the study being inducible wall motion abnormalities. Dobutamine is a potent β agonist with positive inotropic and chronotropic properties which help in mimicking 'exercise-like' cardiac stimulation. Dobutamine stress echocardiography has comparable accuracy to exercise with a sensitivity ranging from 85–90% and a specificity of ∼90% respectively [30]. Its reliability is increased when ischemia is detected in the territory of the left anterior descending artery and is somewhat less reliable in patients with DM. However, a normal dobutamine echocardiogram is associated with a low annual risk of death or adverse cardiac events (1–2%) [31]. Ultrasound contrast agents can improve endocardial border definition and improve diagnostic accuracy [32]. They should be used whenever >2 of the 17 wall segments to be visualized are not adequately seen. The appropriate use criteria (AUC) for stress echocardiography are listed below.

Appropriate use criteria for stress echocardiography

Patients with no known CAD: Stress echocardiography is appropriate for symptomatic and asymptomatic patients with intermediate or high PTP of CAD and who cannot complete an exercise stress test adequately. On the other hand, for asymptomatic patients with low global CAD risk, stress echocardiography is rarely appropriate [33].

Patients with prior CAD: For patients with worsening symptoms, stress echocardiography is appropriate. For asymptomatic patients who had an abnormal stress test >2 years ago and have not undergone coronary revascularization, a repeat stress echocardiogram may be appropriate. Stress echocardiography is appropriate for patients who have only had incomplete revascularization; however, for asymptomatic patients who underwent PCI >2 years before or CABG >5 years before, the value of repeat stress echocardiography is uncertain [33].

Pharmacological myocardial perfusion imaging Pharmacological stress is generally induced by vasodilator agents (e.g. adenosine, dipyridamole or regadenoson). The diagnostic endpoint of nuclear MPI is evaluation of myocardial perfusion after stress. The diagnostic accuracy for detection of obstructive CAD for pharmacological MPI is very good with a diagnostic sensitivity ranging from 88–91% and specificity of ~90% [34]. Diagnostic image quality can be reduced in obese patients, women and men with large breasts. In addition, global and balanced reductions in myocardial perfusion in the setting of left main or multivessel CAD can result in false-negative results. The patient with left bundle branch block (LBBB) or with a pacemaker would benefit from pharmacological stress, because they do not have false reversible results in the inferior wall area due to bundle branch block or pacing. Limitations of the pharmacologic agents (adenosine or regadenoson) are the precipitation of bronchospasm in asthmatic individuals by activating the A1, A2B and A3 receptors in addition to activation of the A2A adenosine receptor, which produces hyperemia [35]. The AUC for myocardial perfusion imaging are listed below.

Appropriate use criteria for myocardial perfusion imaging

Patients with no known CAD: MPI is appropriate for **symptomatic** patients with intermediate or high PTP of CAD, and also for patients with low PTP if the ECG is uninterpretable or patient is unable to exercise. On the other hand, for **asymptomatic patients**, radionuclide imaging is inappropriate for patients with low global CAD risk, while it may be appropriate for patients with high global CAD risk or patients with intermediate global CAD risk who cannot complete an exercise stress test adequately.

Patients with prior CAD: For patients with **new or worsening symptoms**, radionuclide imaging is appropriate, as it is for asymptomatic patients who have had incomplete revascularization only. For

asymptomatic patients who have had an abnormal stress imaging study >2 years ago and have not undergone coronary revascularization, radionuclide imaging may be appropriate. However, in asymptomatic patients who underwent PCI >2 years ago, the value for radionuclide imaging is uncertain. In contrast to stress echocardiography, it is appropriate to perform radionuclide imaging for asymptomatic patients more than 5 years after CABG surgery [36]

ANATOMICAL ASSESSMENT OF ISCHEMIC RISK

Coronary angiography

In general, patients with >85% PTP benefit from coronary angiography for anatomical assessment of atherosclerosis burden. Coronary angiography quantifies risk on the basis of an anatomic prognostic index, incorporating the number of vessels (1, 2 or 3) involved and also on the basis of the degree of stenosis [37]. In general, >70% in any major epicardial coronary artery (>50% in the left main coronary artery) is considered hemodynamically obstructive. Angiography is limited by the fact that it only provides anatomic data and is not a reliable indicator of the functional significance of a given coronary stenosis.

A 'Class I' recommendation for coronary angiography is for patients with presumed CAD who have unacceptable ischemic symptoms despite optimal guideline-directed medical therapy and who are amenable to, and candidates for, coronary revascularization. The other indications of coronary angiography are listed in Table 3.5.

Coronary angiography is also not able to provide assessment of the instability of plaque (vulnerable plaque). However, more complicated lesions with a greater number of vessel involvement is associated with

---

Table 3.5 Indications for coronary angiography

1. Ascertain the cause of chest pain or anginal equivalent symptoms.
2. Define coronary anatomy in patients with 'high-risk' non-invasive stress test findings as a requisite for revascularization.
3. Determine whether severe coronary artery disease may be the cause of depressed left ventricular ejection fraction.
4. Assess for possible ischemia-mediated ventricular arrhythmia.
5. Evaluate cardiovascular risk among certain recipient and donor candidates for solid-organ transplantation.

worsened outcome. Although coronary angiography has evolved, it should not be test of initial choice, except in reduced LVEF (<50%), high pretest probability, or in special professions (such as pilots). Patient refusal for invasive assessment or for revascularization is also a contraindication for coronary angiography. The AUC for coronary angiography are listed below.

Appropriate use criteria for coronary angiography

For **symptomatic** patients with high pretest probability for CAD, coronary angiography without any preceding stress testing is appropriate, as it is for patients with resting LV dysfunction (LVEF <40%). In symptomatic patients, if there are intermediate risk findings on radionuclide imaging, or stress positron emission tomography (PET) scan (5–10% ischemic myocardium), or a single area of stress-induced wall motion abnormality, proceeding with coronary angiography is appropriate. For a high-risk treadmill stress test (Duke score >−11) or high-risk findings on radionuclide imaging, or stress PET scan (>10% ischemic myocardium), or ≥2 areas of regional wall motion abnormalities, proceeding with coronary angiography is appropriate regardless of whether the patient is symptomatic or asymptomatic.

For **asymptomatic patients** with intermediate-risk stress test results, the value of pursuing coronary angiography is uncertain. Coronary angiography solely based on calcium scoring is inappropriate. If a coronary stenosis of >50% is discovered on coronary computed tomography angiography (CTA), proceeding with coronary angiography is appropriate if the patient is symptomatic. Coronary angiography is also appropriate if the severity of a lesion is unclear on CTA [38].

Coronary computed tomographic angiography In general, patients with an estimated risk of 10–29% would benefit from coronary computed tomographic angiography (CCTA), mainly because CCTA has a high negative predictive value and is able to provide better anatomical definition non-invasively [39]. Besides anatomical definition and plaque burden assessment, CCTA provides useful prognostic information. Higher plaque burden and presence of low attenuation plaque is strongly correlated with a risk of future ACS. CCTA can qualitatively visualize arterial remodeling and non-obstructive plaque, including calcified, non-calcified, or mixed plaque [40]. The clinical effectiveness of CTA was recently tested in the Prospective Multicenter Imaging Study for Evaluation of Chest Pain (PROMISE) trial, the results of which are shown below [41].

EVIDENCE-BASED MEDICINE

The PROMISE Trial 10,003 symptomatic patients were randomly assigned to a strategy of initial anatomical testing with the use of CTA or to functional testing (exercise electrocardiography, nuclear stress testing, or stress echocardiography). The composite primary endpoint was death, MI, hospitalization for unstable angina, or major procedural complication. Secondary endpoints included invasive cardiac catheterization that did not show obstructive CAD and level of radiation exposure. The results showed that the mean age of the patients was 60.8 ± 8.3 years, 52.7% were women, and 87.7% had chest pain or dyspnea on exertion. The mean pretest likelihood of obstructive CAD was 53.3 ± 21.4%. Over a median follow-up period of 25 months, a primary endpoint event occurred in 164 of 4996 patients in the CTA group (3.3%) and in 151 of 5007 (3.0%) in the functional-testing group (adjusted hazard ratio, 1.04; 95% confidence interval, 0.83 to 1.29; $P = 0.75$). CTA was associated with fewer catheterizations showing no obstructive CAD than was functional testing (3.4% vs. 4.3%, $P = 0.02$), although more patients in the CTA group underwent catheterization within 90 days after randomization (12.2% vs. 8.1%). The median cumulative radiation exposure per patient was lower in the CTA group than in the functional-testing group (10.0 mSv vs. 11.3 mSv), but 32.6% of the patients in the functional-testing group had no exposure, so the overall exposure was higher in the CTA group (mean, 12.0 mSv vs. 10.1 mSv; $P < 0.001$). In conclusion, for symptomatic patients with suspected CAD who required non-invasive testing, a strategy of initial CTA, as compared with functional testing, did not improve clinical outcomes over a median follow-up of 2 years.

Technical considerations of CTA   The diagnostic accuracy of CCTA with 64-slice CT, yields a sensitivity ranging from 93–97% and specificity values ranging from 80–90% [42, 43]. Diagnostic accuracy is limited by favorable imaging requirements, so only patients with adequate breath-holding capabilities, without severe obesity, with a calcium score <40, in sinus rhythm at a rate of 60 beats per minute should be considered. It should be emphasized that CCTA carries a risk of contrast allergy and can induce renal failure in patients with underlying renal insufficiency. The test is also limited by high false-positive rates in patients with increasing calcification and a positive predictive value of only 44% when compared with functional ischemia assessment, and therefore should not be performed in patients with a greater than intermediate likelihood of stable CAD [44, 45].

For asymptomatic patients with type 1 or type 2 diabetes, CCTA did not reduce the composite rate of all-cause mortality, non-fatal MI, or unstable angina requiring hospitalization at four years, and is therefore not used in this patient population. The AUC for coronary CT angiography are listed below.

Appropriate use criteria for coronary CT angiography

Coronary CT angiography is appropriate when performed for symptomatic patients with intermediate pretest probability of CAD if the ECG in un-interpretable or the patient is unable to exercise. Coronary CTA can also be performed in place of invasive coronary angiography with previously abnormal stress testing as long as the patient has not been revascularized. Of note, coronary CTA is rarely appropriate in patients with prior revascularization with either CABG or PCI. Calcium scoring is generally not recommended for any symptomatic patient, but may be appropriate in asymptomatic patients with intermediate to high global CAD risk [46].

DIAGNOSIS

After all the clinical, non-invasive and invasive investigations, stable CAD represents a wide spectrum of ischemic conditions with a common denomination: imbalance between oxygen supply and demand. They range from the classic fixed lesion in the epicardial coronary artery to the functional lesion due to transient spasm of these widely patent arteries (Table 3.6). This list is important to guide the management of stable CAD according to its etiologies.

Table 3.6 Wide spectrum of stable coronary artery disease

1. Stable intermediate or severe lesion (>70% narrowing of minimal luminal diameter).
2. Stabilized post-ACS patient.
3. Intermittent ischemic state related to spontaneous coronary vasospasm or provoked by chemical including cocaine, etc [53, 54].
4. Coronary artery ectasia and/or aneurysms causing ischemia due to platelet or thrombotic emboli to the distal peripheries.
5. Myocardial bridging.

Table 3.7 Questions to discuss with clinicians before treatment

1. What are the levels of certainty of evidence regarding risks and benefits?
2. How do these risks and benefits compare with potential alternatives?
3. What are the treatment options available?
4. What are the rates of success or failure of these treatment options?
5. What kind of side-effects or complications occur with these treatment options?
6. What would be the comparative cost or cost-effectiveness of the treatment?
7. What happens if this treatment approach does not work for me?
8. How will you help me balance my treatment with the demand of active life?

MANAGEMENT

The goals of treatment in stable CAD are (1) to prevent MI or death with disease modification (increase the 'quantity of life') and (2) to reduce ischemia and relieve angina symptoms (improve the quality of life). The optimal medical treatment includes anti-anginal medication, beta-blockers and antiplatelet therapy. A well-informed patient should ask about treatment options and question the success and complications of the proposed treatment. The detailed questions are listed in Table 3.7.

Optimal medical therapy

Optimal medical therapy (OMT) is defined as pharmacologic intervention resulting in symptom alleviation and prevention of further CV events. To that effect, there is a need for immediate relief of angina and then prolonged therapy for long-term symptom alleviation. CV event reduction focuses on reducing incidence of acute thrombotic events and plaque stabilization and development of ventricular dysfunction.

CLINICAL PEARLS
How to achieve optimal medical therapy The first caveat is that the definition of OMT is very fluid. In 2015, the list of medications of OMT includes antiplatelets, beta-blockers, statins, angiotensin converting enzyme

inhibitor/angiotensin receptor blockers (ACEI/ARB) if indicated. ACEI and ARB are anti-atherosclerotic drugs; however they are more appropriate for use in HF. The second caveat is that OMT does not equal maximal therapy. The reason is that OMT needs a delicate balance between the benefits of treatment and its side-effects: The higher the dosage, the higher the numbers of side-effects. According to the Courage trial, the end-goals of OMT are listed in Table 3.8.

Table 3.8 The end-goals of OMT at 5 years

1. Low density lipoprotein <100 mg%, median = 71 mg%.
2. Systolic and diastolic blood pressure <130/85 mmHg.
3. HbA1c <7% for patients with diabetes.
4. High adherence to diet, exercise, smoking cessation, losing weight and medication.

In order to achieve OMT, there is a need of administering a well-maintained infrastructure (mostly by nurses who call, check and remind patients on adhering a healthy lifestyle and taking medications). Not surprisingly, the patients have higher adherence to OMT after a percutaneous coronary intervention (PCI) event so PCI seems to become a focal point that allows patients to enter the world of OMT.

Anti-anginal drugs

Nitroglycerin Short acting anti-anginal agents include sublingual nitroglycerin at doses of 0.3–0.6 mg every 5 minutes until cessation of angina or a maximal dose of 1.2 mg in 15 minutes. Nitroglycerin spray acts more rapidly. Either formulation can be used for symptom resolution or prophylactically prior to activity that triggers symptoms [47]. Isosorbide dinitrate (5 mg sublingually) aborts angina attacks and its effects last for a few hours. However, unlike sublingual nitroglycerin, it requires a few minutes to initiate effect due to hepatic conversion. Oral preparations including isosorbide dinitrate (15–120 mg daily) or mononitrate can be used for prophylaxis of angina, and have been shown to reduce incidence of angina and increased exercise capacity for up to 8 hours. However, long-term administration of nitrate formulations is limited because of significant side-effects such as hypotension and headache or tachyphy-laxis. Recently, a new study showed that the patients with heart failure and preserved ejection fraction were less active and did not have better quality of life when receiving isosorbide mononitrate [47]. Combination of these agents with sildenafil and other prostaglandin D-5 inhibitors can lead to precipitous hypotension. These agents should also not be used with tamsulosin and other alpha-blockers in patients with prostatic problems (because of combined hypotensive side-effect). While nitrates are excellent in symptom relief, they have never demonstrated mortality benefit for patients with stable CAD.

Beta-blockers (BB)   These reduce heart rate and contractility and increase perfusion to ischemic areas by prolonging diastole and increasing arteriolar resistance in non-ischemic areas. BBs are effective in controlling exercise-induced events and improving exercise capacity by limiting both symptomatic and asymptomatic ischemic episodes. Although BBs reduce risk of CV related death and MI by 30% in post-MI patients, their role in patients with CV risk factors, but without prior MI or known CAD (primary prevention) has not been demonstrated [48, 49]. However BBs prevent worsening HF and may be used for this indication in patients with stable CAD and LV dysfunction [50]. The most commonly used BBs are metoprolol, carvedilol, bisoprolol, atenolol and nebivolol. All agents can be used as first line anti-anginal therapy targeting a resting heart rate less than 60 beats per minute [51, 52]. Carvedilol and metoprolol are metabolized by the liver and may be safer in patients with renal dysfunction.

CLINICAL PEARLS
Differences between cardioselective and non-cardioselective beta-blockers Blockade of non-cardiac beta$_2$ receptors inhibits catecholamine-induced glycogenolysis, so non-cardioselective beta blockers can mask the premonitory signs of hypoglycemia. Nevertheless, BBs are generally well-tolerated by patients with DM. Moreover, carvedilol has been shown to exhibit modest insulin-sensitizing properties and can relieve some manifestations of the metabolic syndrome.

Blockade of beta$_2$ receptors also inhibits the vasodilating effects of catecholamines in peripheral vasculature and leaves the constrictor (alpha-adrenergic) receptors unopposed, thereby enhancing vasoconstriction, including coronary vasculature. This is why BBs are avoided in patients with Prinzmetal's angina, PAD, or Raynaud's disease. BBs should usually be avoided in patients with a history of significant depressive illness and should be prescribed cautiously for patients with sexual dysfunction, sleep disturbance, nightmares, fatigue, or lethargy.

Abrupt withdrawal of beta-adrenergic blocking agents after prolonged administration can result in increased total ischemic activity in patients with chronic stable angina. This increased ischemia may be caused by a return to the previously high levels of myocardial O_2 demand while the underlying atherosclerotic process has progressed, but a rebound phenomenon resulting in increased beta-adrenergic sensitivity probably occurs in some patients. Occasionally, such withdrawal can precipitate unstable angina and may, in rare cases, even provoke MI. Chronic BB therapy can be safely discontinued by slowly withdrawing the drug in a stepwise manner over the course of 2 to 3 weeks. If abrupt withdrawal of BBs is required, patients should be instructed to reduce exertion and manage angina episodes with sublingual nitroglycerin and/or substitute a calcium antagonist.

Calcium channel blockers These are selective L-channel inhibitors in the vascular smooth muscle and act chiefly by vasodilation and reduction of peripheral vascular resistance. They are classified into dihydropyridine and non-dihydropyridine groups. The non-dihydropyridine (verapamil and diltiazem) agents show benefit in all varieties of angina by reducing heart rate, atrioventricular conduction and blood pressure. Verapamil has shown similar efficacy to metoprolol and demonstrated fewer anginal attacks, glucose intolerance and psychological depression compared to atenolol [53]. Diltiazem has similar vasodilatory and cardioinhibitory properties as verapamil but there are no head-to-head comparisons.

Nifedipine and amlodipine are the dihydropyridine calcium channel blockers with more potent vasodilatory effects than non-dihydropyridine agents. Nifedipine reduces anginal episodes and the need for revascularization compared to placebo. Amlodipine has a longer half-life and is administered once a day [54]. Short-acting nifedipine should not be used because the reflex-mediated tachycardia may aggravate ischemia. Dihydropyridine calcium channel blockers in combination with beta-blockers are more effective in controlling angina symptoms than monotherapy.

Calcium antagonists are clearly preferred for patients with suspected Prinzmetal (variant) angina.

Ranolazine   Despite the use of the above mentioned (BB, CCB, NTG) anti-anginal agents, up to 25% of patients with stable CAD remain symptomatic. Ranolazine is a selective inhibitor of late sodium current with anti-ischemic and anti-anginal properties without negative chronotropic and blood pressure reduction. Ranolazine reduces angina and increase exercise capacity in patients with chronic angina, especially after CABG and diabetes when administered at doses of 500 to 2000 mg daily. Recently, the results of the Ranolazine for Incomplete Vessel Revascularization (RIVER-PCI) trial showed that in patients with prior angina who underwent PCI but with incomplete revascularization, ranolazine made no difference on quality of life or angina improvement compared with placebo [55].

Ranolazine is metabolized by the cytochrome P3A (CYP3A) system and its level increases with renal and hepatic impairment or concomitant use of CYP3A inhibitors like diltiazem, verapamil, macrolide antibiotics, and grapefruit juice. This can lead to increased QTc, and should therefore be used carefully in patients with QT prolongation or on QT-prolonging drugs (e.g. tikosyn) [55].

Event prevention
Antiplatelet therapy   Aspirin (ASA) remains the cornerstone of pharmacological prevention of arterial thrombosis. It acts via irreversible inhibition of platelet cyclooxygenase-1 and thus thromboxane production. Most studies demonstrate its efficacy at doses between 75–150 mg/day and greater risk of gastrointestinal and hemorrhagic side-effects in higher doses [56]. The role of P2Y12 inhibitor as monotherapy is only limited to patients with intolerance to or non-responders to ASA. Clopidogrel has shown benefit compared to ASA (81 mg/day) in patients with stable CAD although the results were driven by patients with underlying PAD. Ticagrelor and prasugrel, despite being more efficacious than clopidogrel in patients with ACS, have not exhibited additional benefit in patients with stable CAD and should not be administered for this indication.

Lipid modification   Patients with stable CAD are considered high risk for adverse CV events and statin therapy is recommended both for cholesterol modification and plaque stabilization. Current guidelines recommend initiation of high-dose statin therapy aimed at reducing serum low density lipoprotein (LDL) levels by 50% from baseline. Previous goals of targeting LDL <70 mg/dL may still be valuable for metric assessment of response, but are not required for modulation of therapy [1]. Based on current evidence, high-dose rosuvastatin (>20 mg daily) or atorvastatin (80 mg daily) is the recommended maintenance dose for stable CAD. In intolerant and inadequate responders (<50% LDL reduction from baseline), non-statin therapy including ezetimibe may be used for further LDL reduction. Although non-statins were proven beneficial in the pre-statin era, their role in mortality reduction is limited and they should only be employed in combination with statins for further LDL reduction. Modulating non-LDL cholesterol with non-statin therapy or with therapy combining statins and non-statins has not demonstrated mortality reduction [57].

Lipid-lowering with statins has been shown to reduce circulating levels of hsCRP, decrease thrombogenicity, and favorably alter the collagen and inflammatory components of arterial atheroma; these effects do not appear to correlate well with the change in serum LDL cholesterol levels and suggest anti-atherothrombotic properties of statins. These properties may contribute to improvement in blood flow, reduction in inducible myocardial ischemia, and the reduction in coronary events in patients treated with statins [58].

Renin-angiotensin-aldosterone system blockers Angiotensin converting enzyme inhibitors (ACEI) mitigate reverse myocardial remodeling and reduce mortality in patients with stable CAD with reduced (<40%) LV dysfunction [59]. Although ACEIs are advisable in patients with stable CAD and preserved LV function, their role in mortality reduction is not unanimously proven [60]. In patients with stable CAD and HTN, the combination of an ACEI and a dihydropyridine CCB is proven effective in BP control and mortality reduction [61, 62]. Angiotensin receptor blockers (ARBs) have demonstrated similar mortality benefit when compared to ACEIs in patients with stable CAD [63]. Combination of both (ACEI and ARB) demonstrated no additional benefit and was associated with more adverse outcomes including electrolyte abnormalities and renal complications [64]. ARB treatment may be an alternative therapeutic option for patients with stable CAD when ACEIs are not tolerated. Post-MI patients with a reduced LV function with optimized doses of ACEI or ARB therapy and a beta blocker benefit from the addition of spironolactone or eplerenone, especially if they have DM [65]. This combination is not recommended for patients with renal dysfunction and hyperkalemia.

Although inhibitors of the renin-angiotensin-aldosterone system are not indicated for the treatment of CAD, these drugs appear to have important benefits in reducing the risk of future ischemic events in some patients with CV disease. An unexpected finding from randomized trials of ACEI in post-infarction and other patients with ischemic and non-ischemic causes of LV dysfunction was a significant reduction in the incidence of subsequent coronary ischemic events.

CLINICAL PEARLS
Inter-exchange between ACEI and ARB ARBs are generally recommended to be used only in ACE-intolerant patients due to cough. There is an approximately 10% incidence of cross-reactivity of angioedema in patients who receive an ARB after experiencing ACEI-associated angioedema. Reports of angioedema related to ARBs show that it is less severe and occurs earlier compared to angioedema which develops as a result of ACEI. Therefore, in patients who develop angioedema on ACEI, ARBs should only be used in those with a strong therapeutic need for close observation and education on signs of angioedema and its management.

Polypharmacy

HTN, chronic obstructive pulmonary disease (COPD), DM and arthritis are the most common co-morbidities in elderly patients with CAD. Medications given to patients with these conditions can interfere with those used for CV disease and, in some cases, even pose serious health risks.

Revascularization

The role of revascularization for patients with stable CAD optimized on medical therapy has been a source of great controversy. Seven major randomized trials have assessed the utility of revascularization versus medical therapy in chronic stable CAD in the past 10 years [66–68]. Revascularization remains a useful option for unstable angina and angina refractory to medical therapy when there is evidence of significant obstructive coronary artery stenosis, large amounts of reversible ischemia on non-invasive imaging, and sufficient life expectancy (>1 year). Decision to revascularize should be individualized and based on a multidisciplinary approach.

Single vessel disease In stable asymptomatic patients with single vessel CAD, preserved LV function and small (<10%) area of myocardial ischemia, the strategy of initial OMT is safe and should be the default approach. Patients who develop angina or angina equivalent symptoms, worsening LV function or large (>10%) areas of ischemia may be considered for revascularization. When a period of OMT has not been adequately conducted, physicians should be more conservative when making a decision over revascularization, especially in case of high-risk comorbidities, difficult anatomies, mildly symptomatic patients or in patients without large areas of ischemia. The results of the Clinical Outcomes Utilizing Revascularization and Aggressive Drug Evaluation (COURAGE) trial served as evidence supporting the above strategy [69].

EVIDENCE-BASED MEDICINE
The COURAGE Trial 2287 patients with stable CAD and Canadian Cardiovascular Society (CCS) class II–III angina, ≥70% single vessel CAD and ischemia or ≥80% and classic angina without provocable ischemia. 1149 patients underwent PCI with OMT (PCI group) and 1138 received OMT alone (medical-therapy group). There were no significant differences between the PCI group and the medical-therapy group in the composite of death, MI and stroke (20.0% vs. 19.5%; HR 1.05; (*P* = 0.62); hospitalization for ACS (12.4% vs. 11.8%; (HR 1.07; *P* = 0.56); or MI (13.2% vs. 12.3%; HR 1.13; 95% *P* = 0.33). As an initial management strategy in patients with stable CAD, PCI did not reduce the risk of death, MI, or other major CV events when added to OMT [69].

How long antiplatelet therapy after PCI? Dual antiplatelet therapy (DAPT) following second-generation drug-eluting stent (DES) implantation appears to be acceptable at 12 months with regard to incidences of cardiac death, MI, stroke, definite/probable stent thrombosis, and Bleeding Academic Research Consortium (BARC) type 3 or 5 bleeding. In a randomized, multicenter, international study, patients were randomized to receive for six-months (*n* = 682) vs. 12-months (*n* = 717) in the Dual Antiplatelet Therapy (DAPT) study. The results are shown below [70].

EVIDENCE-BASED MEDICINE
The DAPT Study A total of 9961 patients were enrolled after they had undergone a coronary stent procedure in which a DES was placed. After 12 months of treatment with a thienopyridine drug (clopidogrel or prasugrel) and ASA, patients were randomly assigned to continue receiving thienopyridine treatment or to receive placebo for another 18 months; all patients continued receiving ASA. The co-primary efficacy endpoints were stent thrombosis and major adverse CV and cerebrovascular events (a composite of death, MI, or stroke) during the period from 12 to 30 months. The primary safety endpoint was moderate or severe bleeding. The results of the study showed that continued treatment with thienopyridine, as compared with placebo, reduced the rates of stent thrombosis (0.4% vs. 1.4%; hazard ratio, 0.29 [95% confidence interval {CI}, 0.17 to 0.48]; P <0.001) and major adverse CV and cerebrovascular events (4.3% vs. 5.9%; hazard ratio, 0.71 [95% CI, 0.59 to 0.85]; P <0.001). The rate of MI was lower with thienopyridine treatment than with placebo (2.1% vs. 4.1%; hazard ratio, 0.47; P <0.001). The rate of death from any cause was 2.0% in the group that continued thienopyridine therapy and 1.5% in the placebo group (hazard ratio, 1.36 [95% CI, 1.00 to 1.85]; P = 0.05) while there was no difference in cardiovascular death. The rate of moderate or severe bleeding was increased with continued thienopyridine treatment (2.5% vs. 1.6%, P = 0.001). An elevated risk of stent thrombosis and MI was observed in both groups during the 3 months after discontinuation of thienopyridine treatment. According to this study, DAPT beyond 1 year after placement of a DES, as compared with ASA therapy alone, significantly reduced the risks of stent thrombosis and major adverse CV and cerebrovascular events, but was associated with an increased risk of bleeding (possibly leading to higher mortality) [70].

The DAPT bleeding calculator Based on the cohort from the DAPT study, a scoring system has been created to help determine who should and should not receive DAPT for more than 1 year after stenting. The DAPT scores are calculated based on the data in Table 3.9.

The DAPT Score calculator is available at www.daptstudy.org/for-clinicians/score_calculator.htm. From the results, the DAPT calculator

Table 3.9 The DAPT bleeding score calculator

For age 75 years or older	2 points
For age 65 to 74 years	1 point
For age <65 years	0 point
Diabetes	1 point
Current smoking	1 point
Prior MI or PCI	1 point
Congestive HF or LVEF <30%	2 points
MI at presentation	1 point
Vein graft PCI	2 points
Stent diameter <3 mm	1 point

could predict four numbers for each patient:

1. Predicted ischemic event rate with placebo.
2. Predicted ischemic event rate with treatment.
3. Predicted bleeding event rate with placebo.
4. Predicted bleeding event rate with treatment.

In patients who have not had a major bleeding event or ischemic event in the first year after PCI with stenting, a score of less than 2 indicates that bleeding risk may outweigh ischemic benefit of long-term DAPT, and a score of 2 or more indicates that ischemic benefit may outweigh bleeding risk [71]. So the decision of stopping or prolonging DAPT in each individual patient could be based on the above results.

CAD and LV dysfunction Left ventricular dysfunction is an independent predictor of mortality and patients with three vessel CAD and LV dysfunction have shown improved survival with revascularization. The greatest benefit in survival is derived in patients with an EF of 35–49%. Recent data from the Surgical Treatment for Ischemic Heart Failure (STICH) trial demonstrated no improvement in overall mortality in patients with severe LV dysfunction (EF <35%) based on viability testing [72]. However, there was improvement in CV morbidity and mortality and due to the high crossover rate in both treatment arms, readjustment of data based on type of treatment received showed a significant improvement in overall mortality after revascularization [72].

EVIDENCE-BASED MEDICINE
The STICH trial A total of 1212 patients with CAD and LV dysfunction were enrolled in a randomized trial of medical therapy with or without CABG. A total of 601 underwent assessment of myocardial viability using either single-photon-emission computed tomography (SPECT), dobutamine echocardiography, or both on the basis of pre-specified thresholds. 37% patients with viable myocardium and 51% patients without viable myocardium died (HR for death among patients with viable myocardium 0.64 (95% CI 0.48–0.86; $P = 0.003$). However, after adjustment for other baseline variables, this association with mortality was not significant ($P = 0.21$). There was no significant interaction between viability status and treatment assignment with respect to mortality for patients with CAD and LV dysfunction undergoing CABG ($P = 0.53$) [72].

CAD and multi-vessel disease   Symptom and disease severity are also critical predictors of outcome. Patients with triple vessel disease or those with either >50% left main stenosis or >70% proximal left anterior descending artery involvement have exhibited survival advantage with revascularization irrespective of symptoms [73]. However, recent evidence also suggests that asymptomatic patients with multi-vessel CAD only exhibit survival advantage if they have associated LV dysfunction (EF <35%) [73]. Alternatively patients with preserved LV function with severe angina and ischemia have exhibited survival benefit with revascularization even with two or more vessel involvement [74]. This suggests that patients with severe angina or ischemia (>10% myocardial involvement) benefit from revascularization. The currently underway International Study of Comparative Health Effectiveness with Medical and Invasive Approaches (ISCHEMIA) study aims to assess the therapeutic utility of revascularization in patients with severe (>10%) ischemia on non-invasive testing. The role of revascularization based on myocardial viability testing is not proven as in the STICH trial above.

PCI versus CABG   Choice of revascularization depends on the severity of CAD, number of coronary arteries involvement, associated LV dysfunction and risk of the procedure. Although most of the initial studies with revascularization utilized CABG, PCI for patients with stable CAD has a proven safety with an overall complication rate of <0.5% [75]. CABG and

PCI showed similar survival and incidence of MI over 5 years in a composite analysis of 22 studies [75]. However CABG was associated with higher stroke, improved angina and lower target vessel revascularization. CABG was associated with better outcomes in patients with diabetes mellitus and in those ≥65 years of age. Of interest, the relative outcomes of CABG and PCI were not influenced by other patient characteristics, including the number of diseased coronary arteries. These conclusions result from the Synergy between Percutaneous Coronary Intervention with Taxus and Cardiac Surgery (SYNTAX) trial [76].

EVIDENCE-BASED MEDICINE

The SYNTAX trial at 5 years This is the analysis comparing 5-year clinical outcomes in PCI- and CABG-treated LM patients in the SYNTAX trial. 1800 LM and/or 3-vessel disease patients were randomized to receive either PCI (with TAXUS Express paclitaxel-eluting stents) or CABG. The unprotected LM cohort ($N = 705$) was predefined and powered. MACCE at 5 years was 36.9% in PCI patients and 31.0% in CABG patients (hazard ratio (HR) 1.23 [0.95, 1.59]; $P = 0.12$). Mortality was 12.8% and 14.6% in PCI and CABG patients, respectively (HR 0.88 [0.58, 1.32], $P = 0.53$). Stroke was significantly increased in the CABG group (PCI 1.5% vs. CABG 4.3%, HR 0.33 [0.12, 0.92], $P = 0.03$) and repeat revascularization in the PCI arm (26.7% vs. 15.5%, HR 1.82 [1.28, 2.57], $P <0.01$). MACCE was similar between arms in patients with low/intermediate SYNTAX Scores but significantly increased in PCI patients with high scores (≥33). At 5 years, there was no difference in overall MACCE between the two treatment groups. PCI-treated patients had a lower stroke but higher revascularization rate versus CABG. These results suggest that both treatments are valid options for LM patients. The extent of disease should be accounted for when choosing between surgery and PCI, as patients with high SYNTAX scores seem to benefit more from surgery compared to the lower terciles [76].

Although the results were robust, SYNTAX trial's comparison of CABG with drug eluting stents (DES) has not been reproduced in other studies. Recent comparison of CABG with sirolimus-coated DES in the Premier of Randomized Comparison of Bypass Surgery vs. Angioplasty Using Sirolimus-Eluting Stent in Patients with Left Main Coronary Artery Disease (PRECOMBAT) has shown similar composite endpoints of death, cerebrovascular accident and MI between both groups (4.7% vs. 4.4%) [77]. In fact, the incidence of stroke was also lower than reported with SYNTAX. However, this study was underpowered and the left main cohort was also an underpowered subsegment of SYNTAX. Therefore, until further evidence is available, left main revascularization remains a 'heart team' dictated approach.

PCI for patient after CABG   Use of DES in PCI of SVG was associated with lower mortality than BMS (hazard ratio [HR]: 0.72; 95% confidence interval [CI]: 0.57 to 0.89) and similar rates of MI (HR: 0.94; 95% CI: 0.71 to 1.24) [78]

CAD in diabetic patients   While aggressive glycemic control in diabetic patients has demonstrated a significant reduction in microvascular complications of DM such as retinopathy, nephropathy and neuropathy, trials have failed to directly show a similar reduction in development of epicardial CAD and its complications such as ACS [79, 80]. The large UK prospective diabetes study did not demonstrate any impact of diabetes treatment on end points of CV disease.

In another prospective study to evaluate predictors of the first incidence of stable or unstable CAD, it was determined that microvascular complications markedly enhance the risk of incident symptomatic CAD [81]. There was a >60% increased relative risk for acute MI and an almost 40% increased relative risk of stable CAD. This risk if higher in women, compared to men with microvascular complications from diabetes. The proposed mechanisms included oxidative stress, endothelial dysfunction and subclinical inflammation. It can be indirectly inferred that poor hyperglycemic control over a period of time, is a potential precursor for CAD as well. These conclusions resulted from the Future Revascularization Evaluation in Patients with Diabetes Mellitus: Optimal Management of Multivessel Disease (FREEDOM) trial [82].

EVIDENCE-BASED MEDICINE
The FREEDOM Trial A total of 1900 patients with DM and multi-vessel CAD on OMT were randomized to undergo CABG or PCI. At 5 years, cardiac death was lower (18.7 vs. 26.6%; *P* <0.001) with CABG while all-cause mortality was similar (*P* = 0.049) between both treatment arms. CABG was associated with higher major stroke events (5.2 vs. 2.4%;

$P = 0.03$). These findings suggests that diabetics with multivessel disease benefit greater with CABG but at a higher cost of stroke [82].

ACTION POINTS

The diagnosis and management of stable CAD could be summarized as follows:

1 Identify and treat precipitating factors such as anemia, uncontrolled HTN, thyrotoxicosis, tachyarrhythmias, uncontrolled HF, and concomitant valvular heart disease.

2 Initiate risk factor modification, physical exercise, diet, and lifestyle counseling. Initiate therapy with a statin, as needed, to reduce the LDL cholesterol level.

3 Initiate pharmacotherapy with low-dose aspirin and a beta-blocker. Initiate an ACE inhibitor in all patients with an LV ejection fraction of 40% or lower and in those with HTN, diabetes, or chronic kidney disease. In addition, an ACE inhibitor should be considered for all other patients.

4 If angina persists, the next step is usually the addition of a calcium antagonist or long-acting nitrate via dosing schedules to prevent nitrate tolerance. The decision to add a calcium antagonist or long-acting nitrate is not based entirely on the frequency and severity of symptoms. The need to treat concomitant HTN or the presence of LV dysfunction and symptoms of HF may be an indication for the use of one of these agents, even in patients in whom episodes of symptomatic angina are infrequent.

5 If angina persists despite two anti-anginal agents (a beta-blocker with a long-acting nitrate preparation or calcium antagonist), add a third anti-anginal agent. The selection of the agent will be guided by potential side-effects and the presence or absence of concomitant HTN, relative hypotension, conduction system disease, tachyarrhythmias, or LV dysfunction.

6 Stress testing or coronary angiography, with a view to considering coronary revascularization, is indicated for patients with refractory symptoms or ischemia despite optimal medical therapy. It should also be carried out in patients with high-risk non-invasive test results and in those with occupations or lifestyles that require a more aggressive approach [44].

REFERENCES

1. Genders TS, Steyerberg EW, Alkadhi H, et al. A clinical prediction rule for the diagnosis of coronary artery disease: validation, updating, and extension. *Eur Heart J*. 2011;32:1316–1330.

2. Stone NJ, Robinson J, Lichtenstein AH, et al. 2013 ACC/AHA Guideline on the Treatment of Blood Cholesterol to Reduce Atherosclerotic Cardiovascular Risk in Adults: A Report of the American College of Cardiology/American Heart Association Task Force on Practice Guidelines. *Circulation*. 2013.

3. http://www.cardiosource.org/Science-And-Quality/Practice-Guidelines-and-Quality-Standards/2013-Prevention-Guideline-Tools.aspx.

4. Hubbard BL, Gibbons RJ, Lapeyre AC III, et al. Identification of severe coronary artery disease using simple clinical parameters. *Arch Intern Med*. 1992;152:309–311.

5. Morrow DA. Risk prediction in cardiovascular medicine: cardiovascular risk prediction in patients with stable and unstable coronary heart disease. *Circulation*. 2010;121:2681–2691.

6. Shaw LJ, Peterson ED, Shaw LK, Kesler KL, DeLong ER, Harrell FE Jr, Muhlbaier LH, Mark DB. Use of a prognostic treadmill score in identifying diagnostic coronary disease subgroups. *Circulation*. 1998;98:1622–1630.

7. Ridker PM, Cannon CP, Morrow D, Rifai N, Rose LM, McCabe CH, Pfeffer MA, Braunwald E. C-reactive protein levels and outcomes after statin therapy. *N Engl J Med*. 2005;352:20–28.

8. Kragelund C, Gronning B, Kober L, Hildebrandt P, Steffensen R. N-terminal pro-B-type natriuretic peptide and long-term mortality in stable coronary heart disease. *N Engl J Med*. 2005;352:666–675.

9. Diamond GA. A clinically relevant classification of chest discomfort. *J Am Coll Cardiol*. 1983;1:574. Letter.

10. Li XK, Nguyen T, Sim KH. Stable coronary artery disease. In T Nguyen, et al. *Evidence based Cardiology Practice*. PMPH, USA, 2011, pp. 376–408.

11. Lyngbæk S, Winkel P, Gøtze JP, Kastrup J, Gluud C, Kolmos HJ, Kjøller E, Jensen GB, Hansen JF, Hildebrandt P, Hilden J; the CLARICOR Trial Group. Risk stratification in stable coronary artery disease is possible at cardiac troponin levels below conventional detection and is improved by use of N-terminal pro-B-type natriuretic peptide. *Eur J Prev Cardiol*. 2013, May 30.

12. www.cardiosource.org/en/News-Media/Publications/Cardiology-Magazine/2014/09/AHA-ACC-HHS-Release-Strategies-to-Enhance-CVD-and-Comorbid-Condition-Guidelines.aspx.

13. D'Andrea A, Nistri S, Castaldo F, Galderisi M, Mele D, Agricola E, Losi MA, Mondillo S, Marino PN; Working Group Nucleus on Echocardiography of Italian Society of Cardiology. The relationship between early left ventricular myocardial alterations and reduced coronary flow reserve in non-insulin-dependent diabetic patients with microvascular angina. *Int J Cardiol*. 2012 Feb 9;154(3):250–255.

14. Sox HC Jr., Hickam DH, Marton KI, et al. Using the patient's history to estimate the probability of coronary artery disease: a comparison of primary care and referral practices. *Am J Med*. 1990;89:7–14.

15. Avogaro A, Giorda C, Maggini M, et al. Incidence of coronary heart disease in Type 2 diabetic men and women: Impact of microvascular complications, treatment, and geographic location. *Diabetes Care* 2007;30(5):1241–1247.

16. Kwok Y, Kim C, Grady D, et al. Meta-analysis of exercise testing to detect coronary artery disease in women. *Am J Cardiol.* 1999;83:660–666.

17. Mark DB, Hlatky MA, Harrell FE Jr., Lee KL, Califf RM, Pryor DB. Exercise treadmill score for predicting prognosis in coronary artery disease. *Ann Intern Med.* 1987;106:793–800.

18. Miller TD, Roger VL, Hodge DO, Gibbons RJ. A simple clinical score accurately predicts outcome in a community-based population undergoing stress testing. *Am J Med.* 2005;118:866–872.

19. Shaw LJ, Peterson ED, Shaw LK, et al. Use of a prognostic treadmill score in identifying diagnostic coronary disease subgroups. *Circulation.* 1998;98:1622–1630.

20. Gulati M, Black HR, Shaw LJ, Arnsdorf MF, Merz CN, Lauer MS, Marwick TH, Pandey DK, Wicklund RH, Thisted RA The prognostic value of a nomogram for exercise capacity in women. *N Engl J Med.* 2005 Aug 4;353(5):468–475.

21. CR, Blackstone EH, Pashkow FJ, Snader CE, Lauer MS. Heart-rate recovery immediately after exercise as a predictor of mortality. *N Engl J Med.* 1999 Oct 28;341(18):1351–1357.

22. Leischik R, Dworrak B, Littwitz H, et al. Prognostic significance of exercise stress echocardiography in 3329 outpatients (5-year longitudinal study). *Int J Cardiol.* 2007;119:297–305.

23. McCully RB, Roger VL, Mahoney DW, et al. Outcome after normal exercise echocardiography and predictors of subsequent cardiac events: follow-up of 1,325 patients. *J Am Coll Cardiol.* 1998;31:144–149.

24. Marwick TH, Mehta R, Arheart K, Lauer MS. Use of exercise echocardiography for prognostic evaluation of patients with known or suspected coronary artery disease. *J Am Coll Cardiol.* 1997;30:83–90.

25. Marwick TH, Case C, Vasey C, Allen S, Short L, Thomas JD. Prediction of mortality by exercise echocardiography: a strategy for combination with the duke treadmill score. *Circulation.* 2001;103:2566–2571.

26. Hachamovitch R, Rozanski A, Shaw LJ, et al. Impact of ischemia and scar on the therapeutic benefit derived from myocardial revascularization vs. medical therapy among patients undergoing stress-rest myocardial perfusion scintigraphy. *Eur Heart J.* 2011;32:1012–1024.

27. Cerqueira MD, Allman KC, Ficaro EP, et al. Recommendations for reducing radiation exposure in myocardial perfusion imaging. *J Nucl Cardiol.* 2010;17:709–718.

28. Hachamovitch R, Hayes SW, Friedman JD, Cohen I, Berman DS. Comparison of the short-term survival benefit associated with revascularization compared with medical therapy in patients with no prior coronary artery disease undergoing stress myocardial perfusion single photon emission computed tomography. *Circulation.* 2003;107:2900–2907.

29. Hachamovitch R, Rozanski A, Hayes SW, et al. Predicting therapeutic benefit from myocardial revascularization procedures: are measurements of both

resting left ventricular ejection fraction and stress-induced myocardial ischemia necessary? *J Nucl Cardiol.* 2006;13:768–778.

30. Picano E, Molinaro S, Pasanisi E. The diagnostic accuracy of pharmacological stress echocardiography for the assessment of coronary artery disease: a meta-analysis. *Cardiovasc Ultrasound.* 2008;60:30.

31. Kamalesh M, Matorin R, Sawada S. Prognostic value of a negative stress echocardiographic study in diabetic patients. *Am Heart J.* 2002;143:163–168.

32. Senior R, Becher H, Monaghan M, Agati L, Zamorano J, Vanoverschelde JL, Nihoyannopoulos P. Contrast echocardiography: evidence-based recommendations by European Association of Echocardiography. *Eur J Echocardiogr.* 2009;10:194–212.

33. Douglas PS, Ragosta S, Ward RP, et al. ACCF/ASE/AHA/ASNC/HFSA/ HRS/SCAI/SCCM/SCCT/SCMR 2011 Appropriate Use Criteria for Echocardiography. *J Am Coll Cardiol.* 2011; 57, 1126–1166.

34. Mahajan N, Polavaram L, Vankayala H, et al. Diagnostic accuracy of myocardial perfusion imaging and stress echocardiography for the diagnosis of left main and triple vessel coronary artery disease: a comparative meta-analysis. *Heart.* 2010;96:956–966.

35. Al Jaroudi W, Iskandrian AE. Regadenoson: a new myocardial stress agent. *J Am Coll Cardiol.* 2009;54:1123–1130.

36. Hendel RC, Henkin RE, Pellikka PA, et al. ACCF/ASNC/ACR/AHA/ASE/ SCCT/SCMR/SNM 2009 Appropriate Use Criteria for Cardiac Radionuclide Imaging. JACC 2009, 53: 2201-29.

37. Harris PJ, Harrell FE Jr., Lee KL, et al. Survival in medically treated coronary artery disease. *Circulation.* 1979;60:1259–1269.

38. Patel MR, Dehmer GJ, Hirshfeld JW, et al. ACCF/SCAI/STS/AATS/AHA/ ASNC/HFSA/SCCT 2012 Appropriate Use Criteria for Coronary Revascularization Focused Update. *J Am Coll Cardiol.* 2012;59(9):857–881.

39. Miller JM, Rochitte CE, Dewey M, Arbab-Zadeh A, Niinuma H, Gottlieb I, Paul N, Clouse ME, Shapiro EP, Hoe J, Lardo AC, Bush DE, de Roos A, Cox C, Brinker J, Lima JA. Diagnostic performance of coronary angiography by 64-row CT. *N Eng J Med.* 2008;359:2324–2336.

40. Motoyama S, Sarai M, Harigaya H, et al. Computed tomographic angiography characteristics of atherosclerotic plaques subsequently resulting in acute coronary syndrome. *J Am Coll Cardiol.* 2009;54:49–57.

41. Shaw LJ, Min JK, Narula J, et al. Sex differences in mortality associated with computed tomographic angiographic measurements of obstructive and nonobstructive coronary artery disease: an exploratory analysis. *Circ Cardiovasc Imaging.* 2010;3:473–481.

42. Miller JM, Rochitte CE, Dewey M, et al. Diagnostic performance of coronary angiography by 64-row CT. *N Engl J Med.* 2008;359:232–236.

43. Budoff MJ, Dowe D, Jollis JG, et al. Diagnostic performance of 64-multidetector row coronary computed tomographic angiography for evaluation of coronary artery stenosis in individuals without known coronary artery disease: results from the prospective multicenter ACCURACY (Assessment by Coronary Computed Tomographic Angiography of Individuals Undergoing

Invasive Coronary Angiography) trial. *J Am Coll Cardiol.* 2008;52:1724–1732.

44. Meijboom WB, Meijs MF, Schuijf JD, Cramer MJ, Mollet NR, van Mieghem CA, Nieman K, van Werkhoven JM, Pundziute G, Weustink AC, de Vos AM, Pugliese F, Rensing B, Jukema JW, Bax JJ, Prokop M, Doevendans PA, Hunink MG, Krestin GP, de Feyter PJ. Diagnostic accuracy of 64-slice computed tomography coronary angiography: a prospective, multicenter, multivendor study. *J Am Coll Cardiol.* 2008;52:2135–2144.

45. Di Carli MF, Dorbala S, Curillova Z, et al. Relationship between CT coronary angiography and stress perfusion imaging in patients with suspected ischemic heart disease assessed by integrated PET-CT imaging. *J Nucl Cardiol.* 2007;14:799–809.

46. Wolk MJ, Kamer CM, Min JK, et al. ACCF/AHA/ASE/ASNC/HFSA/HRS/SCAI/SCCT/SCMR/STS 2013 Multimodality Appropriate Use Criteria for the Detection and Risk Assessment of Stable Ischemic Heart Disease. *J Am Coll Cardiol.* 2014.

47. Lanza GA, Crea F. Primary coronary microvascular dysfunction: clinical presentation, pathophysiology, and management. *Circulation* 2010;121:2317–2325.

48. Yusuf S, Wittes J, Friedman L. Overview of results of randomized clinical trials in heart disease. I. Treatments following myocardial infarction. *JAMA.* 1988 Oct 14;260(14):2088–2093.

49. Bangalore S, Steg G, Deedwania P, Crowley K, Eagle KA, Goto S, Ohman EM, Cannon CP, Smith SC, Zeymer U, Hoffman EB, Messerli FH, Bhatt DL; REACH Registry Investigators. β-Blocker use and clinical outcomes in stable outpatients with and without coronary artery disease. *JAMA.* 2012 Oct 3;308(13):1340–1349.

50. Hjalmarson A, Goldstein S, Fagerberg B, Wedel H, Waagstein F, Kjekshus J, Wikstrand J, El Allaf D, Vítovec J, Aldershvile J, Halinen M, Dietz R, Neuhaus KL, Jánosi A, Thorgeirsson G, Dunselman PH, Gullestad L, Kuch J, Herlitz J, Rickenbacher P, Ball S, Gottlieb S, Deedwania P. Effects of controlled-release metoprolol on total mortality, hospitalizations, and well-being in patients with heart failure: the Metoprolol CR/XL Randomized Intervention Trial in congestive heart failure (MERIT-HF). MERIT-HF Study Group. *JAMA.* 2000 Mar 8;283(10):1295–1302.

51. Diaz A, Bourassa MG, Guertin MC, Tardif JC. Long-term prognostic value of resting heart rate in patients with suspected or proven coronary artery disease. *Eur Heart J.* 2005 May;26(10):967–974.

52. Ho JE, Bittner V, Demicco DA, Breazna A, Deedwania PC, Waters DD. Usefulness of heart rate at rest as a predictor of mortality, hospitalization for heart failure, myocardial infarction, and stroke in patients with stable coronary heart disease (Data from the Treating to New Targets [TNT] trial). *Am J Cardiol.* 2010 Apr 1;105(7):905–911.

53. Pepine CJ, Handberg EM, Cooper-DeHoff RM, Marks RG, Kowey P, et al. INVEST Investigators. A calcium antagonist vs a non-calcium antagonist hypertension treatment strategy for patients with coronary artery disease. The

International Verapamil-Trandolapril Study (INVEST): a randomized controlled trial. *JAMA*. 2003 Dec 3;290(21):2805–2816.

54. Nissen SE, Tuzcu EM, Libby P, Thompson PD, Ghali M, Garza D, Berman L, Shi H, Buebendorf E, Topol EJ; CAMELOT Investigators. Effect of antihypertensive agents on cardiovascular events in patients with coronary disease and normal blood pressure: the CAMELOT study: a randomized controlled trial. *JAMA*. 2004 Nov 10;292(18):2217–2225.

55. Morrow DA, Scirica BM, Chaitman BR, McGuire DK, Murphy SA, Karwatowska-Prokopczuk E, McCabe CH, Braunwald E. Evaluation of the glycometabolic effects of ranolazine in patients with and without diabetes mellitus in the MERLIN-TIMI 36 randomized controlled trial. *Circulation* 2009;119:2032–2039.

56. Collaborative meta-analysis of randomised trials of antiplatelet therapy for prevention of death, myocardial infarction, and stroke in high risk patients. *BMJ* 2002;324:71–86.

57. AIM-HIGH Investigators. Niacin in patients with low HDL cholesterol levels receiving intensive statin therapy. *N Engl J Med* 2011;365:2255–2267.

58. Ray KK, Cannon CP: The potential relevance of the multiple lipid-independent (pleiotropic) effects of statins in the management of acute coronary syndromes. *J Am Coll Cardiol*. 2005;46:1425.

59. Yusuf S, Sleight P, Pogue J, Bosch J, Davies R, Dagenais G. Effects of an angiotensin-converting-enzyme inhibitor, ramipril, on cardiovascular events in high-risk patients. *The Heart Outcomes Prevention Evaluation Study Investigators. N Eng J Med*. 2000;342:145–153.

60. Braunwald E, Domanski MJ, Fowler SE, Geller NL, Gersh BJ, Hsia J, Pfeffer MA, Rice MM, Rosenberg YD, Rouleau JL, Investigators PT. Angiotensin-converting-enzyme inhibition in stable coronary artery disease. *N Eng J Med* 2004;351:2058–2068.

61. Dahlof B, Sever PS, Poulter NR, Wedel H, Beevers DG, Caulfield M, Collins R, Kjeldsen SE, Kristinsson A, McInnes GT, Mehlsen J, Nieminen M, O'Brien E, Ostergren J. Prevention of cardiovascular events with an antihypertensive regimen of amlodipine adding perindopril as required versus atenolol adding bendroflumethiazide as required, in the Anglo-Scandinavian Cardiac Outcomes Trial-Blood Pressure Lowering Arm (ASCOT-BPLA): a multicentre randomised controlled trial. *Lancet* 2005;366:895–906.

62. Jamerson K, Weber MA, Bakris GL, Dahlof B, Pitt B, Shi V, Hester A, Gupte J, Gatlin M, Velazquez EJ. Benazepril plus amlodipine or hydrochlorothiazide for hypertension in high-risk patients. *N Eng J Med*. 2008;359:2417–2428.

63. Yusuf S, Teo KK, Pogue J, Dyal L, Copland I, Schumacher H, Dagenais G, Sleight P, Anderson C. Telmisartan, ramipril, or both in patients at high risk for vascular events. *N Engl J Med*. 2008;358:1547–1559.

64. Mann JF, Schmieder RE, McQueen M, Dyal L, Schumacher H, Pogue J, Wang X, Maggioni A, Budaj A, Chaithiraphan S, Dickstein K, Keltai M, Metsarinne K, Oto A, Parkhomenko A, Piegas LS, Svendsen TL, Teo KK, Yusuf S. Renal outcomes with telmisartan, ramipril, or both, in people at high vascular risk (the

ONTARGET study): a multicentre, randomised, double-blind, controlled trial. *Lancet.* 2008;372: 547–553.

65. Pitt B, Remme W, Zannad F, Neaton J, Martinez F, Roniker B, Bittman R, Hurley S, Kleiman J, Gatlin M. Eplerenone, a selective aldosterone blocker, in patients with left ventricular dysfunction after myocardial infarction. *N Eng J Med.* 2003;348:1309–1321.

66. Erne P, Schoenenberger AW, Burckhardt D, Zuber M, Kiowski W, Buser PT, Dubach P, Resink TJ, Pfisterer M. Effects of percutaneous coronary interventions in silent ischemia after myocardial infarction: the SWISSI II randomized controlled trial. *JAMA.* 2007;297:1985–1991.

67. Nishigaki K, Yamazaki T, Kitabatake A, Yamaguchi T, Kanmatsuse K, Kodama I, Takekoshi N, Tomoike H, Hori M, Matsuzaki M, Takeshita A, Shimbo T, Fujiwara H. Percutaneous coronary intervention plus medical therapy reduces the incidence of acute coronary syndrome more effectively than initial medical therapy only among patients with low-risk coronary artery disease a randomized, comparative, multicenter study. *JACC Cardiovasc Interv.* 2008;1:469–479.

68. Hueb W, Lopes NH, Gersh BJ, Soares P, Machado LA, Jatene FB, Oliveira SA, Ramires JA. Five-year follow-up of the Medicine, Angioplasty, or Surgery Study (MASS II): a randomized controlled clinical trial of 3 therapeutic strategies for multivessel coronary artery disease. *Circulation.* 2007;115:1082–1089.

69. Boden WE, O'Rourke RA, Teo KK, et al. for the COURAGE Trial Research Group Optimal Medical Therapy with or without PCI for Stable Coronary Disease. *N Engl J Med.* 2007;356:1503–1516.

70. Mauri L, Kereiakes D, Yeh R, et al. on behalf of the DAPT investigators, Twelve or 30 Months of Dual Antiplatelet Therapy after Drug-Eluting Stents. *N Engl J Med.* 2014;371:2155–2166.

71. www.acc.org/latest-in-cardiology/clinical-trials/2014/09/13/23/29/isar-triple

72. Velazquez EJ, Lee KL, Marek A. Deja coronary-artery bypass surgery in patients with left ventricular dysfunction. *N Engl J Med.* 2011;364:1607–1616.

73. Bonow RO, Maurer G, Lee KL, Holly TA, Binkley PF, Desvigne-Nickens P, Drozdz J, Farsky PS, Feldman AM, Doenst T, Michler RE, Berman DS, Nicolau JC, Pellikka PA, Wrobel K, Alotti N, Asch FM, Favaloro LE, She L, Velazquez EJ, Jones RH, Panza JA. Myocardial viability and survival in ischemic left ventricular dysfunction. *N Eng J Med.* 2011;364:1617–1625.

74. Dzavik V, Ghali WA, Norris C, Mitchell LB, Koshal A, Saunders LD, Galbraith PD, Hui W, Faris P, Knudtson ML. Long-term survival in 11,661 patients with multivessel coronary artery disease in the era of stenting: a report from the Alberta Provincial Project for Outcome Assessment in Coronary Heart Disease (APPROACH) Investigators. *Am Heart J.* 2001;142:119–126.

75. De Bruyne B, Fearon WF, Pijls NH, et al. Fractional flow reserve-guided PCI for stable coronary artery disease. *N Engl J Med.* 2014;371:1208–1217.

76. Marie-Claude Morice MC, Serruys P, Kappetein AP, et al. Five-year outcomes in patients with left main disease treated with either percutaneous coronary intervention or coronary artery bypass grafting in the SYNTAX Trial. *Circulation.* 2010;121:2645–2653.

77. Park SJ, Kim YH, Park DW, Yun SC, Ahn JM, Song HG, Lee JY, Kim WJ, Kang SJ, Lee SW, Lee CW, Park SW, Chung CH, Lee JW, Lim DS, Rha SW, Lee SG, Gwon HC, Kim HS, Chae IH, Jang Y, Jeong MH, Tahk SJ, Seung KB. Randomized trial of stents versus bypass surgery for left main coronary artery disease. *N Eng J Med.* 2011;364:1718–1727.

78. Aggarwal V, Stanislawski M, Maddox T, et al. Safety and effectiveness of drug-eluting versus bare-metal stents in saphenous vein bypass graft percutaneous coronary interventions insights from the veterans affairs CART Program. *J Am Coll Cardiol.* 2014;64(17):1825–1836.

79. Sorajja P, Chareonthaitawee P, Rajagopalan N, Miller TD, Frye RL, Hodge DO, Gibbons RJ. Improved survival in asymptomatic diabetic patients with high-risk SPECT imaging treated with coronary artery bypass grafting. *Circulation.* 2005;112:311–316.

80. The Diabetes Control and Complications Trial Research Group. The effect of intensive treatment of diabetes on the development and progression of long-term complications in insulin-dependent diabetes mellitus. *N Engl J Med.* 1993 Sep 30;329(14):977–986.

81. Turner RC, Millns H, Neil HAW, Stratton IM, Manley SE, Matthews DE. Risk factors for coronary artery disease in non-insulin dependent diabetes mellitus: United Kingdom Prospective Diabetes Study (UKPDS: 23). *BMJ.* 1998;316:823–828.

82. Farkouh ME, Domanski M, Sleeper LA, Siami FS, Dangas G, Mack M, Yang M, Cohen DJ, Rosenberg Y, Solomon SD, Desai AS, Gersh BJ, Magnuson EA, Lansky A, Boineau R, Weinberger J, Ramanathan K, Sousa JE, Rankin J, Bhargava B, Buse J, Hueb W, Smith CR, Muratov V, Bansilal S, King S 3rd, Bertrand M, Fuster V; FREEDOM Trial Investigators. Strategies for multivessel revascularization in patients with diabetes. *N Engl J Med.* 2012;367:2375–2384.

CHAPTER 4

Acute Coronary Syndrome

Udho Thadani, Quang Tuan Nguyen and Han Yaling

Management of Complex Cardiovascular Problems, Fourth Edition. Edited by Thach N. Nguyen, Dayi Hu, Shao Liang Chen, Moo Hyun Kim and Cindy L. Grines.
© 2016 John Wiley & Sons, Ltd. Published 2016 by John Wiley & Sons, Ltd.

BACKGROUND

The term acute coronary syndrome (ACS) is defined arbitrarily as one or more episodes of chest pain (angina) at rest, usually lasting more than ten minutes, and is due to acute myocardial ischemia [1]. Patients with ACS, without electrocardiographic (EKG) evidence of ST elevation myocardial infarction (STEMI), are considered to have non-ST segment elevation (NSTE)-ACS, which on further blood work up, can be divided into patients with NSTEMI (elevated troponin values) or unstable angina (normal troponin values) [2, 4].

CHALLENGES

Once the diagnosis of ACS is entertained, it is imperative to obtain a 12-lead electrocardiogram (ECG), as soon as possible, but no later than 10 minutes [2, 3], to make sure that the patient is not having an acute STEMI. This is the **first challenge** at the beginning of the work-up of a patient with ACS. The reason is that the patients with an acute STEMI require immediate triage at an appropriate facility for consideration of urgent reperfusion therapy [2, 4]. In addition to classical ST segment elevation, if the ECG shows marked ST segment depression in the chest leads, it is imperative to obtain ECG leads V7 to V9, so as not to miss a true posterior STEMI, which becomes an indication for reperfusion strategy [2].

The **second challenge** is to risk stratify the ACS patients into high-, intermediate- or low-risk by demographic, clinical and laboratory data. There are no controversies in the management of high- or low-risk patients. The problem is for the low- and intermediate-risk group: there are no published reports to substantiate the current guideline recommendations of routine stress testing to identify those at high risk.

The third challenge is that besides ACS, elevated troponin values have been reported in normal subjects and in many other conditions such as renal failure or heart failure (HF), so it is recommended that a rising or falling value of 20% or greater in serial measurements to establish a diagnosis of acute myocardial infarction (MI). **The fourth challenge** is to have a cost-effective and patient-centered treatment strategy for the ACS patients who are very different from each other because not all patients have ACS due to coronary plaque erosions.

STRATEGIC MAPPING

At the initial evaluation of the ACS patient in the emergency room, a detailed history and thorough physical examination is essential. Then an ECG is carried out. Once the patient is considered to have NSTE-ACS, the patient should receive regular 325 mg of aspirin (ASA), either 80 mg atorvastatin or 20 to 40 mg rosuvastatin (most potent statin: recommended in the 2014 Guidelines) [5] and have blood taken for measurement of high sensitive troponin I or T at the time of presentation and 3 or 6 hours thereafter [2, 4, 6, 7]. Either intravenous fractionated heparin (UFH) or subcutaneous low molecular weight heparin (LMWH) should also be given while waiting for the troponin results [2]. Sublingual nitroglycerin (NTG) should be given for angina relief and repeated if necessary, 5 minutes later [2], provided the patient has not taken a phosphodiesterase type 5 inhibitor in the previous 24 to 48 hours for erectile dysfunction. If chest pain persists, intravenous nitroglycerin should be started and dose titrated upwards as necessary to relieve chest pain [8]. This strategy is usually effective in overcoming nitrate tolerance during the acute phase of NSTE-ACS [8]. Oral dose of a beta-blocker (BB) should also be started provided there are no contraindications [2].

Patients with ECG evidence of ST segment depression of 2 mm or greater, and those with dynamic ST-T changes [9], hemodynamic compromise, signs of left ventricular (LV) failure, or acute mitral regurgitation should be considered for an invasive strategy, and sent either directly to the catheterization laboratory or admitted to the cardiac intensive care unit waiting for the earliest opportunity at the cardiac catheterization laboratory for urgent coronary angiography and possible revascularization [2, 10].

Others should be observed closely in the emergency department until the results of high sensitive troponin become available. For these patients, either clopidogrel or ticagrelor can be started if the patient is not being considered for immediate invasive strategy. Those with elevated and or rising troponin levels should be hospitalized and referred for coronary angiography during the next 24 to 48 hours, and possible revascularization if indicated.

With the demographic data, clinical and laboratory results, the patients considered to be not at a high risk can be managed conservatively [2] with dual antiplatelet treatment (DAPT), a potent high-dose statin, and aggressive lifestyle modification including no smoking, regular exercise and treatment with antianginal drugs as indicated.

In patients showing high-risk features such as an early positive stress test, with multiple areas of ischemia or wall motion abnormalities or LV cavity dilation, coronary angiography and revascularization should be performed, if there is no contraindication.

All other low-risk patients can be safely discharged on daily ASA, clopidogrel or ticagrelor and a high-dose statin and a BB if tolerated, and sublingual NTG on an 'as needed' basis for angina relief. Further risk stratification can be done as an outpatient on an individual basis by obtaining a stress test and LV function.

All patients should receive counseling for aggressive risk factor modification, including cessation of smoking, and regular exercise. Those with reduced LV ejection fraction (LVEF) should also receive guideline based treatment with a BB (carvedilol or metoprolol succinate or bisoprolol) and an ACE inhibitor. Patients should continue low-dose ASA for life and DAPT for 11 to 12 months [2].

 CLINICAL PEARLS
Acute coronary syndrome due to and not due to coronary plaque erosion In patients with NSTE-ACS, the underlying mechanism of myocardial ischemia is invariably an acute reduction in coronary blood flow (oxygen supply) due to either a spontaneous plaque rupture or endothelial erosion, with superimposed platelet and thrombus formation on the exposed sub-endothelial surface, resulting in acute reduction of coronary blood flow [2, 3, 11]. However, NSTE-ACS may also be due to coronary artery spasm, spontaneous coronary artery dissection, distal coronary embolism, worsening of known underlying coronary artery disease (CAD), endothelial dysfunction, severe hypotension, and myocardial muscle bridge, which can reduce perfusion to the distal coronary bed [4]. Yet many patients may present with NSTE-ACS due to an increase in myocardial oxygen demand, due to an acute increase in heart rate caused by sepsis, acute illness, anxiety, atrial or ventricular tachyarrhythmias, severe anemia, markedly elevated blood pressure; severe aortic stenosis; or thyrotoxicosis, rather than due to a decrease in coronary blood flow from plaque rupture [2]. Other patients may present with NSTE-ACS due to non-ischemic myocardial injury due to myocarditis, cardiotoxic drugs, or following cardiac contusion. This distinction is important as management strategies differ widely in this group of patients compared to those with classical NSTE-ACS due to plaque disruption or endothelial erosion.

HIGH-RISK PROFILING

Once it has been established that the patient has NSTE-ACS, the next step is to risk stratify these patients. Those at high risk need to be considered for coronary angiography and revascularization, if indicated, in addition to institution of antiplatelet, anticoagulation and anti-anginal/anti-ischemic treatment. Several risk models (Thrombolysis in Myocardial Infarction (TIMI) RISK score [12]; Global Registry of Acute Coronary Events (GRACE) RISK score [13]; Controlled Abciximab and Device Investigation to Lower Late Angioplasty Complications (CADILLAC) score [14]; Synergy Between PCI With Taxus and Cardiac Surgery (SYNTAX) Risk score [15]; the Erlanger HEART # Score [16]) have incorporated clinical and laboratory variables to stratify patients into high-, intermediate- and low-risk groups to determine the treatment options [9, 12–17]. However, in the authors' opinion, routine management of NSTE-ACS does not require calculations of these scores to determine management options on an individual basis. Furthermore, none of the publications have randomized patients on the basis of risk scores alone.

HIGH-RISK PREDICTORS

The factors predicting high risk NSTE-ACS are listed in Table 4.1 [9].

In addition to the above risk factors, the presence of established clinical risk factors, including age, family history of CAD, known previous history of CAD, previous history of coronary artery bypass surgery or percutaneous revascularization, peripheral arterial disease, carotid artery disease as well as other co-morbid conditions (diabetes mellitus [DM], chronic kidney disease, severe pulmonary obstructive disease, pneumonia, severe anemia, uncontrolled hypertension [HTN], history of bleeding, and cerebrovascular disease, untreatable cancer), influence management decisions. Baseline levels of hemoglobin, serum creatinine and effective glomerular filtration rate (eGFR), are also important in management planning and decision-making. Although other cardiac biomarkers besides troponins have been correlated with short- and long-term prognosis,

---

Table 4.1 Factors indicating of high-risk NSTE-ACS patients

1. Presence of 2 mm or greater ST segment depression.
2. Fluctuating ST-T wave changes.
3. Elevated and or rising cardiac troponin levels.
4. Signs of circulatory or hemodynamic instability.
5. Left heart failure.
6. Acute mitral regurgitation.
7. Ventricular arrhythmias.

routine measurements of these biomarkers are not recommended to define treatment strategies [2].

CLINICAL PEARLS
Evidence-based medicine work-up for low and intermediate risk NSTE-ACS patients In clinical practice, patients with high-risk features, outlined above, require hospitalization, and on an individual basis, consideration for treatment with an anti-ischemic, antiplatelet and anticoagulant treatment, and possible revascularization if indicated. All other patients fall into the low- and intermediate-risk NSTE-ACS categories and usually can be managed with anti-ischemic, antiplatelet therapy, and aggressive lifestyle modifications. Further risk stratified by non-invasive testing or by coronary CT angiography has been advocated in the current guidelines [2, 6], but is merely an expert opinion and not based on the results of any randomized controlled trials.

INVESTIGATIONS

Symptoms to look for
Chest pain may radiate to the left arm, neck, jaw, back or to the epigastric area. Many patients complain of chest tightness rather than chest pain. Some patients, especially the elderly, and women [18] may present with acute shortness of breath, dizziness, pre-syncope, or syncope, nausea and vomiting, (due to the consequences of acute myocardial ischemia) rather than classical angina [19]. Yet others (4% to 16%) may present with an atypical location of chest or arm pain or rarely sharp pain rather than the classical squeezing chest pain [20].

At the time of initial presentation, one must exclude non-ischemic causes of chest pain, such as pleurisy and musculoskeletal pain; and chest pain due to pericarditis or an acute aortic dissection. ACS may be the initial presentation or may present in patients with known CAD [6].

Signs to look for
There are no specific physical findings for ACS, so often the goal of the physical examination is to detect possible precipitating factors or identify clues of alternative diagnoses. However, several related physical findings could rank the patients in a higher risk category (such as pulmonary edema, a new or worsening mitral regurgitation murmur, a third or fourth

heart sound, hypotension, bradycardia, tachycardia or signs of circulatory or hemodynamic instability, left HF).

Smart testing

The selection of a diagnostic test depends on the level of certainty of evidence regarding risks and benefits, how these risks and benefits compared with potential alternatives, and what the comparative cost or cost-effectiveness of the diagnostic test would be.

Biomarkers

All patients presenting with NSTE-ACS should have high sensitivity cardiac troponin T or I determined at the time of presentation [2, 21]. The values of troponin vary from assay to assay used by different laboratories; it is therefore imperative that each laboratory establish its 99th percentile values in order to make an accurate diagnosis of MI [23]. If the high sensitive troponin is elevated above the 99th percentile values for that laboratory, it is often indicative of myocardial injury with a 95% positive predictive value and 92% negative predictive value for myocardial infarction (MI) [7, 22–24]. However, if the initial troponin value is normal, a repeat measurement at 3 to 6 hours should be performed [7]. In these patients, a 20% rise in troponin value from baseline value in the presence of a good clinical history is indicative of NSTEMI [7, 25].

One needs to be aware that elevated troponin values have been reported in normal subjects and in many other conditions (chronic kidney disease or HF) and it is recommended that one documents a rising or falling value of 20% or greater in serial measurements to establish a diagnosis of acute MI [2, 7, 24, 25].

CLINICAL PEARLS
Discriminating values between biomarkers Cardiac troponin I and T are highly specific for cardiac injury and thus diagnostic of an MI. The current American Heart Association (AHA) and American College of Cardiology (ACC) [2, 6] and European guidelines [21] recommend only initial and 3 to 6 hour later measurement of this biomarker. Routine measurements of total CPK, CKMB and other biomarkers are not necessary.

MANAGEMENT

In the management of the acute phase of ACS, the first strategy is to combat the consequences of platelet deposition and superimposed

Table 4.2 Questions to discuss with clinicians before treatment

1. What are the level of certainty of evidence regarding risk and benefits?
2. How do these risks and benefits compare with potential alternatives?
3. What are the treatment options available?
4. What are the rates of success or failure of these treatment options?
5. What kind of side effects or complications with these treatment options?
6. What would be the comparative cost or cost-effectiveness of the treatment?
7. What happens if this treatment approach does not work for me?
8. How will you help me balance my treatment with the demand of active life?

non-occlusive thrombus formation at the site of the culprit coronary lesion responsible for NSTE-ACS. The second strategy is to increase coronary blood flow to the ischemic area and to reduce myocardial oxygen demand. The patient should have a good discussion with the clinician about the treatment plan. A well-informed patient should ask about treatment options and question the success, complication of the proposed treatment. The detailed discussion is listed in Table 4.2.

Antiplatelet agents

The decision to give antiplatelet or anticoagulant therapy depends on the patient risk profile (gastrointestinal, ischemic stroke, or intracranial bleeding), timing of PCI, or decision to pursue ischemia-guided medical management. At the beginning, the patient should be checked for adequate platelet counts – so as not to be at higher bleeding risk – and is not actively bleeding. Then creatinine clearance should be measured because patients with clearance of <30 mL/min have a greater risk of bleeding. The patients with a high risk of bleeding are listed in Table 4.3.

Aspirin ASA reduces thromboxane levels and reduces platelet aggregation by blocking the enzyme cyclooxygenase. The role of ASA in reducing major adverse cardiac events after STEMI-ACS and in patients with known CAD is well-established [26]. Earlier studies in patients with NSTE-ACS were done with much higher doses of ASA than are currently recommended [26]. Only a small European study has evaluated low dose of 75 mg daily ASA in patients with unstable angina [27].

Given the overall beneficial effect of ASA in CAD patients, it is recommended that all patients with NSTE-ACS receive a 325 mg of chewable

Table 4.3 Patients with a high risk of bleeding while on antiplatelet therapy

1. Previous history of ulcer or bleeding.
2. Advanced age.
3. Symptom of dyspepsia or gastro-esophageal reflux (GERD).
4. Multiple medical comorbidities (history of heart failure, diabetes, liver disease, history of alcohol abuse, smoking).
5. Concomitant medication use: non-steroidal anti-inflammatory drugs (NSAIDs), steroids, anticoagulants.
6. *Helicobacter pylori* infection.
7. Chronic kidney disease (CKD 4 or greater).

ASA, at initial presentation, followed by a daily low dose of 81 to 162 mg daily (75 to 150 mg in European countries), provided there are no absolute contraindications, such as known anaphylaxis to ASA or ongoing major active bleeding [2, 27].

 CLINICAL PEARLS
Correct dosage of aspirin Low-dose (81 to 162 mg) ASA, rather than a high-dose (325 mg), for daily use, is recommended due to the lower incidence of gastrointestinal side-effects and lower rates of bleeding especially when ASA is given concomitantly with other antiplatelet agents [28–30].

Thienopyridines Currently clopidogrel, prasugrel and ticagrelor are approved by the Federal Drug Administration (FDA) for treating patients with NSTE-ACS. These agents reduce platelet aggregation by interfering with adenosine diphosphate (ADP) mediated platelet activation. Only clopidogrel and ticagrelor have been shown to reduce adverse clinical outcomes (when added to ASA) at the time of initial presentation (upstream treatment) in patients presenting with NSTE-ACS, whether subsequent coronary angiography and revascularization is performed or not [31–33]. (Class IIa, Level of Evidence: B by the AHA/ACC 2014 guidelines) In contrast, prasugrel is only approved for patients requiring percutaneous coronary intervention (PCI) at the time of coronary angiography [34, 35].

The benefits of clopidogrel plus ASA were proved in the Clopidogrel in Unstable Angina to Prevent Recurrent Events (CURE) trial [28]. Clopidogrel is recommended in addition to low-dose ASA, provided there is no clinical contraindication, or an immediate need for a coronary angiogram and possible revascularization. In those patients requiring PCI, a loading dose of 300 mg to 600 mg followed by 75 mg daily dose of clopidogrel is recommended.

Ticagrelor Ticagrelor is a more potent antiplatelet agent than clopidogrel. A combination of ticagrelor plus ASA was compared to clopidogrel plus ASA, in over 17,000 patients with NSTE-ACS in the Platelet Inhibition and Patient Outcomes (PLATO) trial [32]. Ticagrelor was superior to clopigogrel in reducing the composite endpoints of death, nonfatal MI, and stroke, including a reduction in total mortality at 30 days, with benefit maintained for up to 12 months. This benefit was especially seen in patients who received low-dose ASA [32]. There was an increased rate of bleeding in the ticagrelor group, and a higher incidence of symptomatic bradycardia and breathlessness [32, 33]. A subgroup of patients who needed subsequent percutaneous revascularization improved to a greater extent in the ticagrelor plus ASA group compared to the clopidogrel plus ASA group [32].

Thus ticargrelor is currently approved as an alternative to clopidogrel; to be given at the time of presentation in patients with a NSTE-ACS, provided there are no contraindications to dual antiplatelet therapy, and urgent coronary angiogram and possible revascularization is not already planned.

In both the CURE and PLATO trials, routine coronary angiography and revascularization was not mandated even in high-risk patients. In both trials, the patients who underwent either an elective or emergent revascularization continued to show benefit compared to ASA treatment alone. Patients who require CABG need to have clopidogrel discontinued for at least 5 to 7 days, and ticagrelor for at least 3 to 5 days before CABG in order to minimize the risk for postoperative bleeding.

Prasugrel Prasugrel is more potent than clopidogrel in preventing platelet aggregation, and is associated with minimal variations in patient response compared to clopidogrel [34]. Prasugrel plus ASA was superior to clopidogrel plus ASA in a large TIMI trial in NSTE-ACS patients requiring PCI [34]. However, with upstream use in patients with NSTE-ACS, prasugrel plus ASA and was not superior to clopidogrel plus ASA, and there were increased rates of bleeding [35]. Thus prasugrel is not currently approved for upstream use in patients with NSTE-ACS.

CLINICAL PEARLS
Differences in use of new antiplatelet agents
Ticagrelor and clopidogrel, but not prasugrel, given in addition to ASA, have FDA approved for upstream use to treat patients with NSTE-ACS in the emergency department. Prasugrel is recommended ONLY when the coronary anatomy is defined and stenting is planned (right before PCI in the cardiac catheterization laboratories).

Because all antiplatelets could cause bleeding, prasugrel should not be used in patients with a prior stroke or TIA, age older than 75, or weight lower than 60 kg. Prasugrel causes intracranial bleeding (ICH) more than clopidogrel, but not in patients with prior transient ischemic attack (TIA) or stroke. Ticagrelor causes increased bleeding only in non-CABG related situations, but not during CABG or when total fatal bleeding is counted.

Glycoprotein 2b3a inhibitors   Glycoprotein 2b3a inhibitors (GPI) include abciximab, eptifibatide and tirofiban. They block circulating fibrinogen from binding to the receptor located on the activated platelets, and thus inhibit platelet aggregation. These agents have potent effects on platelet aggregation and increase bleeding when used in addition to ASA and anticoagulants. Without concomitant thienopyridines, eptifibatide, when given in addition to ASA and heparin, reduced the composite endpoints of death, non-fatal MI, need for repeat revascularization, compared with treatment with ASA and heparin alone [36, 37]. In an early invasive strategy, tirofiban given in addition to ASA and heparin reduced adverse clinical outcomes, but did not reduce mortality [38]. Abciximab is a very potent drug but can cause prolonged thrombocytopenia and is associated with increased bleeding when used in addition to ASA and other anticoagulants [39, 40].

CLINICAL PEARLS
When to use glycoprotein 2b3a inhibitors Due to current routine use of thienopyridines in addition to ASA and heparin, GPIs are no longer used routinely to treat NSTE-ACS patients. These agents are reserved for patients who continue to experience ischemic chest pain despite conventional medical treatment or at the time of PCI when the clot burden is high [2, 40].

Anticoagulants

Unfractionated heparin Smaller trials in NSTE-ACS patients have shown the benefit of unfractionated heparin (UFH) compared to placebo [41]. Some of these trials were done prior to the routine use of ASA, which is now approved for this indication. In a meta-analysis Oler et al. reported a 33% reduction in death or MI in those treated with UFH and ASA, compared to treatment with ASA alone [40]. Currently, routine use of UFH in addition to heparin with an initial bolus of 4000 IU, followed by an infusion, 1000 IU per hour, with dose titration to aPTT of 1.5 to 2.0 times control is recommended [2]. Careful monitoring, every 4 to 6 hours and after dose adjustment is important due to a marked inter- and intra-patient variability in response. Even in well-controlled randomized trials, less than 60% patients are at therapeutic goal during a 24 to 48-hour period [43].

Low molecular weight heparin Enoxaparin was shown to be superior to UFH in the Efficacy and Safety of Subcutaneous Enoxaparin in Non-Q Wave Coronary Events (ESSENCE) trial [43]. In 3171 patients with NSTEMI and unstable angina, enoxaparin reduced composite endpoint of death, MI or recurrent angina at day 14, and at one year also reduced the need for subsequent revascularization. However, in the Superior Yield of the New Strategy of Enoxaparin, Revascularization and Glycoprotein IIb/IIIa Inhibitors (SYNERGY) trial in patients with NSTE-ACS, patients managed with an intended early invasive strategy, enoxaparin was not superior to UFH.

CLINICAL PEARLS
Preferential uses of heparin and low molecular weight heparin Currently both UFH and LMWH, enoxaparin and deltaparin have approval for the upstream treatment of NSTE-ACS. LMWH has an advantage over UFH as there is no need for routine monitoring of aPTT; but UFH should be used when there is evidence of severe renal impairment (CKD stage 4 and lower), as enoxaparin is primarily cleared by the kidney.

Direct thrombin inhibitors These agents provide stable and predictable levels of anticoagulation by working directly against free and clot-bound thrombin. Bivalirudin plus GPI was not shown to be superior to UFH with planned GPI [52]. In a large randomized trial in 13,800 patients [45] there was no difference in composite endpoint of death, MI, unplanned revascularization for ischemia and major bleeding at 30 days between UFH or enoxaparin plus GPI vs. bivalirudin and elective GPI vs. bivalirudin plus elective GPI. But bleeding was reduced with bivalirudin plus elective GPI. At present DTI are not routinely used in the initial phase of NSTE-ACS, but their use has increased in patients who are directly referred for angiography and PCI if indicated.

Factor Xa inhibitors   Currently these agents are not used to treat patients with NSTE-ACS. Fondaparinux was shown to be superior to enoxaparin in the Optimal Antiplatelet Strategy for Interventions (OASIS) 5 trial [46], but patients who underwent PCI did not show a greater benefit with fondaparinux, and required additional UFH for coronary clots at the site of intervention [46]. Although approved, this agent is not used routinely in the US. Newer agents, apixaban and rivaroxaban, have been studied in NSTE-ACS patients, but were not approved by the FDA for clinical use due to higher rates of bleeding [47, 48].

Lipid lowering agents

High-dose treatment with atorvastatin (80 mg daily) compared to the weaker statin pravastatin (40 mg daily), reduced the composite endpoint of death and MI in the Pravastatin or Atorvastatin Evaluation and Infection Therapy–Thrombolysis in Myocardial Infarction (PROVE-IT-TIMI) 22 trial (3.0% vs. 4.2%), without a decrease in total or CV mortality [5].

The current 2014 AHA/ACC guidelines recommend treatment with a high-dose potent statin (atorvastatin 80 mg or rosuvastatin 40 mg) for all patients with known CAD as well as those with NSTE-ACS at the time of presentation [2]. This simplifies treatment as no further dose titration or measurement of blood lipids is needed. Use of either nicotinic acid or a fibrate is not recommended due to the lack of additive effects in recent trials in patients with CAD [49, 50]. These guidelines are likely to be revised, as a recent trial in more than 18,000 NSTE-ACS patients lasting 9 years, showed a reduction in non-fatal MI and ischemic stroke during treatment with simvastatin 40 mg (increased to 80 mg if needed) plus ezetimibe 10 mg daily compared to treatment alone with 40 mg simvastatin (titrated to 80 mg if needed) [49]. There was no reduction in either CV mortality or total mortality in the 9-year trial. But the trials did show that lowering LDL to values lower than 70 mg/dL may be more effective in reducing non-fatal MI and ischemic stroke than in the currently recommendations in the guidelines.

The trial has limitations; only a small number of patients received the higher dose of 80 mg simvastatin, as this dose is not currently recommended by the FDA due to higher incidence of rhabdomyolysis and drug–drug interactions. It is likely that a more potent statin such as atorvastatin 80 mg or rosuvastatin 40 mg by itself would have achieved the same results with the combination of simvastatin plus ezetimibe reported in the *IMProved* Reduction of Outcomes: Vytorin Efficacy International (IMPROVE IT) trial [51]. At present, given the lack of effects on mortality, we would recommend the additional use of ezetimibe only in those patients who are unable to tolerate the higher doses of a potent statin such as atorvastatin or rosuvastatin. More studies are required to address the low threshold for LDL values needed for best outcomes in patients with NSTE-ACS patients.

SYMPTOM RELIEF AND REDUCTION OF MYOCARDIAL ISCHEMIA

Nitroglycerin   NTG is a potent venodilator and reduces venous return to the heart and thus left ventricular end diastolic pressure and also dilates coronary stenosis and prevents coronary artery spasm. At higher doses it is also an arterial dilator and reduces blood pressure. The net effect is improved subendocardial perfusion and relief of chest pain due to its anti-ischemic effects [8]. At the beginning, 0.4 mg sublingual NTG may suffice to relieve chest pain. For recurrent chest pain or pain not relieved with the initial sublingual dose, we prefer intravenous NTG with dose titration to override tolerance, which can develop rapidly [55]. Often intravenous NTG to control angina is required in a small number of patients and for usually no more than 24 to 48 hours [8, 52]. There is no evidence that nitrates reduce either the mortality or other major adverse outcomes, but NTG is still highly effective in relieving angina in these patients [8]. Intermittent oral use of nitrates, as recommended in the current guidelines is not recommended in the acute phase of NSTE-ACS [8].

NTG should not be given to patients who have consumed sildenafil or vardenafil within the previous 24 hours, or tidalafil within the previous 48 hours, as it may produce a marked reduction in blood pressure [8].

Beta-blockers   Beta-blockers (BB) reduce myocardial oxygen demand by reducing the heart rate, cardiac contractility, and blood pressure. These agents have not been shown to improve survival in NSTE-ACS patients or stable angina [53]. An older meta-analysis prior to routine use of ASA and thienopyridines showed a reduction in progression to acute MI with the use of BB in patients with ACS [54]. Thus at present BBs are routinely used to treat NSTE-ACS patients provided there are no absolute contraindications such as sinus bradycardia, AV block, hypotension or active bronchospasm.

> **CLINICAL PEARLS**
> **Roles of nitroglycerin and beta-blockers in the context of contemporary management** Both NTG and BBs reduce myocardial ischemia and relieve treat angina. Both agents are routinely used in the management of patients with NSTE-ACS, provided there are no contraindications to their use. However these agents have not been shown to reduce mortality or MI with the concurrent use of antiplatelet agents or following coronary artery revascularization.

Supplemental oxygen Routine use of supplemental oxygen has not been shown to improve adverse outcomes in patients with NSTE-ACS and may be even detrimental [55].

Angiotensin converting inhibitors and angiotensin receptor blockers Currently there are no randomized trials with either the ACE inhibitors or angiotensin (AT2) receptor antagonists in NSTE-ACS patients. ACE inhibitors have been shown to improve survival in patients with STEMI and in patients with ischemic dialed cardiomyopathy [56, 57]. At present these agents are recommended for routine use in NSTE-ACS patients who have reduced LV function and those who have diabetes with proteinuria [2]. In contrast to the US Guidelines, the European guidelines recommend routine use of ACE inhibitors in all patients with CAD [3].

Invasive versus conservative strategy

Current guidelines recommend invasive strategy in high-risk NSTE-ACS patients [2, 6]. These include patients with electrocardiographic evidence of myocardial ischemia, elevated high sensitivity troponin values, signs of hemodynamic instability, evidence of left HF, acute ischemic mitral regurgitation and recurrent or continuous chest pain despite medical therapy. These recommendations are on the basis of many randomized trials and meta-analysis showing that an invasive strategy reduces the composite endpoint of death, MI and need for urgent revascularization [58–64]. The only divergent results are from the Dutch Invasive versus Conservative

Treatment in Unstable coronary Syndromes (ICTUS) trial, in 1200 patients with NSTE-ACS and elevated troponin T values, showing no benefit of early invasive strategy on composite endpoint of mortality, MI, and need for urgent revascularization, compared to a selective invasive strategy (22.7% vs. 21.2%, $P = 0.33$) [61]. None of the trials have shown a survival benefit either short-term or during long-term follow-up [63]. Published data from large national registries show a survival benefit of an invasive strategy in high-risk group patients, including elderly patients with NSTE-ACS [65]. However, an invasive strategy may not be an initial choice if there is evidence of active ongoing bleeding, or serious co-morbidities such as pneumonia, or acute renal failure.

Early invasive strategy involves a coronary angiogram to define the culprit lesion and assess the extent of CAD. Forty to 60% of patients undergoing coronary angiography have significant obstructive CAD requiring either a PCI with a stent (stents) or coronary artery bypass surgery. Others have either non-obstructive CAD (less than 50% stenosis) or normal coronary arteries and need to be managed conservatively.

MANAGEMENT OF PATIENTS WITH MAJOR CO-MORBIDITIES

Diabetes mellitus   In published reports and registry data, 20 to 30% of patients presenting with NSTE-ACS have DM. There are no large randomized trials in patients with NSTE-ACS who also have DM. However, a subgroup analysis of reported randomized trials and registry data show that patients with high-risk NSTE-ACS who had DM derive the same short-term benefit from revascularization as other patients [66]. Long-term outcomes remain far from ideal following PCI. Diabetic patients who have left main or triple disease or proximal LAD disease should be considered for surgical revascularization including an arterial graft to the LAD. This recommendation is based on better long-term results from recent trials in patients with known CAD [67].

Anemia and active bleeding   Patients with evidence of active ongoing bleeding need to be treated medically without the use of antiplatelet and anticoagulants, unless one can identify a correctable source of bleeding. Those with chronic anemia pose an issue and one should try to identify the underlying cause of anemia. If no cause can be found, and the patient is considered a high-risk NSTE-ACS, one may consider an invasive strategy and use of a bare metal stent for revascularization and shorter term dual antiplatelet therapy, and sparing use of blood transfusions if indicated.

Chronic kidney disease Patients with chronic disease often have persistent elevations of high sensitivity troponin values [25], and in these patients a 20% rise in value over a 3 to 6 hour presentation for NSTE-ACS is considered to be diagnostic of NSTEMI. Patients with high-risk NSTE-ACS, who also have chronic kidney disease, need special attention to minimize contrast induced renal injury during invasive studies and percutaneous intervention. Outcomes of patients with renal disease after PCI are not as good as in patients with normal renal function [2]. Patients with renal disease tend to have higher rates of bleeding during dual antiplatelet and anticoagulant treatment, and need a careful follow-up with judicious use of medications.

Acute illnesses Often initial conservative medical treatment is the best option in this group of patients. Once the active process resolves, one can individualize decisions based on symptoms and stress testing if clinically indicated.

Chronic heart failure Patients with chronic HF presenting with NSTE-ACS may have elevated values of high sensitivity troponin due to underlying HF. Serial measurements documenting an increase in values over a 3 to 6-hour period is indicative of a NSTEMI and carries an adverse prognosis. These patients need to be considered for an invasive strategy on an individual basis. Those patients who have reduced LVEF should also continue to receive guideline-based treatment of HF, which has been shown to reduce mortality and need for hospitalizations for HF.

Chronic atrial fibrillation Patients with chronic atrial fibrillation are often already receiving an oral anticoagulant and need long-term treatment with an anticoagulant to reduce the incidence of thromboembolism. These patients presenting with NSTE-MI need special attention, as dual antiplatelet treatment (DAPT) is often indicated and prescribed as in other patients with NSTE-ACS. Those undergoing PCI often have a bare metal stent placed; and DAPT is needed for at least one month and preferably for three months. Patients should then continue treatment with a low dose ASA or clopidogrel and anticoagulation for life.

SPECIAL SITUATIONS

NSTE-ACS and non-significant obstructive CAD Nearly 30% of patients with NSTE-ACS will have non-obstructive CAD, but this does not mean that these patients are not at risk for future events such as acute MI, sudden ischemic death or recurrence of NSTE-ACS [2]. Non-obstructive lesions are prone to unpredictable rupture. Disease progression over time is also unpredictable and varies from patient to patient. Aggressive risk factor modification includes cessation of smoking, treatment with a potent and high-dose statin and DAT with ASA plus clopidogrel or ticagrelor for at least 11 to 12 months, and then daily ASA indefinitely. Control of blood pressure to 140/90 mmHg and better control of diabetes if present to HbA1C levels of 7 to 7.5%, regular exercise and diet including daily fruits and vegetables are also very important in preventing disease progression and minimizing future serious adverse cardiac events [2].

NSTE-ACS and normal coronary arteries   In nearly 8 to 20% of patients presenting with NSTE-ACS, one finds that coronary arteries are entirely normal [2]. Some of these patients have subclinical atherosclerosis, but others may have endothelial dysfunction or transient coronary artery spasm to explain the symptoms. If coronary artery spasm is confirmed or suspected, empirical treatment with long acting nitrates and a calcium channel blocker is worth a trial. In other patients no specific treatment has been shown to be effective in relieving recurrent chest pain which these patients often experience. The role of daily ASA, statins and antianginal medications is also not well-studied. Response to antianginal drugs is also highly variable. Those with elevated LDL levels are candidates for treatment with a statin, but the most appropriate dose is not well-defined. A low to moderate dose of a statin as used in large outcome studies in patients without CAD may suffice.

NSTE-ACS and illicit drugs   Cocaine is a potent vasoconstrictor and its use may lead to chest pain and typical ACS presentation. Management is similar to other patients with NSTE-ACS, with the exception that instead of a beta-blocker, treatment with a calcium channel blocker is often needed. Early use of benzodiazepines is also recommended [2].

Duration of dual antiplatelet therapy   Based on the results of published randomized trials, all patients with NSTE-ACS should receive DAPT with low-dose daily ASA (81 to 162 mg) for life and 75 mg clopidogrel daily for 11 months or daily 81 mg ASA for life plus 90 mg twice daily ticagrelor for 12 months. Those undergoing PCI need to be treated in a similar way with the exception if patients receiving ASA plus prasugrel, when a 14-month duration of treatment is indicated, based on the reported results of the large TIMI trial. In special situations such as in patients with increased risk for bleeding and those needing an elective

Table 4.4 Length of dual antiplatelet therapy

A Patients with 1 to 3 months of DAPT (presuming these patients receive bare metal stents)
1. Patients at bleeding risk due to prior bleeding events
2. Advanced age
3. Need for surgery
4. Nuisance bleeding events
5. Need for anticoagulation due to atrial fibrillation or other reasons
6. Co-morbidities that put patients at risk (such as due to gastrointestinal problems or stroke).

B Patients to consider for more than 12 months of DAPT
1. Drug eluting stent in left main lesion
2. Paclitaxel-eluting or other first-generation stent
3. History of prior stent thrombosis or myocardial infarction
4. Extensive coronary artery disease or stenting, or other diseased territories
5. Patients at high ischemic risk? (Diabetes, smoking, strong family history, statin intolerance, chronic kidney disease).

non-cardiac surgery in the near future, bare metal stents are often used to treat the culprit lesion and DAPT needs to be continued for at least 1 month and preferably for three months.

Duration of DAPT to prevent stent thrombosis   Current recommendations based on published randomized trials are to continue DAPT for at least 12 months in patients who have received a stent following an episode of NSTE-ACS. With the newer generation of stents incidence of stent thrombosis is less than 1% and there is no certainty that if longer periods of treatment are justified because of the increased risk of bleeding during DAPT. With the older generation of stents, the DAPT study reported that a 36 months of DAPT prevented late stent thrombosis compared to treatment for a period of 12 months [68]. However, in this trial there was an increased rate of bleeding and total mortality during prolonged DAPT, and in many patients in whom older DES were used, now known to be associated with higher rates of restenosis and stent thrombosis. Thus the results of this trial may not be clinically relevant with newer 3rd generation DES. Suggestions for patients with 1–3 months or 12 months DAPT are listed in Table 4.4 [69, 70].

Prevention of gastrointestinal bleeding while on DAPT   If a patient wants to reduce the risk of ulcer-related bleeding, the patient needs to be 80% compliant in taking the proton-pump inhibitor (PPI) ordered (8 out of 10 doses in a given 10-day period). Enteric-coated ASA did not prevent GI bleeding [71–73]. If the patient is on DAPT and needs oral anticoagulant therapy, then vitamin K antagonist (VKA) is a better choice with clopidogrel for 6 week as in the ISAR-TRIPLE study [74].

Clinical relevance of aspirin and clopidogrel resistance Patients with NSTE-ACS may already be taking daily ASA. An important question arises if these patients are truly ASA resistant or non-responders to ASA or neither. Some of these patients have true ASA resistance as determined by platelet aggregation studies. This could be minimized by using higher doses of ASA, but such doses are not recommended due to increased gastrointestinal toxicity and increased rates of bleeding. Furthermore, the clinical relevance of ASA resistance remains unclear as these patients initially also receive a thienopyridine agent.

Resistance to clopidogrel has also been reported, but seems to be of no clinical relevance and thus routine testing of platelet aggregation during dual antiplatelet therapy is not recommended. Prasugrel and ticagrelor are more potent agents than clopigogrel and exert a more uniform effect in different patients, but clinical relevance of this is far from clear in individual patients.

ACTION POINTS

1 Emergency Room management Patients initially seen in the emergency room and confirmed to have a diagnosis of NSTE-ACS, by history, physical examination and a 12-lead ECG, should receive regular 325 mg of ASA and either 80 mg atorvastatin or 20 to 40 mg rosuvastatin. They should also have blood taken for measurement of high sensitive troponin I or T at the time of presentation and 3 or 6 hours after the presentation. Either intravenous UFH or subcutaneous LMWH should also be given while waiting for the troponin results. Sublingual NTG should be given for angina relief and repeated if necessary, 5 minutes later, provided the patient has not taken a PDE5 inhibitor in the previous 24 to 48 hours for erectile dysfunction. If chest pain persists, intravenous NTG should be started and dose titrated upwards as necessary to relieve chest pain. This strategy usually is effective in overcoming nitrate tolerance. Oral dose of a beta-blocker should also be started provided there are no contraindications. Morphine should not be used routinely as it may mask pain and one may miss conversion of

NSTE-ACS to a STEMI, which requires immediate revascularization. Routine use of supplemental oxygen is not recommended.

2 **Invasive management** Patients with ECG evidence of ST segment depression of 2 mm or greater, and those with dynamic ST-T changes, hemodynamic compromise, signs of left ventricular failure, or acute mitral regurgitation should be considered for an invasive strategy, and sent either directly to the catheterization laboratory or admitted to the CICU, until the availability of the catheterization laboratory for possible revascularization.

3 **Medical management** Others should be observed closely in the emergency department until the results of high sensitive troponin become available. In these patients either clopigogrel or ticagrelor can be started if the patient is not being considered for immediate invasive strategy. Those with elevated and or rising troponin levels should be hospitalized and referred for coronary angiography during the next 24 to 48 hours, and possible revascularization if indicated. Prasugrel could be given in the CCL prior to PCI, if indicated.

4 **Discharge from Emergency Room** All other patients can be safely discharged on daily DAPT, a high-dose statin and a beta-blocker if tolerated, and sublingual NTG on a PRN basis for angina relief. Further risk stratification can be done as an outpatient on an individual basis by obtaining a stress test and LV function.

5 **Long-term management** All patients should receive counseling for aggressive risk factor modification, including cessation of smoking, and regular exercise. Those with reduced LVEF should also receive Guideline based treatment with a beta-blocker (carvedilol or metoprolol succinate or bisoprolol) and an ACE inhibitor. Patients should continue low dose ASA for life and dual antiplatelet treatment for 11 to 12 months.

6 Patients who receive BMS due to an increased risk of bleeding or need for chronic anticoagulation treatment should receive DAPT for at least one month and preferably for 3 months.

REFERENCES

1. Braunwald E. Unstable angina: a classification. *Circulation*. 1989;80:410–4.
2. Amsterdam EA, Wenger NK, et al. 2014 AHA/ACC Guideline for the Management of Patients With Non-ST-Elevation Acute Coronary Syndromes: A Report of the American College of Cardiology/American Heart Association

Task Force on Practice Guidelines. *J Am Coll Cardiol*. 2014: doi:10.1016/j.jacc.2014.09.017.

3. Steg PG, James SK, Atar D, et al. ESC Guidelines for the management of acute MI in patients presenting with ST-segment elevation. The Task Force on the management of ST-segment elevation acute MI of the European Society of Cardiology. *Eur Heart J*. 2012;33(20):2569–2619.

4. O'Gara PT, Kushner FG, Ascheim DD, Casey DE Jr, et al. 2013 ACCF/AHA guideline for the management of ST-elevation myocardial infarction: a report of the American College of Cardiology Foundation/American Heart Association Task Force on Practice Guidelines. *Am Coll Cardiol*. 2013;61(4):e78–e140.

5. Cannon CP, Braunwald E, McCabe CH, et al. Intensive versus moderate lipid lowering with statins after acute coronary syndromes. *N Engl J Med*. 2004;350(15):1495–1504.

6. Jneid H, Anderson JL, Wright RS, et al. 2012 ACCF/AHA Focused Update of the Guideline for the Management of Patients With Unstable Angina/Non-ST-Elevation Myocardial Infarction (Updating the 2007 Guideline and Replacing the 2011 Focused Update). A Report of the American College of Cardiology Foundation/American Heart Association Task Force on Practice Guidelines. *J Am Coll Cardiol*. 2012;60(7):645–681.

7. Thygesen K, Mair J, Giannitsis E, et al. How to use high-sensitivity cardiac troponins in acute cardiac care. *Eur Heart J*. 2012;33:2252–2257.

8. Thadani U, Opie LH. Nitrates for unstable angina. *Cardiovasc Drugs Ther*. 1994;8(5):719–726.

9. Boersma E, Pieper KS, Steyerberg EW, *et al*. Predictors of outcome in patients with acute coronary syndromes without persistent ST-segment elevation: results from an international trial of 9461 patients. *Circulation*. 2000;101:2557–2567.

10. Savonitto S, Ardissino D, Granger CB, et al. Prognostic value of the admission electrocardiogram in acute coronary syndromes. *JAMA*. 1999;281(8):707–713.

11. Libby P. Current concepts of the pathogenesis of the acute coronary syndromes. *Circulation*. 2001;104(3):365–372. plibby@rics.bwh.harvard.edu.

12. Antman EMI, Cohen M, Bernink PJ, et al. The TIMI risk score for unstable angina/non-ST elevation MI: A method for prognostication and therapeutic decision making. *JAMA*. 2000;284:835–842.

13. Lyon R, Morris AC, Caesar D, *et al*. Chest pain presenting to the emergency department to stratify risk with GRACE or TIMI? *Resuscitation*. 2007;74:90–93.

14. Granger CB, Goldberg RJ, Dabbous OM, Pieper KS, Eagle KA, Goodman SG, et al. Predictors of hospital mortality in the global registry of acute coronary events. *Arch Int Med*. 2003;163:2345–2353.

15. Zhang YJ1, Iqbal J2, Campos CM2, Klaveren DV3, et al. Prognostic value of site SYNTAX score and rationale for combining anatomic and clinical factors in decision making: insights from the SYNTAX trial. *J Am Coll Cardiol*. 2014;64(5):423–432.

16. Fesmire FM, Martin EJ, Cao Y, Heath GW. Improving risk stratification in patients with chest pain: the Erlanger HEARTS3 score. *Am J Emerg Med*. 2012;30(9):1829–1837.

17. Savonitto S, Ardissino D, Granger CB, et al. Prognostic value of the admission electrocardiogram in acute coronary syndromes. *JAMA.* 1999;281:707–713.

18. Alexander KP, Newby LK, Armstrong PW, et al. Acute Coronary Care in the Elderly, Part II: ST-Segment-Elevation Myocardial Infarction: A Scientific Statement for Healthcare Professionals From the American Heart Association Council on Clinical Cardiology: In Collaboration With the Society of Geriatric Cardiology. *Circulation.* 2007;115:2570–2589.

19. Culić V, Eterović D, Mirić D, Silić N. Symptom presentation of acute myocardial infarction: influence of sex, age, and risk factors. *Am Heart J.* 2002 Dec;144(6):1012–1217.

20. Canto JG, et al. Atypical presentations among Medicare beneficiaries with unstable angina pectoris. *Am J Cardiol.* 2002;90:248–253.

21. Hamm CW, Bassand JP, Agewall S, et al. ESC Guidelines for the management of acute coronary syndromes in patients presenting without persistent ST-segment elevation: The Task Force for the management of acute coronary syndromes (ACS) in patients presenting without persistent ST-segment elevation of the European Society of Cardiology (ESC). *Eur Heart J.* 2011;32(23):2999–3054.

22. Thygesen K, Alpert JS, Jaffe AS, et al. Third universal definition of myocardial infarction. *J Am Coll Cardiol.* 2012;60:1581–1598.

23. Sandoval Y, Apple FS. The global need to define normality: the 99th percentile value of cardiac troponin. *Clin Chem.* 2014;60(3):455–462.

24. Diercks DB, Peacock WFT, Hollander JE, et al. Diagnostic accuracy of a point-of-care troponin I assay for acute myocardial infarction within 3 hours after presentation in early presenters to the emergency department with chest pain. *Am Heart J.* 2012;163:74–80.

25. Freda BJ, Tang WH, Van Lente F, Peacock WF, Francis GS. Cardiac troponins in renal insufficiency. *J Am Coll Cardiol.* 2002;40:2065–2071.

26. Baigent C, Blackwell L, et al. Antithrombotic Trialists (ATT) Collaboration. Aspirin in the primary and secondary prevention of vascular disease: collaborative meta-analysis of individual participant data from randomised trials. *Lancet.* 2009;373(9678):1849–1860.

27. Wallentin LC. Aspirin (75 mg/day) after an episode of unstable coronary artery disease: Long-term effects on the risk for myocardial infarction, occurrence of severe angina and the need for revascularization. *J Am Coll Cardiol.* 1991;18(7):1587–1593.

28. Yusuf S, Zhao F, Mehta SR, Chrolavicius S, et al. Effects of clopidogrel in addition to aspirin in patients with acute coronary syndromes without ST-segment elevation. *N Engl J Med.* 2001;345(7):494–502.

29. The CURRENT–OASIS 7 Investigators. Dose comparisons of clopidogrel and aspirin in acute coronary syndromes. *N Engl J Med.* 2010;363:930–942.

30. Berger JS1, Sallum RH, Katona B, Maya J, et al. Is there an association between aspirin dosing and cardiac and bleeding events after treatment of acute coronary syndrome? A systematic review of the literature. *Am Heart J.* 2012;164(2):153–162.

31. Mehta SR, Yusuf S, Peters RJG. Effects of pretreatment with clopidogrel and aspirin followed by long-term therapy in patients undergoing percutaneous coronary intervention: the PCI-CURE study. *Lancet.* 2001;358:527–533.

32. Wallentin L, Becker RC, Budaj A, et al. Ticagrelor versus clopidogrel in patients with acute coronary syndromes. *N Engl J Med.* 2009;361:1045–1057.

33. Becker RC, Bassand JP, Budaj A, et al. Bleeding complications with the P2Y12 receptor antagonists clopidogrel and ticagrelor in the PLATelet inhibition and patient Outcomes (PLATO) trial. *Eur Heart J.* 2011;32(23):2933–2944.

34. Wiviott SD, Braunwald E, McCabe CH, et al. Prasugrel versus clopidogrel in patients with acute coronary syndromes. *N Engl J Med.* 2007;357:2001–2015.

35. Roe MT, Armstrong PW, Fox KA, et al. Prasugrel versus clopidogrel for acute coronary syndromes without revascularization. *N Engl J Med.* 2012;367:1297–1309.

36. Giugliano RP, White JA, Bode C, et al. Early versus delayed, provisional eptifibatide in acute coronary syndromes. *N Engl J Med.* 2009;9;360:2176–2190.

37. The PURSUIT Trial Investigators. Inhibition of platelet glycoprotein IIb/IIIa with eptifibatide in patients with acute coronary syndromes. *N Engl J Med.* 1998;339:436–443.

38. Cannon CP, Weintraub WS, Demopoulos LA, et al. Comparison of early invasive and conservative strategies in patients with unstable coronary syndromes treated with the glycoprotein IIb/IIIa inhibitor tirofiban. *N Engl J Med.* 2001;344(25):1879–1887.

39. Ottervanger JP, Armstrong P, Barnathan ES, et al. Long-term results after the IIb/IIIa inhibitor abciximab in unstable angina: 1-year survival in the GUSTO IV-ACS Trial. *Circulation.* 2003;107:437–442.

40. Stone GW, Bertrand ME, Moses JW, et al. Routine upstream initiation vs deferred selective use of glycoprotein IIb/IIIa inhibitors in acute coronary syndromes: the ACUITY Timing trial. *JAMA.* 2007;297(6):591–602.

41. Théroux P, Ouimet H, McCans J, et al. Aspirin, heparin, or both to treat acute unstable angina. *N Engl J Med.* 1988;319(17):1105–1511.

42. Oler A, Whooley MA, Oler J, Grady D. Adding heparin to aspirin reduces the incidence of myocardial infarction and death in patients with unstable angina. A meta-analysis. *JAMA.* 1996;276(10):811–815.

43. Goodman SG, Cohen M, Bigonzi F, Gurfinkel EP, et al. Randomized trial of low molecular weight heparin (enoxaparin) versus unfractionated heparin for unstable coronary artery disease: one-year results of the ESSENCE Study. Efficacy and Safety of Subcutaneous Enoxaparin in Non-Q Wave Coronary Events. *J Am Coll Cardiol.* 2000;36(3):693–698.

44. Ferguson JJ, Califf RM, Antman EM, et al. Enoxaparin vs unfractionated heparin in high-risk patients with non-ST-segment elevation acute coronary syndromes managed with an intended early invasive strategy: primary results of the SYN-ERGY randomized trial. *JAMA.* 2004;292(1):45–54.

45. Lincoff AM, Kleiman NS, Kereiakes DJ, et al. Long-term efficacy of bivalirudin and provisional glycoprotein IIb/IIIa blockade vs heparin and planned glycoprotein IIb/IIIa blockade during percutaneous coronary revascularization: REPLACE-2 randomized trial. *JAMA.* 2004;292(6):696–703.

46. Yusuf S, et al. Comparison of fondaparinux and enoxaparin in acute coronary syndromes. *NEJM.* 2006;354:1465–1472.

47. The Apixaban for Prevention of Acute Ischemic Events 2 (APPRAISE-2) trial Alexander JH, Lopes RD, James S, et al. Apixaban with antiplatelet therapy after acute coronary syndrome. *N Engl J Med.* 2011;365(8):699–708.

48. Mega JL, Braunwald E, Wiviott SD, et al. Rivaroxaban in patients with a recent acute coronary syndrome. *N Engl J Med.* 2012;366(1):9–19.

49. The AIM-HIGH Investigators. Niacin in patients with low HDL cholesterol levels receiving intensive statin therapy. *N Engl J Med.* 2011;365:2255–2267.

50. The ACCORD Study Group. Effects of combination lipid therapy in type 2 diabetes mellitus. *N Engl J Med.* 2010;362:1563–1574.

51. Cannon CP, Blazing MA, Giugliano RP, et al. for the IMPROVE-IT Investigators. Ezetimibe added to statin therapy after acute coronary syndromes. *N Engl J Med.* 2015;372:2387–2397. OI: 10.1056/NEJMoa1410489.

52. Kaplan K, Davison R, Parker M, et al. Intravenous nitroglycerin for the treatment of angina at rest unresponsive to standard nitrate therapy. *Am J Cardiol.* 1983;51(5):694–698.

53. de Peuter OR, Lussana F, Peters RJ, et al. A systematic review of selective and non-selective beta-blockers for prevention of vascular events in patients with acute coronary syndrome or heart failure. *Neth J Med.* 2009;67:284–294.

54. Yusuf S, Peto R, Lewis J, Collins R, Sleight P. Beta blockade during and after myocardial infarction: An overview of the randomized trials. *Progr Cardiovasc Dis.* 1985;27(5):335–371.

55. Shuvy M, Atar D, Steg PG, et al. Oxygen therapy in acute coronary syndrome: are the benefits worth the risk? *Eur Heart J.* 2013;34(22):1630–1635.

56. Ryden L, Ariniego R, Amman K, et al. A double-blind trial of metoprolol in acute myocardial infarction – effects on ventricular tachyarrhythmias. *NEJM.* 1983;308:614–618.

57. Garg R, Yusuf S. Overview of randomized trials of angiotensin-converting enzyme inhibitors on mortality and morbidity in patients with heart failure. Collaborative Group on ACE Inhibitor Trials. *JAMA.* 1995;273(18):1450–1456.

58. de Winter RJ1, Windhausen F, et al. Early invasive versus selectively invasive management for acute coronary syndromes. *N Engl J Med.* 2005;353(11):1095–1104.

59. Fox KA, Poole-Wilson PA, Henderson RA, et al. Interventional versus conservative treatment for patients with unstable angina or non-ST-elevation myocardial infarction: the British Heart Foundation RITA 3 randomised trial. Randomized Intervention Trial of unstable Angina. *Lancet.* 2002;360(9335):743–751.

60. FRagmin and Fast Revascularisation during InStability in Coronary artery disease Investigators. Invasive compared with non-invasive treatment in unstable coronary-artery disease: FRISC II prospective randomised multicentre study. *Lancet.* 1999;354(9180):708–715.

61. Damman P, et al. 5-year clinical outcomes in the ictus (invasive versus conservative treatment in unstable coronary syndromes) trial: a randomized comparison of an early invasive versus selective invasive management in patients with non-ST-segment elevation acute coronary syndrome. *JACC.* 2010;55:858–864.

62. Mehta SR, Cannon CP, Fox KA, et al. Routine vs. selective invasive strategies in patients with acute coronary syndromes: a collaborative meta-analysis of randomized trials. *JAMA.* 2005;293(23):2908–2917.

63. Fox KA, Poole-Wilson P, Clayton TC, et al. 5-year outcome of an interventional strategy in non-ST-elevation acute coronary syndrome: the British Heart Foundation RITA 3 randomised trial. *Lancet.* 2005;366(9489):914–920.

64. Navarese EP, Gurbel PA, Andreotti F, et al. Optimal timing of coronary invasive strategy in non-ST-segment elevation acute coronary syndromes: a systematic review and meta-analysis. *Ann Intern Med.* 2013;158(4):261–270.

65. Ramanathan KB, Weiman DS, Sacks J, et al. Percutaneous intervention versus coronary bypass surgery for patients older than 70 years of age with high-risk unstable angina. *Ann Thorac Surg.* 2005;80(4):1340–1346.

66. O'Donoghue ML, Vaidya A, Afsal R, et al. An invasive or conservative strategy in patients with diabetes mellitus and non-ST-segment elevation acute coronary syndromes: a collaborative meta-analysis of randomized trials. *J Am Coll Cardiol.* 2012;60(2):106–111.

67. Farkouh ME1, Domanski M, Sleeper LA, et al. Strategies for multivessel revascularization in patients with diabetes. *N Engl J Med.* 2012;367(25):2375–2384.

68. Mauri L, Kereiakes DJ, Yeh RW, et al. on behalf of the DAPT Investigators. Twelve or 30 months of dual antiplatelet therapy after drug-eluting stents. *N Engl J Med.* 2014;371:2155–2166.

69. www.daptstudy.org/for-clinicians/score_calculator.htm.

70. www.acc.org/latest-in-cardiology/clinical-trials/2014/11/18/16/27/dapt-study? w_nav=LC

71. Goldstein JL, Howard KB, Walton SM, McLaughlin TP, Kruzikas DT. Impact of adherence to concomitant gastroprotective therapy on nonsteroidal-related gastroduodenal ulcer complications. *Clin Gastroenterol Hepatol.* 2006;4:1337.

72. Bhatt DL, Cryer BL, Contant CF, et al. for the COGENT Investigators. Clopidogrel with or without omeprazole in coronary artery disease. *N Engl J Med.* 2010;363:1909–1907.

73. Kelly JP, Kaufman DW, Jurgelon JM, Sheehan J, Koff RS, Shapiro S. Risk of aspirin-associated major upper-gastrointestinal bleeding with enteric-coated or buffered product. *Lancet.* 1996;348:1413–1416.

74. Fiedler KA, Maeng M, Mehilli J, et al. Duration of triple therapy in patients requiring oral anticoagulation after drug-eluting stent implantation. The ISAR-TRIPLE Trial. *J Am Coll Cardiol.* 2015;65(16):1619–1629. doi:10.1016/j.jacc.2015.02.050

CHAPTER 5

ST Segment Elevation Myocardial Infarction

Thach Nguyen, Xu Bo, Faisal Latif, Ho Thuong Dung, Duane Pinto, Pham Manh Hung, Michael Gibson and Runlin Gao

Management of Complex Cardiovascular Problems, Fourth Edition. Edited by Thach N. Nguyen, Dayi Hu, Shao Liang Chen, Moo Hyun Kim and Cindy L. Grines.
© 2016 John Wiley & Sons, Ltd. Published 2016 by John Wiley & Sons, Ltd.

BACKGROUND

The diagnosis of ST segment elevation myocardial infarction (STEMI) is made in patients presenting with ischemic chest pain and a 12-lead electrocardiogram (ECG) showing new ST segment elevation at the J point in at least two contiguous leads of >2 mm in men or >1.5 mm in women in leads V2–V3 and/or of >1 mm in other contiguous chest leads or the limb leads [1].

CHALLENGES

The **first challenge** in the treatment of STEMI is to achieve at the earliest successful reperfusion which is defined as early and complete restoration of coronary blood flow of the infarct-related artery (IRA) leading to prompt resolution of chest pain, ST segment elevation and achieving Thrombolysis In acute Myocardial Infarction (TIMI) 3 flow and TIMI myocardial perfusion grade 3. The **second challenge** is that timely reperfusion will limit myocardial necrosis but still 10% of patients will go on to develop heart failure (HF) in 2 years [2].

STRATEGIC MAPPING

At the first encounter in the emergency room (ER), **the first step** is to do a quick history interview and physical examination in order to confirm the diagnosis of STEMI and to rule out other severe conditions mimicking symptoms or EKG changes of STEMI such as aortic dissection, myocarditis, pericarditis or impending stroke, acute abdomen, cholecystitis or pancreatitis or mechanical complication of MI. Then **the next step** is to identify the high-risk patients and factors predicting poor outcome so aggressive care can be committed and more resources allocated for these patients. The strategies which guide the cardiologist for the next 120 minutes from the first medical contact with the patient are listed in Table 5.1.

HIGH-RISK MARKERS

The high-risk patients are predicted to have higher mortality and complication rates despite appropriate guideline directed optimal therapy. The high-risk markers based on demographic data or co-morbidities are listed in the first part of Table 5.2. These patients should be identified and provided special attention and pathway so that their care can be more intensively managed and specifically focused.

HIGH-RISK PREDICTORS

At the first encounter with patients, relevant signs or symptoms predicting a bad prognosis such as the signs heralding the appearance of cardiogenic shock are listed in Table 5.3. Other signs suggesting extensive myocardial injuries include high white blood cell count and elevated brain natriuretic peptide level (BNP).

Table 5.1 **Management strategies for patients with STEMI**

1. Quickly screen patients for indication and risks of thrombolytic therapy or primary coronary intervention.
2. Be sure that there is no severe anemia, no high protime and prothrombin time, no elevated blood urea nitrogen (BUN) and creatinine level.
3. Check the status of allergy to contrast media.
4. Start thrombolytic therapy or send the patient quickly to the cardiac catheterization laboratory for emergent primary coronary intervention.
5. Open the infarct-related artery and its distal microvasculature with minimal incidence of stroke (<1%) by the fastest (<90 minutes: door to-balloon time) and most effective way (<3% 30-day mortality, <4% reinfarction, <2% restenosis in 1 year).
6. Prevent left ventricular remodeling (i.e., left ventricular dilation).
7. Watch for and prevent re-infarction, mechanical complication: new ventricular septal defect, perforation, rupture of the papillary muscle etc.

Table 5.2 **The high-risk markers**

Based on demographic data and co-morbidities
1. Elderly patients (>75 years of age)
2. Female gender
3. Patients with anemia
4. Diabetes mellitus
5. Chronic kidney disease
6. Lower weight <67 kg
7. Delay in treatment >4 hours from the onset of symptoms.

Based on cardiovascular data
8. Aortic stenosis
9. Peripheral arterial disease
10. Cardiogenic shock
11. Heart failure
12. Hemodynamically compromising ventricular arrhythmias
13. Anterior myocardial infarction
14. Inferior myocardial infarction with right ventricular involvement or diffuse precordial ST segment depression or ST segment elevation in lead aVR.

Table 5.3 **Factors requiring immediate attention and correction**

1. Hypotension (blood pressure <100 mmHg)
2. Sinus tachycardia (heart rate >100)
3. Killip class II–IV pulmonary edema

CLINICAL PEARLS
Which STEMI patients will not die in the next 24 hours? In patients with STEMI, if the heart rate is below 100 and the blood pressure is above 100, then the probability of death in the near future is low. Even when these patients may develop ischemia, reinfarction etc, however, mortality is still minimal in the next 24 hours [3]. A very low heart rate (<50) might be detrimental because it can represent advanced atrioventricular block or agonal rhythm [4].

CRITICAL THINKING
False alarms Rarely, the ST-elevation might return to baseline along with the resolution of chest pain with no intervention. This could represent Prinzmetal's angina, even though the possibility of a spontaneous recanalization of a thrombotic occlusion secondary to a plaque rupture cannot be ruled out. If the ST-segment elevation lasts less than 20 minutes, the emergent treatment can be delayed as long as the EKG signs of ST elevation do not recur. Patients with Takotsubo cardiomyopathy come to the hospital with severe chest pain, ST segment elevation, and elevated troponin level. Their coronary angiograms show no significant obstructive lesion and the left ventricular (LV) angiogram shows localized hypokinesis not uniquely corresponding to an anatomical coronary distribution.

INVESTIGATIONS

Symptoms to look for

Chest pain may radiate to the left arm, neck, jaw, back or to the epigastric area. Many patients complain of chest tightness rather than chest pain. Some patients, especially the elderly, and women may present with acute shortness of breath, dizziness, pre-syncope, or syncope, nausea and vomiting, (due to the consequences of acute myocardial ischemia) rather than classical angina. Yet others (4% to 16%) may present with an atypical location of chest or arm pain or rarely sharp pain rather than the classical squeezing chest pain.

At the time of initial presentation, one must exclude non-ischemic causes of chest pain, such as pleurisy and musculoskeletal pain; and chest pain due to pericarditis, pulmonary embolism or an acute aortic dissection.

Signs to look for

There are no specific physical findings for STEMI, so often the goal of the physical examination is to detect possible precipitating factors or identify clues of alternative diagnoses. However, several related physical findings could rank the patients in a higher risk category (such as pulmonary edema, a new or worsening mitral regurgitation murmur, a third or fourth heart sound, hypotension, bradycardia, tachycardia or signs of circulatory or hemodynamic instability, or left HF).

SMART TESTING

In the acute setting of STEMI, only the ECG, and basic blood tests of complete blood count and electrolytes (sodium, potassium), blood urea nitrogen, creatinine level, protime and prothrombin time are needed before the patient receives thrombolytic therapy or undergoes urgent coronary angiogram for possible angioplasty.

MANAGEMENT

Upstream management

In the ER, once STEMI is identified, the patient should be given a tablet of high-dose non-enteric-coated aspirin (ASA) (325–500 mg) to chew (not to swallow). A bolus of 60 unit/kg of unfractionated heparin (UFH) also could be given, if the patients is planned for PCI and will receive bivalirudin in the cardiac catheterization laboratories (CCL). The UFH may prevent thrombus formation in the guide or stent thrombosis, and may prompt earlier reperfusion in a substantial number of patients especially in the laboratories where bivalirudin is not commonly used.

The European Society of Cardiology (ESC) guidelines suggest ticagrelor and clopidogrel as preferred agents and prasugrel is reserved once coronary anatomy is known [5, 6]. Once the patient receives the basic medications at the ER (ASA, morphine for pain, beta-blockers (if no low blood pressure or bradycardia), the patient may be screened for thrombolytic therapy (TT), primary PCI or medical therapy. High-dose oxygen does not convey better outcome to patients with STEMI and causes more major cardiovascular events (MACE). The results of the Air Verses Oxygen In

---

Table 5.4 Questions to discuss with clinicians before treatment

1. What are the level of certainty of evidence regarding risk and benefits?
2. How do these risks and benefits compare with potential alternatives?
3. What are the treatment options available?
4. What are the rates of success or failure of these treatment options?
5. What kind of side effects or complications with these treatment options?
6. What would be the comparative cost or cost-effectiveness of the treatment?
7. What happens if this treatment approach does not work for me?

---

myocarDial infarction (*AVOID) study are shown below* [7]. Even in this urgent situation, the patient and family should have a frank discussion with the clinician about a treatment plan. A well-informed patient should ask about treatment options and question the success, complication of the proposed treatment. The detailed questions are listed in Table 5.4.

 EVIDENCE-BASED MEDICINE
The AVOID Study This was a multicenter, prospective, randomized, controlled trial comparing oxygen (8 L/min) with no supplemental oxygen in patients with STEMI diagnosed on paramedic 12-lead electrocardiogram. Of 638 patients randomized, 441 were confirmed STEMI patients who underwent primary endpoint analysis. The primary endpoint was myocardial infarct size as assessed by cardiac enzymes, troponin (cTnI) and creatine kinase (CK). Secondary endpoints included recurrent MI, cardiac arrhythmia and myocardial infarct size assessed by cardiac magnetic resonance (CMR) imaging at 6 months. The results of the study showed that there was a significant increase in mean peak CK in the oxygen group compared to the no oxygen group (1948 U/L vs. 1543 U/L; means ratio, 1.27; 95% CI,1.04 to 1.52; $P = 0.01$). Mean peak troponin was similar in the oxygen and no oxygen groups (57.4 mcg/L vs. 48.0 mcg/L; ratio, 1.20; 95% confidence interval [CI], 0.92 to 1.56; $P = 0.18$).There was an increase in the rate of recurrent MI in the oxygen group compared to the no oxygen group (5.5% vs. 0.9%, $P = 0.006$) and an increase in frequency of cardiac arrhythmia (40.4% vs. 31.4%; $P = 0.05$). At 6-months the oxygen group had an increase in myocardial infarct size on CMR $n = 139$; 20.3 g vs. 13.1 g; $P = 0.04$) [7].

CAVEAT: PHARMACOKINETICS OF TICAGRELOR AND MORPHINE

A randomized, double-blind study evaluating the influence of morphine on pharmacokinetics and pharmacodynamics of ticagrelor and its active metabolite (AR-C124910XX) was carried out. In the IMPRESSION study on patients with ST-segment elevation myocardial infarction and non-ST-segment elevation myocardial infarction, 70 patients with STEMI received IV morphine 5 mg or placebo followed by ticagrelor (Brilinta, AstraZeneca) 180 mg, and the pharmacokinetics and pharmacodynamics of ticagrelor were assessed. In all three platelet function tests, the placebo group had a stronger antiplatelet effect and the morphine group had a higher rate of high platelet reactivity. However further clinical studies did not show the clinical impact on patients with STEMI [8].

Thrombolytic therapy

The advantage of thrombolytic therapy (TT) is the earlier restoration of flow due to its quick and simple intravenous administration (door-to-needle <30 minutes). It does not, however, restore normal epicardial or microvascular flow in a large proportion of patients, and reocclusion rate is high. The contraindications of TT are listed in Table 5.5 [1].

Various thrombolytic agents have been developed over the last few decades. They are non-fibrin specific (streptokinase) or fibrin-specific (tenecteplase, alteplase, reteplase). Due to a lower price-tag, streptokinase remains the most commonly used thrombolytic, however the IRA patency rate is only 60%. With the most fibrin-specific characteristics, tenecteplase achieves the highest patency rate of the IRA at 85%, and is administered in a single bolus dose, as compared to reteplase (2 doses, 30 minutes apart) and alteplase (infused over 1.5 hours) [9].

If TT is not successful i.e., persistent ST-elevation or continued chest pain, the patient should undergo urgent coronary angiography and rescue PCI, as appropriate. If TT is successful, coronary angiography is still appropriate and can be performed up to 24 hours later [10]. However, as per the ACC/AHA guidelines, PCI should be performed only if there is evidence of HF, recurrent ischemia, unstable ventricular arrhythmias, reduced LV EF, or multi-vessel CAD [11]. If the angiography is performed >3 days after STEMI and the IRA is totally occluded, then PCI does not provide any incremental benefit in the asymptomatic patient compared to medical therapy alone [12].

Table 5.5 Contraindications of thrombolytic therapy

Absolute contraindications
1. Any prior intracranial bleeding.
2. Known structural cerebral vascular lesion (e.g. arteriovenous malformations).
3. Known malignant intracranial neoplasm (primary or metastatic).
4. Ischemic stroke within 3 months, EXCEPT ischemic stroke within 3 hours.
5. Suspected aortic dissection.
6. Active bleeding or bleeding diathesis (excluding menses).
7. Significant closed head or facial trauma within 3 months.

Relative contraindications
1. History of chronic, severe, poorly controlled hypertension.
2. Severe uncontrolled hypertension on presentation (systolic blood pressure >180 mmHg, diastolic blood pressure >110 mmHg).
3. History of prior ischemic stroke >3 months, dementia, or known intracranial pathology (not covered in absolute contraindications).
4. Traumatic (greater than 10 minutes) cardiopulmonary resuscitation or major surgery (<3 weeks).
5. Non-compressible vascular puncture.
6. For streptokinase/anistreplase: prior exposure (more than 5 days ago) or prior allergic reaction to these agents.
7. Pregnancy.
8. Active peptic ulcer.
9. Current use of anticoagulants such as warfarin (the higher the INR, the higher the risk of bleeding) or newer oral anticoagulants (dabigatran, apixaban or rivaroxaban).

Anticoagulants following thrombolytic therapy

Unfractionated heparin (UFH) is used after TT with tPA or reteplase to prevent the propagation of the thrombus, formation of new mural thrombosis, systemic embolism, and coronary reocclusion. The aPTT is maintained at 1.5–2 times control (50–70 seconds). There is no need to use UFH after streptokinase. Low-molecular weight heparin (LMWH) (enoxaparin), can also be used in patients receiving fibrin-specific TT, and has proven to be of equivalent efficacy and safety profile when compared to UFH, with the benefit of not having to monitor the aPTT.

Primary percutaneous coronary intervention

Percutaneous interventions include percutaneous plain balloon angioplasty (POBA), bare-metal stenting (BMS) or drug-eluting stenting (DES), drug coated stent *or* drug-eluting bioresorbable vascular scaffold without prior TT. The efficacy of POBA was limited with recurrent ischemia

Table 5.6 Angiographic exclusions precluding performance of PCI in STEMI

1. The infarct-related artery supplies a small amount of myocardium, in which the risk of PCI may outweigh the benefit.
2. Inability to clearly identify the infarct-related artery.
3. Caution if etiology of STEMI is spontaneous coronary artery dissection.

Note: PCI: percutaneous coronary interventions; STEMI: ST segment elevation myocardial infarction.

in 10% to 15%, early reocclusion in 4% and late restenosis in 31% to 45 %. Even in the DES era, not every STEMI patient was eligible for stenting because the artery could be too small or too large with a diameter >4.0 mm. Contraindications for PCI are listed in Table 5.6.

Anticoagulants during primary PCI

In patients undergoing primary PCI, with the concomitant use of glycoprotein 2b3a inhibitor (GPI), 60 U/kg of UFH are given to achieve an activated clotting time (ACT) of 200–250 seconds. If GPI are not used, high-dose UFH to achieve ACT >350 seconds has been associated with reduced subacute thrombosis. UFH is not continued after the procedure because it has not been proven to decrease the rate of reocclusion or ischemia, unless there are a lot of residual thrombi.

Direct thrombin inhibitor (DTI), mainly bivalirudin is conveniently given to patients undergoing primary PCI because of the small bolus dose and the short infusion time. DTI is found to be beneficial, due to reduced bleeding without causing a higher rate of complications compared to UFH, though increased rate of stent thrombosis has been observed [13]. While bivalirudin is an accepted treatment modality for primary PCI, however, recently the efficacy and safety of bivalirudin was challenged against UFH in the HEAT PPCI trial [14].

 EVIDENCE-BASED MEDICINE
The HEAT PPCI Trial In an open-label, randomized controlled trial, 1829 consecutive adults with STEMI were enrolled. The primary efficacy outcome was a composite of all-cause mortality, cerebrovascular accident,

reinfarction, or unplanned target lesion revascularization. The primary safety outcome was incidence of major bleeding (type 3–5 as per Bleeding Academic Research Consortium [BARC] definitions). 83% patients randomized in the bivalirudin group and 82% patients in the UFH group had a PCI. The rate of GPI use was similar between the two groups [13% vs. 15%]. The primary efficacy outcome occurred in 8.7% of patients in the bivalirudin group and 5.7% of patients in the UFH group (absolute risk difference 3.0%; relative risk [RR] 1.52, 95% CI 1.09–2.13, $P = 0.01$). The primary safety outcome occurred in 3.5% of patients in the bivalirudin group and 3.1% of patients in the UFH group (0.4%; 1.15, 0.70–1.89, $P = 0.59$). Compared with bivalirudin, the HEAT PPCI trial showed that UFH reduces the incidence of major adverse ischemic events without increase in bleeding complications [14].

However, the HEAT PPI trial is a single center trial, so the evidence level may be not very strong until other centers could duplicate its results. There is another anticoagulant, enoxaparin, which is used frequently in France. In the ATOLL trial, the results showed no significant difference in the primary endpoints, with favoring trends in mortality and MI and no excess bleeding [15]. However, another challenge to the interventional cardiologists is when the patient presents with STEMI while on a maintenance dose of oral anticoagulants. How does one carry out PPCI in these patients?

CRITICAL THINKING
PCI while on a therapeutic level of oral anticoagulants If the patient arrives while on a maintenance dose of vitamin K antagonist (VKA) warfarin and with therapeutic international ratio (INR), the patient should be given one bolus dose UFH (5000 units) to maintain therapeutic pTT during PCI. If the patient arrives while on a maintenance dose of new oral anticoagulants (OAC) such as dabigatran, rivaroxaban, apixaban, these patients should receive standard medications and one single dose of UFH as above and then continue to PCI if indicated. There is not much information about the safety of dabigatran or apixaban in primary PCI. Rivaroxaban was found to be safe after PCI for acute coronary syndrome (ACS) patients in the ATLAS ACS 2 TIMI 51 trial [16].

Table 5.7 Indicators of excellence in providing interventional service for STEMI

1. Door to balloon time <90 minutes
2. TIMI 2 or 3 flow attained in >90% of patients
3. Emergency coronary artery bypass surgery <2%
4. Actual performance of PCI in >95% appropriate for it
5. 30-day all cause risk-standardized mortality rate following PCI for patients with STEMI or cardiogenic shock (National Quality Forum #0536)

Indicators of excellence

Even with the best and most expensive equipment and pharmaceutical products available in the CCL, the results of PCI in STEMI are operator-dependent and institution-related. The indicators of excellent interventional service of a CCL are listed in Table 5.7. If the data of a particular hospital are worse than the national benchmarks, then the treatment for patients with STEMI in that particular hospital should be TT, with further referral for PCI to other nearby hospitals when indicated.

Thrombectomy

The new updated guidelines list routine thrombus aspiration as a class III indication in patients with STEMI undergoing PPCI. The question is whether aspiration thrombectomy as an adjunct to primary PCI resulted in superior outcomes as compared with primary PCI alone in patients presenting with STEMI. Therefore, selective aspiration thrombectomy received only a class IIb indication with the results of the Thrombus Aspiration in ST-Elevation Myocardial Infarction in Scandinavia (TASTE) trial [17, 18].

Adjunctive medical management

P2 Y12 inhibitors As the first P2 Y12 inhibitor on the market, clopidogrel has a clear safety profile and it may be given on the table as the loading dose and continued as the maintenance dose. Ticagrelor may be given before or after PCI according to the PLATO trial [19]. Prasugrel may be given only after the coronary angiogram and before patient is planned for PCI [20]. The effects of prasugrel and ticagrelor are evidenced in the TRITON-TIMI 38 and Platelet Inhibition and Patient Outcomes Study sub-analysis on STEMI Patients (PLATO) [19] trials.

EVIDENCE-BASED MEDICINE

TRITON TIMI-38 Study In a double-blind, multicenter RCT, 3534 patients with STEMI were randomized to receive either prasugrel (60 mg loading, 10 mg maintenance) or clopidogrel (300 mg loading, 75 mg maintenance). The primary endpoint was CV death, non-fatal MI, or non-fatal stroke. At 30 days, the primary endpoints occurred in 6.5% of patients assigned to prasugrel when compared to 9.5% of patients assigned to receiving clopidogrel (HR 0.68; $P = 0.0017$). The difference persisted at 15 months ($P = 0.022$). There was no difference in TIMI major bleeding unrelated to open heart surgery at 30 days ($P = 0.33$) and at 15 months ($P = 0.6451$). In conclusion, prasugrel was more effective than clopidogrel for prevention of ischemic events, without an apparent excess in bleeding in patients undergoing PCI for STEMI [20].

CLINICAL PEARLS

Caveats in the use of antiplatelets The metabolism of clopidogrel is affected by the patient's genotype, environmental factors, smoking, diabetes and body mass index, or proton pump inhibitor, etc. Clopidogrel and ticagrelor are indicated in patients not treated with PCI (medical treatment only), while prasugrel is not indicated. Clopidogrel is also suitable for elderly patients and the patient with a high risk of bleeding, compared to ticagrelor and prasugrel.

Prasugrel is effective in ACS (including STEMI); however it has increased non-CABG bleeding (2.4% vs. 1.8%). Therefore, prasugrel should not be used in patients with a prior stroke or transient ischemic attack (TIA). Patient of age >75 and weight <60 Kg should have reduced maintenance dose (5 mg) [20]. Ticagrelor decreased CV and all causes mortality while showing increased non-CABG bleeding and no change in CABG-related bleeding or total fatal bleeding. There was increased intracranial bleeding (ICH) while there was no difference in ICH in patients with prior TIA or stroke [19].

Prehospital administration of ticagrelor in patients with acute STEMI appeared to be safe, but did not improve pre-PCI coronary reperfusion [21].

If any of these patients arrives for primary PCI while on a maintenance dose of the above three P2Y12 inhibitors, the patient should be continued with the same medications after PCI. If there is a question of stent thrombosis not due to mechanical problems (poor stent expansion), a new P2Y12 inhibitor should be tried, especially prasugrel which showed a lower rate of acute stent thrombosis. However, if ticagrelor is used prior to STEMI, ticagrelor should be continued after PCI because of increased subsequent CV events if discontinued [22].

 CRITICAL THINKING
P2Y12 inhibitors for patients with prior stroke
In the Clopidogrel for High Atherothrombotic Risk and Ischemic Stabilization Management and Avoidance (CHARISMA) trial, there was a statistically significant reduction in ischemic stroke with clopidogrel while the primary endpoint was not met [23]. These results were counterbalanced by the Management of Atherothrombosis With Clopidogrel in High-Risk Patients With Recent Transient Ischemic Attacks or Ischemic Stroke (MATCH) trial [24], which had a slightly different design of cerebrovascular disease where the randomization was clopidogrel plus aspirin versus clopidogrel alone. The results showed no significant reduction in cerebrovascular events, and worse bleeding including ICH because in these patients, the risk of hemorrhagic conversion was higher [24]. The stroke guidelines of the American Stroke association clearly do not recommend clopidogrel (class III dual-antiplatelet therapy) unless there is a new stent or this is an ACS patient.

Glycoprotein 2b3a inhibitor

Glycoprotein 2b3a inhibitor (GPI) is a strong and effective antiplatelet drug. It affects the platelet aggregation downstream to the ADP inhibitor. Routine use of the GPI abciximab in STEMI patients undergoing PCI does not add any measurable benefit. If the patient has a heavy thrombotic burden after PCI, then the patient may have short-term GPI or UFH to clear the thrombi.

Looking forward: Anticoagulants after primary PCI

The residual risk after antiplatelet therapy   In the CURE trial [25], the residual risk for death, MI, or stroke after 12 months of treatment with clopidogrel together with aspirin was approximately 10%. In the

TRITON [20] and PLATO [19] trials, with new and more potent antiplatelet agents combined with aspirin, there was the same residual risk. As the mechanism of ACS is due to superimposed thrombus, the hypothesis is that anticoagulants might improve the CV outcomes in patients with a recent ACS. In early 2000, this hypothesis was tested in the WARIS trial with warfarin. The results showed that warfarin could decrease MI and reinfarction; however with a higher risk of bleeding [26]. New studies with ASA, P2Y12 inhibitor on top of oral anticoagulants showed minimal decrease of new MI, with a higher bleeding profile [27].

Beta-blockers   The majority of RCT of BB during STEMI was done in the thrombolytic era. The systemic review of RCTs of beta-blockers (BB) in STEMI has found that BB given within hours of infarction reduces both mortality and reinfarction. BB may reduce the rates of cardiac rupture and ventricular fibrillation. In patients with moderate HF (NYHA class II or III), BB were found to decrease readmission, mortality and sudden death [28]. The benefits of BB were evidenced in patients with STEMI after TT or before PCI.

CLINICAL PEARLS
BB for patients with COPD Patients with significant chronic obstructive pulmonary disease (COPD) who may have a component of reactive airway disease should be given beta-blockers very cautiously. The initial selection should favor a short-acting beta-1-specific drug such as metoprolol or esmolol at a reduced dose (e.g., 12.5 mg of metoprolol orally) rather than the complete avoidance of a beta-blocker. Intravenous metoprolol may be given in 5-mg increments by slow intravenous administration (5 mg over 1 to 2 minutes), repeated every 5 minutes for a total dose of 15 mg. In patients who tolerate the total 15-mg IV dose, oral therapy can be initiated 15 minutes after the last intravenous dose at 25 to 50 mg every 6 hours for 48 hours. Thereafter, patients should receive a maintenance dose of up to 100 mg twice daily.

Angiotensin converting enzyme inhibitors and angiotensin II receptor blockers   Angiotensin receptor blocker (ARB) acts on the angiotensin receptor. In the Valsartan in Acute Myocardial Infarction (VALIANT) trial, patients with STEMI complicated by LV dysfunction, ARBs were compared with angiotensin converting enzyme inhibitors (ACEI) [29]. The results showed that there was no difference in fatal or

Table 5.8 High- and moderate-intensity statins

High-intensity statins
Atorvastatin (40–80 mg
Rosuvastatin 20–40 mg
Moderate-intensity statins
Atorvastatin 10 (20) mg
Rosuvastatin (5) 10 mg
Simvastatin 20–40 mg
Pravastatin 40 (80) mg
Lovastatin 40 mg
Fluvastatin XL 80 mg
Fluvastatin 40 mg bid
Pitavastatin 2–4 mg

non-fatal MI between the captopril or valsartan group [30]. Since then, the guidelines allowed the use of ARBs for LV dysfunction after MI in case of intolerance of ACEI. However, these patients need to have blood pressure and renal function monitored closely.

Lipid lowering drugs

Statin therapy is known to decrease mortality in patients with stable angina, ACS or prior MI. RCTs with statin were conducted in order to clarify the benefits of statins on patients in the acute phase of STEMI. It is important to use the high intensity statin in patients with STEMI. The list of high-intensity and moderate-intensity statins is given in Table 5.8.

In a study using IVUS to check the plaque volume, in a patient with AMI when treated with high intensity statin, the volume of atheromatous plaque decreased by 20.9% (95% confidence interval [CI], 21.56-20.25; $P = 0.007$). Patients had regression in at least one non-IRA while there was no change of the number of necrotic core or the number of defined thin-cap fibroatheromas. The failure to reduce the size of the necrotic core and fibroatheroma characteristics may be related to the relatively short follow-up. As in other statin studies, there was an increase in calcium content, which may be a signal of healing and formation of more stable plaques [31].

COMPREHENSIVE MANAGEMENT

For patients with STEMI, comprehensive management requires early administration of antiplatelet agents, early beta-blockade, early medical

Table 5.9 Optimal dosage of medications in clinical randomized trials

Drug	First dose	Maximal dose	RCT
Carvedilol	3.125 mg PO BID	25 mg PO BID	CAPRICORN [32]
Atenolol	25 mg PO BID	200 mg PO QD	ISIS-1 [33]
Metoprolol tartrate	up to 15 mg IV	200 mg PO QD	COMMIT [34]
Valsartan	20 mg PO BID	160 mg PO BID	VALIANT [29]
Captopril	6.25 mg PO TID	50 mg PO TID	VALIANT
Lisinopril	2.5 mg PO QD	5–10 mg PO QD	Meta-analysis [37]
Ramipril	1.25 mg PO BID	5 mg PO BID	AIRE [35]
Trandolapril	1 mg PO QD	4 mg PO QD	TRACE [36]

or mechanical reperfusion, ACE inhibition (if there is LV dysfunction), early cardiac rehabilitation, smoking cessation counseling, and AMI prevention teaching to patients and family. In real life, besides the above measures, the comprehensive management of STEMI patients requires: (1) the prescription of the same dose of benefit proven drug as used in RCT; (2) instruction to the patient to understand the absolute or relative necessity of a particular drug or modality of treatment so that compliance is better. Special emphasis should be given to compliance with double antiplatelet therapy (DAPT) after stenting. The optimal dosages as used in RCT are listed in Table 5.9.

Indicators of excellence

In order to evaluate the completeness in the management of the patients with STEMI, a checklist for excellent performance indicators is shown in Table 5.10. All the benchmarks are set by the Center of Medicare and Medicaid Services.

PREFERENTIAL MANAGEMENT

PCI after thrombolytic therapy

Early transfer after TT to a PCI center and routine angioplasty is recommended according to the results of the STREAM Trial. The rationale is that PCI prevents ischemic events without excess bleeding [38]. If the patient shows persistent chest pain or ST segment elevation after TT, then the patient should be transferred urgently [39]. The list of high-risk patients by CV criteria is given in Table 5.2.

Table 5.10 Performance indicators of comprehensive care for STEMI patients

Indicator		Benchmark Average US Hospital (3rd Quarter of 2015)
ASA administration within 24 hours after arrival	94.45%	95.65%
ASA prescribed at discharge (if no contraindications)	95%	82.5%
Beta-blocker administration within 24 hours after arrival	90.86%	77.78%
Beta-blocker prescribed at discharge	94%	81.92%
ACEI or ARB prescribed at discharge in patients with EF <40%	83%	66.67%
Door to needle time (for TT) <30 minutes	36.41%	70%
Door to balloon time <90 minutes	64.33%	33.33%

Note: STEMI: ST segment elevation myocardial infarction; ACEI: Angiotensin converting enzyme inhibitors; ARB: Angiotensin receptor blockers; TT: thrombolytic therapy.

CLINICAL PEARLS

Who benefits the most or does not benefit from an expeditious PCI? The patients who need an expedited process for PCI are the ones with high risk (Table 5.2) and with a short interval from symptom onset to presentation. The priority ranking of benefits for expedited PCI between high- and low-risk patients are listed in Table 5.11.

Table 5.11 Priority ranking of benefits for preferential expedition of PCI between high- and low-risk patients

High-risk	>>>	Low-risk
High-risk with short presentation time	>>>	Low-risk
Low-risk with short presentation time	>>>	High-risk with long presentation time
High-risk with long presentation time	>>>	Low-risk with long presentation time

The physicians can make a difference in mortality of these patients by focusing and making an effort to shorten the door-to-balloon time. While the patients with low risk and long interval between symptom onset to presentation also need to have a short door to balloon time, they do not benefit from an expedited PCI because the window of myocardial salvage is passed or the MI is too small to benefit from rapidly invasive interventions [40]. To understand this is to rationalize the fairness in triage and to prioritize the patient who should receive PCI first, or be transferred first when two patients arrive at the same time, in the same ER, or are transferred at the same time from different hospitals (Table 5.11).

Thrombolytic therapy or PCI for STEMI patients who arrive to a non-PCI capable facility   Once brought to non-capable PCI centers, the patients who received in situ fibrinolysis had worse prognosis than patients transferred. In the fibrinolysis group, the 30-day mortality was 7.7 and it was 5.1% in the transfer groups ($P = 0.09$). However, patients in the transfer group whose time FMC-device was achieved within 140 min were associated with significantly lower mortality (2.0% for FMC-device <99 min, and 4.6% for FMC-device 99–140 min; P <0.01 and $P = 0.03$, respectively vs. fibrinolysis). Therefore transfer of patients with STEMI to a PCI-capable center seems recommended in patients with first medical contact (FMC)-device delay <140 min [41].

Diabetes mellitus   During STEMI, diabetic patients frequently present with atypical symptoms. Only 77% of these patients complain of chest pain compared with 84% in patients without diabetes. Diabetic patients also complain more of dyspnea, as they incur more acute LV dysfunction compared with non-diabetic patients (26% vs. 13.5%). The in-hospital mortality has been reported to be 8.7% vs. 5.8% for male diabetic and non-diabetic patients, respectively; the mortality of female diabetic patients was 24% compared with 13% in female non-diabetic patients [41]. In a prospective study comparing diabetic patients with non-diabetic patients, even when both groups were treated with the same medications (BB, ACEI, statins) and achieved the same rate of patency after TT, mortality of diabetic patients was still triple the rate of non-diabetics [42].

Renal dysfunction   Renal impairment is a strong independent indicator of increased mortality in patients who are admitted with STEMI. In patients with mild or moderate renal dysfunction and having primary interventions, the early or late outcome depends on the creatinine clearance (less than 75 mL/min) and not on the serum creatinine level. The patients with creatinine clearance <75 mL/min, have more hypotension in the catheterization laboratory (10% vs. 6.5%), intubation (1.3% vs. 0%), in-hospital mortality (5.1% vs. 0.8%), or 6 month-mortality 7.4% vs. 1.1%. However, the overall mortality in STEMI patients on long-term dialysis was much worse at 59% in 1 year, 73% in 2 years, and 89% in 5 years [43].

In a real-world registry analysis of 1064 consecutive STEMI patients, patients with CKD (eGFR <60 mL/min/1.73 m^2) were compared with patients without CKD (eGFR >60 mL/min/1.73 m^2) [43]. In CKD patients, TIMI-3 flow was restored less frequently (79% vs. 87%), in-hospital major adverse cardiac and cerebrovascular events were more frequent (15% vs. 4%) and 30-day mortality was higher than in non-CKD patients (9% vs. 2%). Additionally, lower eGFR was associated with increased risk of major bleeding (HR 1.6; P <0.0005) [44].

In the care of STEMI patients with CKD, clinicians need to be aware that CKD is an independent predictor of decreased procedural success and poorer short-term outcomes in STEMI patients treated with primary PCI or medical therapy alone.

PCI in non-IRA in STEMI patients   In the 2015 ACC/AHA/SCAI updated guidelines, PCI of a noninfarct artery may be considered in selected patients with STEMI and multivessel disease who are hemodynamically stable, either at the time of primary PCI or as a planned staged procedure as IIb indication. The merit of PCI in non-infarct coronary arteries with major stenoses (preventive PCI) was presented in the Randomized Trial of Preventive Angioplasty in Myocardial Infarction (PRAMI) and Complete versus Lesion-only PRimary PCI (CvLPRIT) studies [45]. The best rationale is to do the FFR guided PCI of non-IRA as evidenced in the Primary PCI in Patients With ST-elevation Myocardial Infarction and Multivessel Disease: Treatment of Culprit Lesion Only or Complete Revascularization (DANAMI-3 PRIMULTI) study [46].

EVIDENCE-BASED MEDICINE

The PRAMI Trial 465 patients with STEMI who underwent the infarct-artery PCI were randomly assigned to either preventive PCI or no preventive PCI. Subsequent PCI in the non-preventive group was recommended only for refractory angina with objective evidence of ischemia. The primary outcome was a composite of death from cardiac causes, non-fatal MI, or refractory angina. During a mean follow-up of 23 months, the primary outcome occurred in 21 patients assigned to preventive PCI and in 53 patients assigned to no preventive PCI (infarct-artery-only PCI), which translated into rates of nine events per 100 patients and 23 per 100, respectively (hazard ratio in the preventive-PCI group, 0.35; 95% confidence interval [CI], 0.21 to 0.58; P <0.001). Hazard ratios for the three components of the primary outcome were 0.34 (95% CI, 0.11 to 1.08) for death from cardiac causes, 0.32 (95% CI, 0.13 to 0.75) for non-fatal MI, and 0.35 (95% CI, 0.18 to 0.69) for refractory angina.

According to the PRAMI investigators, for patients with STEMI and multivessel CAD undergoing infarct-artery PCI, preventive PCI in the non-infarct coronary arteries with major stenoses significantly reduced the risk of adverse CV events, as compared with PCI limited to the infarct artery [45]. These results were re-enforced by the results of the CvLPRIT study [47].

EVIDENCE-BASED MEDICINE
Complete versus Lesion-only PRimary PCI Trial (CvLPRIT) The goal of the CvLPRIT trial was to evaluate PCI of the infarct-related artery compared with complete revascularization at the index admission among participants with STEMI. 296 patients were randomized for complete revascularization at the same time as the primary PCI procedure in 59%, and in a staged fashion (median 1.5 days) in 27%. The primary outcome of mortality, MI, HF, and ischemia-driven revascularization at 12 months occurred in 10.0% of the complete revascularization group vs. 21.2% of the culprit-only group (P = 0.009). All-cause mortality: 1.3% vs. 4.1% (P = 0.14), respectively. MI: 1.3% vs. 2.7% (P = 0.39), respectively. Heart failure: 2.7% vs. 6.2% (P = 0.14), respectively. Repeat revascularization: 4.7% vs. 8.2% (P = 0.2), respectively. Major bleeding: 2.2% vs. 4.3% (P = 0.31), respectively.

The CvLPRIT investigators suggested that that among patients with STEMI, complete revascularization appears to be beneficial by reducing major adverse cardiac events [47].

PCI in patients with STEMI, bleeding and thrombotic problems

Bleeding or intra-arterial thrombosis before, during or after PCI of STEMI could be a major (or possibly fatal) problem triggering a small to full scale crisis situation. Different problems and solutions with bleeding or thrombosis are discussed below [48].

STEMI in patients with bleeding   In general, the principle is if the bleeding can be stopped by a mechanical means (compressing or ligating the artery), then the patient could tolerate 4 hours of anticoagulant during PCI. The favorite anticoagulant is UFH because of its short half-life, and it can be reversed by protamine.

If the patient has gastric bleeding and is hemodynamically stable, a gastroenterologist can carry out a gastroscopy and stop the bleeding by stapling the culprit artery. After that, the patient may be treated with H2 antagonist or proton pump inhibitors and could tolerate short-term anticoagulant and oral dual antiplatelet therapy for stenting of the IRA. GP 2b3a inhibitors are to be avoided. If the patient has a fracture in the extremities and AMI at the same time, the orthopedic surgeons may put on splints and stabilize the extremities. Then the patient may undergo the diagnostic coronary angiogram and angiogram of the artery of the fractured limb to check for extravasation of contrast due to injury in the arterial system. If there is no arterial bleed in the extremities, then the patient can undergo plain balloon angioplasty of the IRA (POBA) without stenting under coverage with UFH and clopidogrel. After POBA, the patient only needs ASA, without UFH nor clopidogrel. At this present time, intracranial bleeding or bleeding from the esophageal varices are the real contraindications for PCI. It must be noted that in a bleeding patient, PCI is the preferred treatment and thrombolytic therapy should be avoided.

STEMI patients with very recent non-cardiac surgery   Less than 4 hours after removal of the right kidney because of cancer, a patient developed ST elevation in leads 2,3 AVF. Therefore, the patient was brought to the CCL, had balloon angioplasty of the RCA with a standard dose of heparin to achieve an ACT of 250–300. No stent was used and no heparin given after the procedure. Because of the short-term heparin use, not much bleeding in the surgical area was noted. If the patient has a clean and limited surgery, then the patient may undergo DES stenting, because there is no problem with long-term antiplatelet therapy with clopidogrel.

STEMI patients with concurrent stroke   Stroke during AMI can occur concomitantly or during the 24–48 hours after the catheterization/PCI procedure: global incidence is about 0.88%, 95% being ischemic stroke. If the stroke occurs just before AMI, it is of utmost importance to perform an emergent CT scan of the head to rule out intracranial hemorrhage before giving the patient any anticoagulant or taking the patient to the cardiac catheterization laboratory. If the patient has an ischemic stroke, then with the agreement from the neurologist on the case, the patient may be given thrombolytic therapy for new stroke and STEMI. Then the patient can undergo PCI and stenting if indicated (as by protocol after thrombolytic treatment). A careful judgment about the stent type to be used is probably advisable, as the bare metal stent is easier to manage in respect of the duration of antiplatelet regimen compared to DES after a stroke. The two concerns are: (1) The risk of hemorrhagic conversion of the ischemic stroke with anticoagulant therapy and (2) Risk of cerebral emboli from the protruding plaque in the aortic arch if they were the cause of emboli stroke in the first place. The patient needs to have strong indication for PCI and the family and patient need to understand the benefits and the risks. If the benefits outweigh the risks, then the patient should have PCI.

When a stroke occurs just after or in the subsequent 24–48 hours after a primary angioplasty for AMI, a correlation with the catheterization procedure itself is likely, as the catheterization procedure through the radial artery in particular, but also through the femoral artery, may dislodge plaque debris. In such cases, usually the cerebral event is small in size: systemic thrombolysis can be suggested if symptoms onset in less than 3 hours. Otherwise, a careful monitoring of the ischemic territory with repeated CT scans represents sensible management [48].

ACTION POINTS

1 **Selection of reperfusion modalities**   Based on worldwide scarcity of facilities, logistics, and resource affordability, especially in developing countries, the benchmark reperfusion strategy remains TT. However, in developed countries, given the availability of catheterization laboratories, interventional expertise, rapid restoration of patency by catheter-based reperfusion can result in excellent outcomes. This is certainly the case in institutions with large volume interventional laboratories and experienced operators [48].

2 **Advantages and disadvantages of thrombolytic therapy** Because of the universal access to TT, certain clinical issues must be underscored. More important than pursuing the ideal thrombolytic agent is the need to administer TT at the earliest possible juncture after the onset of symptoms heralding MI. It is important to use those agents that the practitioner knows best. The earliest administration of any agent is better than the delayed administration of the best agent.

3 Advantages and disadvantages of primary PCI Primary mechanical intervention is an emergency procedure that reduces mortality, reinfarction as primary objectives and prevention of recurrent ischemia and early discharge as secondary objectives. If experienced operators are available and if the interval between door and balloon is less than 90 minutes, it is suggested that the patients undergo primary intervention. Early subacute stent thrombosis still needs to be monitored, especially in patients with initial TIMI-0 to TIMI-1 flow. Adjunctive therapies, especially the ACEI, beta-blockers, and statins are needed to improve short- and long-term outcomes. In addition to the clinical indications, accessibility and costs are obviously relevant variables to be taken into account. The choice of any reperfusion strategy is therefore not only related to scientific rationale, but also depends on affordability of available resources.

4 Comprehensive management Recent efforts regarding the implementation of hospital and physician performance measures such as door-to-device times as well as compliance with guideline-directed medical therapies and preventing re-admission within 30 days, will hopefully translate into improved patient outcomes.

REFERENCES

1. O'Gara PT, Kushner, FG, Ascheim DD, et al. 2013 ACCF/AHA Guideline for the Management of ST-Elevation Myocardial Infarction: A Report of the American College of Cardiology Foundation/American Heart Association Task Force on Practice Guidelines. *J Am Coll Cardiol.* 2013 Jan 29;61(4):e78–140.

2. Hellermann JP, Goraya TY, Jacobsen SJ Incidence of heart failure after myocardial infarction: is it changing over time? *Am J Epidemiol.* 2003 Jun 15;157(12):1101–1107.

3. Lee K, Woodlief LH, Topol E, et al. An international randomized trial comparing four thrombolytic strategies for acute myocardial infarction. The GUSTO investigators. *N Engl J Med.* 1993 Sep 2;329(10):673–682.

4. Crimm A, Severance HW Jr, Coffey K, McKinnis R, Wagner GS, Califf RM. Prognostic significance of isolated sinus tachycardia during first three days of acute myocardial infarction. *Am J Med.* 1984 Jun;76(6):983–988.

5. Antman E, Wiviott S, Murphy S, et al. Early and Late Benefits of Prasugrel in Patients With Acute Coronary Syndromes Undergoing Percutaneous Coronary InterventionA TRITON–TIMI 38 (TRial to Assess Improvement in Therapeutic Outcomes by Optimizing Platelet InhibitioN with Prasugrel–Thrombolysis In Myocardial Infarction) Analysis *J Am Coll Cardiol.* 2008;51(21):2028–2033. doi:10.1016/j.jacc.2008.04.00.

6. ESC Clinical Practice Guidelines Management of Acute Myocardial Infarction in patients presenting with ST-segment elevation. *Eur Heart J.* 2012;33:2569–2619.

7. Stub D, Smith K, Bernard B, et al. A Randomised Controlled Trial of Oxygen Therapy in Acute STEMI: The Air Versus Oxygen in Myocardial Infarction (AVOID) Study. Presented at the AHA scientific meeting, November 2014, Chicago.

8. Adamski P, Ostrowska M, Sroka2 W, et al. Does morphine administration affect ticagrelor conversion to its active metabolite in patients with acute myocardial infarction? A sub-analysis of the randomized, double-blind, placebo-controlled IMPRESSION trial. *Folia Medica Copernicana.* 2015;3(3):100–106. doi:10.5603/FMC.2015.0003.

9. Cannon CP, McCabe CH, Gibson CM, et al. TNK-tissue plasminogen activator in acute myocardial infarction: results of the Thrombolysis in Myocardial Infarction (TIMI) 10A dose-ranging trial. *Circulation.* 1997;95:351–356.

10. Armstrong PWI, Gershlick AH, Goldstein P, et al. for STREAM Investigative Team. Fibrinolysis or primary PCI in ST-segment elevation myocardial infarction. *N Engl J Med.* 2013 Apr 11;368(15):1379–1387.

11. Patel MR, Dehmer GJ, Hirshfield JW, et al. ACCF/SCAI/STS/AATS/AHA/ASNC/HFSA/SCCT 2012 Appropriate Use Criteria for Coronary Revascularization Focused Update. *JACC.* 2012;59:857–881.

12. Hochman JS, Gervasio A, Lamas GA, Buller CE, et al. Coronary Intervention for Persistent Occlusion after Myocardial Infarction. *N Engl J Med.* 2006;355;2395–2407.

13. Stone G, Witzenbichler B, Guagliumi G, et al. on behalf of the HORIZONS-AMI Trial Investigators Heparin plus a glycoprotein IIb/IIIa inhibitor versus bivalirudin monotherapy and paclitaxel-eluting stents versus bare-metal stents in acute myocardial infarction (HORIZONS-AMI): final 3-year results from a multicentre, randomised controlled trial. *Lancet.* 2011;377:2193–2204.

14. Shahzad A, Kemp I, Mars C, et al. for the HEAT-PPCI trial investigators Unfractionated heparin versus bivalirudin in primary percutaneous coronary intervention (HEAT-PPCI): an open-label, single centre, randomised controlled trial. *Lancet.* 5 July 2014; DOI: 10.1016/S0140-6736(14)60924–60927.

15. Montalescot G1, Zeymer U, Silvain J, Boulanger B, et al. Intravenous enoxaparin or unfractionated heparin in primary percutaneous coronary intervention for ST-elevation myocardial infarction: the international randomised open-label ATOLL trial. *Lancet.* 2011 Aug 20;378(9792):693–703.

16. Mega JL, Braunwald E, Wiviott SD, et al. Rivaroxaban in patients with a recent acute coronary syndrome. *N Engl J Med.* 2012;366:9–19.

17. Levine GN, O'Gara PT, Bates ER, et al. 2015 ACC/AHA/SCAI focused update on primary percutaneous coronary intervention for patients with ST-elevation myocardial infarction: an update of the 2011 ACCF/AHA/SCAI guideline for percutaneous coronary intervention and the 2013 ACCF/AHA guideline for the management of ST-elevation myocardial infarction: a report of the American College of Cardiology Foundation/American Heart Association Task Force on Clinical Practice Guidelines and the Society for Cardiovascular Angiography and Interventions. *J Am Coll Cardiol.* 2015.

18. Lagerqvist B, Frobert O, Olivecrona GK, et al. Outcomes 1 year after thrombus aspiration for myocardial infarction. *N Engl J Med.* 2014;371:1111–1120.

19. Steg PG, James S, Harrington RA, et al. Ticagrelor versus clopidogrel in patients with ST-elevation acute coronary syndromes intended for reperfusion with primary percutaneous coronary intervention. A Platelet Inhibition and Patient Outcomes (PLATO) Trial Subgroup Analysis. *Circulation.* 2010;122:2131–2141.

20. Wiviott SD, Braunwald E, McCabe CH. Prasugrel versus clopidogrel in patients with acute coronary syndromes. *N Engl J Med.* 2007;357:2001–2015.

21. Montalescot G, van't Hof AW, Lapostolle F, et al. Prehospital ticagrelor in ST-segment elevation myocardial infarction. *N Engl J Med.* 2014;371:1016–1027.

22. www.cardiologyonline.net/articolo/pegasus-timi-54-sub-analysis-long-term-tolerability-for-ticagrelor-in-patients-with-myocardial-infarction.

23. Bhatt DL, Fox KAA, Hacke W, et al. Clopidogrel and aspirin versus aspirin alone for the prevention of atherothrombotic events. *N Engl J Med.* 2006;354:1706–1717.

24. Diener HC1, Bogousslavsky J, Brass LM, et al. Aspirin and clopidogrel compared with clopidogrel alone after recent ischaemic stroke or transient ischaemic attack in high-risk patients (MATCH): randomised, double-blind, placebo-controlled trial. *Lancet.* 2004 Jul 24–30;364(9431):331–337.

25. Mehta SR, Yusuf S, Peters RJG. Effects of pretreatment with clopidogrel and aspirin followed by long-term therapy in patients undergoing percutaneous coronary intervention: the PCI-CURE study. *Lancet.* 2001;358:527–533.

26. Hurlen M, Abdelnoor M, Smith P, et al. Warfarin, aspirin, or both after myocardial infarction. *N Engl J Med.* 2002; 347:969–974.

27. Dewilde WJ, Oirbans T, Verheugt FW, Kelder JC, et al. Use of clopidogrel with or without aspirin in patients taking oral anticoagulant therapy and undergoing percutaneous coronary intervention: an open-label, randomised, controlled trial. *Lancet.* 2013 Mar 30;381(9872):1107–1115.

28. Hjalmarson A1, Goldstein S, Fagerberg B, Wedel H. Effects of controlled-release metoprolol on total mortality, hospitalizations, and well-being in patients with heart failure: the Metoprolol CR/XL Randomized Intervention Trial in congestive heart failure (MERIT-HF). MERIT-HF Study Group. *JAMA.* 2000 Mar 8;283(10):1295–1302.

29. Velazquez EJ, Pfeffer MA, McMurray JV, Maggioni AP, et al. VALsartan In Acute myocardial iNfarcTion (VALIANT) trial: baseline characteristics in context. *Eur J Heart Fail.* 2003 Aug;5(4):537–544.

30. McMurray J1, Solomon S, Pieper K, Reed S. The effect of valsartan, captopril, or both on atherosclerotic events after acute myocardial infarction: an analysis of the Valsartan in Acute Myocardial Infarction Trial (VALIANT). *J Am Coll Cardiol.* 2006 Feb 21;47(4):726–733.

31. Räber L, Taniwaki M, Zaugg S, et al. on behalf of the IBIS-4 (Integrated Biomarkers and Imaging Study-4) Trial Investigators: Effect of high-intensity statin therapy on atherosclerosis in non-infarct-related coronary arteries (IBIS-4): A Serial Intravascular Ultrasonography Study. *Eur Heart J.* 2014 Sep 2. pii: ehu373.

32. Dargie HJ. Effect of carvedilol on outcome after myocardial infarction in patients with left-ventricular dysfunction: the CAPRICORN randomised trial. *Lancet.* 2001 May 5;357(9266):1385–1390.

33. First International Study of Infarct Survival Collaborative Group. Randomised trial of intravenous atenolol among 16,027 cases of suspected acute myocardial infarction: ISIS-1. *Lancet.* 1986 Jul 12;2(8498):57–66.

34. Chen ZM1, Pan HC, Chen YP, Peto R, et al. Early intravenous then oral metoprolol in 45,852 patients with acute myocardial infarction: randomised placebo-controlled trial. *Lancet.* 2005 Nov 5;366(9497):1622–16232.

35. Hall AS1, Winter C, Bogle SM, Mackintosh AF, Murray GD, Ball SG. The Acute Infarction Ramipril Efficacy (AIRE) Study: rationale, design, organization, and outcome definitions. *J Cardiovasc Pharmacol.* 1991;18 Suppl 2:S105–109.

36. Køber L, Torp-Pedersen C, Carlsen JE, et al. A clinical trial of the angiotensin-converting-enzyme inhibitor trandolapril in patients with left ventricular dysfunction after myocardial infarction. Trandolapril Cardiac Evaluation (TRACE) Study Group. *N Engl J Med.* 1995 Dec 21;333(25):1670–1676.

37. de Kam PJ1, Voors AA, van den Berg MP, van Veldhuisen DJ. Effect of very early angiotensin-converting enzyme inhibition on left ventricular dilation after myocardial infarction in patients receiving thrombolysis: results of a meta-analysis of 845 patients. FAMIS, CAPTIN and CATS Investigators. *J Am Coll Cardiol.* 2000 Dec;36(7):2047–2053.

38. Armstrong P, Gershlick A, Goldstein P and the STREAM investigators. Fibrinolysis or primary PCI in ST-segment elevation myocardial infarction. *N Engl J Med.* 2013;368:1379–1387.

39. Dasari TW, Roe MT, Chen AY, et al. Impact of time of presentation on process performance and outcomes in ST-segment–elevation myocardial infarction. A report from the American Heart Association: mission lifeline program. *Circ Cardiovasc Qual Outcomes.* 2014;7:656–663.

40. Brodie BR, Hansen C, Stuckey TD, Richter S, et al. Door to balloon time with primary percutaneous coronary intervention for acute myocardial infarction impacts late cardiac. *J Am Coll Cardiol.* 2006 Jan 17;47(2):289–295.

41. Carrillo X, Fernandez-Nofrerias E, Rodriguez-Leor O, et al. Early ST elevation myocardial infarction in non-capable percutaneous coronary intervention centres: in situ fibrinolysis vs percutaneous coronary intervention transfer. *Eur Heart J.* 2015 Nov 18;[EPub Ahead of Print].

42. Stone PH, Muller JE, Hartwell T, York BJ, et al. The effect of diabetes mellitus on prognosis and serial left ventricular function after acute myocardial infarction: contribution of both coronary disease and diastolic left ventricular dysfunction to the adverse prognosis. The MILIS Study Group. *J Am Coll Cardiol.* 1989 Jul;14(1):49–57.

43. Herzog CA, Ma JZ, Collins AJ. Poor long-term survival after acute myocardial infarction among patients on long-term dialysis. *N Engl J Med.* 1998;339:799–805.

44. Polanska-Skrzypczyk M, Karcz M, Bekta P, et al. Prognostic value of renal function in STEMI patients treated with primary PCI: ANIN Registry. *Br J Cardiol.* 2013;20:65 doi: 10.5837/bjc.2013.17.

45. Wald DS, Morris JK, Wald NJ, et al. for the PRAMI Investigators Randomized Trial of Preventive Angioplasty in Myocardial Infarction. *N Engl J Med*. 2013; 369:1115–1121.

46. Engstrøm T. The third DANish study of optimal Acute treatment of patients with ST-segment elevation Myocardial Infarction: PRImary PCI in MULTIvessel disease. Presented at: American College of Cardiology/i2 Scientific Session; March 16, 2015; San Diego, CA.

47. Kelly DJ, McCann GP, Blackman D, et al. Complete Versus culprit-Lesion only PRimary PCI Trial (CVLPRIT): a multicentre trial testing management strategies when multivessel disease is detected at the time of primary PCI: rationale and design. European Society of Cardiology Congress, Barcelona, Spain.

48. Nguyen J, Nguyen T. Percutaneous coronary intervention in patients with active bleeding or high bleeding risk – Review. *Anadolu Kardiyol Derg* 2012 Dec 17. doi:10.5152/akd.2013.042 (Epub ahead of print).

CHAPTER 6

Heart Failure (Stages A, B and C)

Dan Le, Trong Ha Le, Võ Minh Việt, Bao V. Ho, Tuan D. Nguyen, Khalid Numan Al Azza, Hau Van Tran and Gianluca Rigatelli

Management of Complex Cardiovascular Problems, Fourth Edition. Edited by Thach N. Nguyen, Dayi Hu, Shao Liang Chen, Moo Hyun Kim and Cindy L. Grines.
© 2016 John Wiley & Sons, Ltd. Published 2016 by John Wiley & Sons, Ltd.

STAGE A: ASYMPTOMATIC HEART FAILURE RISK FACTORS

BACKGROUND

Patients in stage A heart failure (HF) are defined as asymptomatic patients at high risk for developing HF, but without structural heart disease or symptoms of HF. This stage includes patients with hypertension (HTN), coronary artery disease (CAD), obesity, diabetes mellitus (DM), history of drug or alcohol abuse, history of rheumatic fever, family history of cardiomyopathy, or history of treatment with cardiotoxins. Patients with stage B are those with structural heart disease but without signs or symptoms of HF. They include patients with previous myocardial infarction (MI) or left ventricular (LV) remodeling (including left ventricular hypertrophy (LVH), dilation, low ejection fraction (EF), or valvular disease. According to the New York Heart Association (NYHA) classifications, these patients are of functional class I, without limitation to physical activity. These two groups of patients are different from the stage C HF group in which the latter had or are having symptoms of HF [1].

CHALLENGES

The **main challenge** is whether intensive treatment of patients of stage A and B prevents their progression into a subsequent higher stage (A to B or B to C). The progression from stage A to B is not a progression to HF. It is a progression from normal LV function (no disease) to structural abnormality (e.g. LV dysfunction) or structural heart disease (e.g. mitral or aortic regurgitation). The progression from stage A or B to C is the appearance of symptoms of HF. In general, for patients with HF stage B or C, the ventricular remodeling is potentially reversed if treated early (Table 6.1). The list of pathological conditions with questionable or negative potential for reversibility following medical treatment is shown in Table 6.2.

STRATEGIC MAPPING

According to guidelines for stage A HF patients, the main focus of management is prevention and treatment of risk factors. In stage B, the goal is the same: prevention of clinical deterioration (progression to stage C) and treatment of risk factors. All preventive and therapeutic modalities of treatment are applied; however, each stage requires a different level of intensive or preventive care. (Table 6.3)

Table 6.1 Conditions in which ventricular remodeling could be reversed

1. Viral cardiomyopathy
2. Post-partum cardiomyopathy
3. Atrial fibrillation induced cardiomyopathy
4. Aortic stenosis with LV hypertrophy
5. Mitral regurgitation with dilated left ventricle
6. ETOH induced dilated cardiomyopathy
7. Dilated left ventricle from metabolic syndrome
8. LV hypertrophy after long standing uncontrolled HTN
9. Stress-induced cardiomyopathy
10. Tachycardia mediated-cardiomyopathy
11. Nutritional deficiency: beriberi, selenium deficiency
12. Metabolic causes: hypocalcemia, hypophosphate
13. Endocrine disorders: hypo- and hyperthyroidism
14. Drugs such as anabolic steroids, chemotherapy

ETOH, alcohol; HTN, hypertension; LV, left ventricular.

Table 6.2 Clinical conditions in which medical treatment of causes may or may not prevent hypertrophy and dilation

Diabetic cardiomyopathy	Control of diabetes does not prevent dilation or reverse dilation of the left ventricle.
Aortic regurgitation	Medical treatment of aortic regurgitation does not prevent dilation or reverse dilation of the left ventricle.
Mitral regurgitation	Medical treatment of mitral regurgitation does not prevent dilation or reverse the dilation of the left atrium or ventricle.
Heart failure with preserved ejection fraction	No treatment prevents or reverses stiffness of the left ventricle causing heart failure with preserved ejection fraction.

Table 6.3 Main strategies for management of stage A and B heart failure

1. Lifestyle modification.
2. Prevent precipitating and aggravating factors.
3. Essential pharmacologic management with angiotensin converting enzyme inhibitors, angiotensin II receptor blockers and beta-blockers.
4. Complimentary treatment with diuretics or vasodilators.
5. Reverse structural abnormalities (remodeling with hypertrophy or dilation).
6. Device therapy including implantable cardioverter defibrillators, bi-ventricular pacing.

HIGH-RISK MARKERS

The risk factors that have been predictive of severe HF in longitudinal studies include uncontrolled HTN, uncontrolled DM, atrial fibrillation (AF) and obesity (body mass index >30 kg/m^2) [2–4]. Frail elderly patients can develop HF more frequently than non-frail persons [5].

HIGH-RISK PREDICTORS

The predictors of high risk for developing HF in patients who do not look clinically different from their average peers are the elderly, male patients compared with female patients of the same age, AF and patients with evidence of clinical atherosclerosis (peripheral arterial disease; PAD); abdominal aortic aneurysm (AAA); elevated level of B-type natriuretic peptide (BNP); and hemoglobin A1c (HbA1c) [3].

INVESTIGATIONS

Symptoms to look for

Patient has no symptom of fluid overload (shortness of breath) or of left HF (fatigue). Patient is asymptomatic for heart problems.

Signs to look for

There are no physical findings for HF, so the goal of the physical examination is to detect or identify clues of underlying disease.

SMART TESTING

The selection of a diagnostic test depends on the level of certainty of evidence regarding risks and benefits, how these risks and benefits compare with potential alternatives, and what the comparative cost or cost-effectiveness of the diagnostic test would be. An informed patient should ask his or her doctor this question: Could you tell me the purpose and the diagnostic accuracy of this test? For patients with stage A and B, an electrocardiogram (EKG) and an echocardiography may serve as a baseline for the rhythm, ST-T changes and LV function. Other tests to detect hypercholesterolemia, diabetes, hypo- or hyperthyroidism, should be done, if the problem is suspected.

MANAGEMENT

The cornerstone in management of stage A is to screen asymptomatic patients at high risk for ventricular remodeling and to treat any underlying clinical diseases while applying all generic preventive measures (lifestyle change, low sodium, low cholesterol diet, exercise, and education). HTN and lipid disorders should be controlled in accordance with contemporary guidelines. Other conditions such as obesity, DM, tobacco use, and use of known cardiotoxic agents, should be controlled or avoided. In high-risk patients (atherosclerosis, HTN, or DM) with associated cardiovascular (CV) risk factors, angiotensin converting enzyme inhibitor (ACEI) or angiotensin receptor blocker (ARB) is indicated [1]. The treatment plan should be discussed in detail with patients. A well-informed patient should ask about treatment options, and question the success and potential complications of the proposed treatment. The detailed questions are listed in Table 6.4.

Indicators of excellence

The pathologic targets for prevention of heart disease in patients at stage A HF are to prevent the occurrence of any atrial or ventricular hypertrophy or dilation, any systolic or diastolic dysfunction, any increase of pressure of the LV end diastolic pressure (LVEDP), or of the pulmonary artery mean pressure (PAM) or the pulmonary artery wedge pressure (PCWP). The ultimate goal is to prevent any remodeling of the LV or right ventricle (RV) which is the most important and clinically relevant end result of any cardiac injury.

Table 6.4 Questions to discuss with clinicians before treatment

1. What is the level of certainty of evidence regarding risks and benefits?
2. How do these risks and benefits compare with potential alternatives?
3. What are the treatment options available?
4. What are the rates of success or failure of these treatment options?
5. What kind of side-effects or complications are associated with these treatment options?
6. What would be the comparative cost or cost-effectiveness of the treatment?
7. What happens if this treatment approach does not work for me?
8. How will you help me balance my treatment with the demands of an active life?

STAGE B: ASYMPTOMATIC LEFT VENTRICULAR REMODELING

BACKGROUND

In stage B, the patient has structural heart abnormality while being asymptomatic. The clinical, ECG, and echocardiographic abnormalities of asymptomatic ventricular dysfunction shown to be predictive of future HF are prior myocardial infarction (MI), left ventricular hypertrophy (LVH), valvular heart disease, regional wall-motion abnormality, LV enlargement, and systolic and diastolic dysfunction [6, 7].

CHALLENGES

Does intensive treatment of stage B with BB and ACEI prevent progression from stage B to C? The answer is not easy because HF is not a single pathological condition. HF is a COMPLEX SYNDROME involving various etiologies of heart dysfunction (myocardium, genes, electric-mechanical and ventricular uncoupling) and leading to symptoms, disability, and death. HF is a systemic disorder with the kidneys retaining salt and water, the skeletal muscle deteriorating and deconditioning, with concomitant involvement of the lung and liver accompanied by cognitive dysfunction. So the prevention of stage B in the HF patient is not limited to the heart, but involves the prevention of disease in the renal, vascular, or skeletal system [8]. In general, the **main challenge** for management of asymptomatic stage B patients is how to prevent them from progressing into symptomatic stage C.

STRATEGIC MAPPING

The first strategy is to identify the high-risk patients and their clinical, non-invasive, or laboratory predictors. Once that is determined, management includes: (1) prevention of clinical worsening; (2) reduction of morbidity and mortality; and (3) reversal of ventricular remodeling (Tables 6.5–6.6).

HIGH-RISK MARKERS

In the first office visit, the asymptomatic patient with stage B HF is evaluated for causes, extent of LV dysfunction, risk of severe arrhythmias, sudden death and chance of relapse.

Table 6.5 Management strategies for asymptomatic heart failure stage B patients

1. Detect and treat the causes of atrial or ventricular remodeling.
2. Maintain asymptomatic status by diet, exercise, and medication.
3. Prevent and treat precipitating and exacerbating factors.
4. Prevent progression of heart failure at the cellular level.
5. Prevent sudden cardiac death with implantable cardiac defibrillators.
6. Reverse ventricular remodeling by diet, exercise, and medications.

Table 6.6 Initial evaluation of patients with stage B heart failure

1. Assess clinical severity of HF by history and physical examination.
2. Assess cardiac structure and function.
3. Determine the etiology of HF.
4. Evaluate for coronary disease and myocardial ischemia.
5. Evaluate the risk of life-threatening arrhythmia.
6. Identify any exacerbating factors for HF.
7. Identify comorbidities which could influence therapy.
8. Identify barriers to adherence and compliance.

HF, heart failure.

HIGH-RISK PREDICTORS

The predictors of high risk for developing symptomatic HF in patients who do not look different from their average peers are the elderly, male patients compared with female patients, those with evidence of atherosclerosis (PAD, AAA), uncontrolled HTN, uncontrolled DM, AF or elevated level of BNP, N-terminal pro-B-type natriuretic peptide (NT-proBNP), and cardiac troponin T (cTnT) [9].

MANAGEMENT

Lifestyle change and education
The first step in the treatment plan for asymptomatic stage B HF patients is lifestyle change including a low sodium, low cholesterol diet, fluid

Table 6.7 Instructions for patients with heart failure

1. Rationale and practical tips for compliance with a low sodium, low cholesterol diet.
2. Rationale and practical tips for compliance with fluid restriction.
3. Rationale and practical tips for compliance with medication, office visits, and blood testing.
4. Rationale and practical tips for a low calorie diet and losing weight.
5. Rationale and practical tips for regular exercise.
6. Keep a daily log of blood pressure and weight.
7. Explanation of signs and symptoms of HF and change due to worsening HF.

HF, heart failure.

restriction (<2000 cc/day), no smoking, and regular exercise. Because the patient is asymptomatic, the main focus is prevention and education of the patient about the disease, disease process, and worsening of symptoms and signs. The instructions for HF are listed in Table 6.7.

Pharmacologic therapy

Angiotensin converting enzyme inhibitor (ACEI) is the main treatment for patients with asymptomatic LV dilation or hypertrophy. The benefits of ACEI were evidenced by the Studies of Left Ventricular Dysfunction (SOLV) trial in which the ACEI enalapril significantly reduced the incidence of HF and the rate of related hospitalizations [10].

Caution should be exercised in prescribing ACEI in patients with marked renal dysfunction who are not dialysis-dependent. Most randomized trials on ACEI in HF excluded patients with significant renal dysfunction (serum creatinine >2.5 mg/dL) [11]. Even though a dearth of solid evidence does not represent a contraindication to the use of ACEI in advanced CKD, close monitoring of glomerular filtration rate (GFR), serum creatinine, and potassium levels is warranted [12].

Besides ACEI, beta-blocker (BB) is the second most important drug for HF. The evidence, which proved the benefits of BB on HF stage B is in the Carvedilol US Heart Failure trial which randomized a large group of patients with mild, moderate, and severe HF. The results showed that carvedilol reduces the risk of death as well as the risk of hospitalization for CV causes in patients with HF who are receiving treatment with digoxin, diuretics, and an ACEI [13].

Table 6.8 Dosage of medications in heart failure clinical trials

Medication	Starting dose	Target dose	Clinical trial
Captopril	6.25–12.5 mg TID	50 mg TID	SAVE [11]
Enalapril	2.5–5 mg BID	10–20 mg BID	SOLV [10]
Ramipril	2.5 mg BID	5 mg BID	AIRE [15]
Trandolapril	1 mg/day	4 mg/day	TRACE [16]
Carvedilol	3.125 mg BID 50 mg BID for >187 lb	25 mg BID	Carvedilol HF [13]
Metoprolol succinct	12.5–25 mg/day	200 mg/day	MERIT-HF [17]
Candesartan	4–8 mg/day	32 mg/day	RESOLVD [18]
Losartan	12.5 mg/day	50 mg/day	ELITE [19]
Valsartan	20 mg/day	160 mg BID	CHARM [20]

Subsequently, BB is recommended even if there is concomitant diabetes (DM), chronic obstructive lung disease (COPD), or peripheral vascular disease. However, BB should be used with caution in patients with asthma, resting limb ischemia, or diabetes with recurrent hypoglycemia. BBs are not recommended in patients with asthma when having active bronchospasm, marked bradycardia (<55 beats/min) or marked hypotension (systolic blood pressure <80 mmHg) [14].

As the benefits of BB or ACEI are supported by reduction of mortality and morbidity from randomized clinical trials (RCT), patients should be given the same dosage at which the benefits were proven (Table 6.8).

Diuretics should not be used in stage B unless the patient has sign of fluid retention. If fluid overload is to be prevented, a low sodium diet and fluid restriction are the first steps. Once there is sign of fluid overload, diuretics can be used intermittently or as needed. Digoxin is not indicated either, unless there are atrial arrhythmias with coexisting low LVEF. In a recent retrospective study in patients with new-onset atrial fibrillation, treating patients with digoxin was an independent predictor of increased mortality when compared to those not treated with digoxin [21].

Prevention and treatment of precipitating factors

With appropriate treatment, the stage B HF patient can be asymptomatic and function normally for a long period of time, especially the patients who did exercise well and regularly before the onset of cardiomyopathy. This asymptomatic condition can change quickly when any precipitating factor tips over the precarious clinical balance (Table 6.9). This is why

Table 6.9 Precipitating factors of heart failure

1. Non-compliance low Na diet (<2 g sodium a day).
2. Non-compliance to fluid restriction (<64 ounces a day).
3. Non-compliance to office visit and follow-up.
4. Infection.
5. Brady- or tachyarrhythmia.
6. Myocardial ischemia or infarction.
7. Physical or emotional stress.
8. Pulmonary embolism.
9. High-output states such as anemia, thyrotoxicosis, Paget's disease, pregnancy, Beriberi, and arteriovenous fistula.
10. Cardiac infection and inflammation (myocarditis, infective endocarditis).
11. Co-morbidities (renal, liver, thyroid, respiratory insufficiency).
12. Cardiac toxin (chemotherapy, cocaine, alcohol etc.)

prevention of any precipitating or aggravating factor is the second most important strategy in stage B HF. The list of medications to be avoided in patients with HF stage B are shown in Table 6.10.

Prevention of heart failure

Besides treating risk factors, the management of stage B HF patients is to prevent progression of HF. There are many questions focused on etiologies, strategies, etc. Does obesity in the childhood cause ventricular remodeling? Do physical exercise, treatment of HTN, DM, no smoking, exercise, or chronic resynchronization therapy (CRT) by bi-ventricular (BiV) pacing prevent development of HF? Could the progression into HF be predicted by levels of highly sensitive troponin T (cTnT) and NT-proBNP? Does ICD prevent sudden cardiac death (SCD)? Based on a similar background of asymptomatic LV dysfunction, the questions listed above were raised and their merits are discussed below.

Table 6.10 Drugs to avoid in patients with stage B heart failure

1. Non-steroidal anti-inflammatory drugs.
2. Most anti-arrhythmics except amiodarone, dofetilide.
3. Most calcium channel blockers (except felodipine and amlodipine).
4. Thiazolidinediones.

CRITICAL THINKING
Does obesity cause left ventricular hypertrophy?
Cardiovascular risk factors are associated with LVH, but little is known regarding the related impact of longitudinal measures of childhood adiposity and LV hemodynamic variables.

In this longitudinal study, 1061 adults, age 24 to 46 years, who had been examined four or more times for body mass index (BMI) and BP starting in childhood, with a mean follow-up of 28.0 years were studied. The area under the curve (AUC) was calculated as a measure of long-term burden (total AUC) and trends (incremental AUC) of BMI and BP from childhood to adulthood. Four LV geometric types were defined – normal, concentric remodeling (CR), eccentric hypertrophy (EH), and concentric hypertrophy (CH) – all on the basis of LV mass indexed for body height (m2.7) and relative wall thickness.

The results showed that higher values of BMI and systolic and diastolic BP in childhood and adulthood, as well as total AUC and incremental AUC, were all significantly associated with higher LV mass index and LVH, adjusted for race, sex, and age. In addition, higher values of BMI and BP in childhood and adulthood, total AUC, and incremental AUC were significantly associated with EH and CH but not with CR. Importantly, all of these measures of BMI had a consistently and significantly greater influence on EH than did measures of BP. These findings indicate that the adverse influence of excessive adiposity and elevated BP levels on LVH begins in childhood [22].

Is the goal of preventing heart failure achievable?

The question is whether measures are effective in preventing HF. The results of the Atherosclerosis Risk in Communities (ARIC) study are shown below [23].

EVIDENCE-BASED MEDICINE
The ARIC Study In the population-based ARIC cohort of 13,462 adults ages 45–64 years in 1987–1989, a Life's Simple 7 scoring system was created for smoking, body mass, physical activity, diet, cholesterol, blood pressure, and

glucose with 2 points for ideal, 1 point for intermediate, and 0 points for poor performance.

After 22 years, in 2011, the results showed that 25.5% participants developed HF through the age of 85 years. This lifetime HF risk was low at 14.4% for those with a middle-age Life's Simple 7 score of 10–14 (optimal), average at 26.8% for a score of 5–9 (average), and high at 48.6% for a score of 0–4 (inadequate). Among those with no clinical cardiovascular event, the prevalence of left ventricular hypertrophy in late life was approximately 40% as common, and diastolic dysfunction was approximately 60% as common, among those with an optimal middle-age score, compared with an inadequate score. Therefore, the positive achievement of the American Heart Association's Life's Simple 7 in middle age is associated with a lower lifetime occurrence of HF and greater preservation of cardiac structure and function (asymptomatic LVH and diastolic dysfunction) [23].

Also, according to the results of the Cardiovascular Health Study, moderate physical activity has protective effects on early HF phenotypes, preventing cardiac injury and neurohormonal activation [24]. Exercise training improves quality of life and exercise capacity, and reduces the risk of HF hospitalization [24]. This conclusion is also supported by the data of 14 small phase II randomized, controlled trials, as well as the landmark HF-ACTION (Heart Failure: A Controlled Trial Investigating Outcomes of Exercise Training) study [25, 26].

However, a lot of key questions remain: How do the benefits of exercise vary according to the stage of HF? How do frequency, intensity, and duration of exercise training influence outcomes? What is the minimum adherence rate necessary to achieve benefit? What is the mechanism of benefit? Can biomarkers be used as reliable surrogate markers of exercise efficacy or as measures of adherence [27]?

The positive effects of a combination of lifestyle factors on incident HF were also evidenced in the WHI (Women's Health Initiative) observational study. The concept that exercise prevents HF was reinforced and proved that an increasingly healthy lifestyle was associated with decreasing HF risk among post-menopausal women, even in the absence of antecedent CAD, HTN, and diabetes [28].

Prevention of heart failure and sudden death

Dilated cardiomyopathy can cause severe or possibly fatal arrhythmias causing sudden cardiac death (SCD). Does ICD or ICD-BiV prevent SCD and recurrence of HF in mild HF patients? The results are shown in the Multicenter Automatic Defibrillator Implantation Trial with Cardiac Resynchronization Therapy (MADIT-CRT) trial.

EVIDENCE-BASED MEDICINE

The MADITT II Trial at 7 years The MADIT-CRT showed that early intervention with CRT therapy with a defibrillator (CRT-D) in patients with an EKG pattern showing LBBB was associated with a significant reduction in HF events over a median follow-up of 2.4 years, as compared with ICD therapy alone. Post-trial follow-up over a median period of 5.6 years was assessed among all 1691 surviving patients (phase 1) and subsequently among 854 patients who were enrolled in post-trial registries (phase 2). The results showed that at 7 years of follow-up after initial enrollment, the cumulative rate of death from any cause among patients with LBBB was 18% among patients randomly assigned to CRT-D, as compared with 29% among those randomly assigned to ICD (adjusted hazard ratio in the CRT-D group, 0.59; 95% confidence interval [CI], 0.43 to 0.80; P <0.001). The long-term survival benefit of CRT-D in patients with LBBB did not differ significantly according to sex, cause of cardiomyopathy, or QRS duration. In contrast, CRT-D was not associated with any clinical benefit and could possibly cause harm in patients without LBBB (adjusted hazard ratio for death from any cause, 1.57; 95% CI, 1.03 to 2.39; P = 0.04; P <0.001 for interaction of treatment with QRS morphologic findings).

Therefore, for patients with mild HF symptoms, LV dysfunction, and LBBB, early intervention with CRT-D was associated with a significant long-term survival benefit [29].

Indicators of excellence

The pathologic targets for prevention of heart disease in patients at stage B HF are to prevent any worsening of atrial or ventricular hypertrophy or dilation, systolic or diastolic dysfunction, increased LVEDP, PAM or PCWP. The ultimate goal is to prevent any symptoms or progression to stage C HF. It seems that this goal is achievable by practicing the seven suggestions of the AHA (no smoking, ideal body mass, moderate physical activity, low sodium diet, control cholesterol level, optimal blood pressure, and control glucose level) in addition to ACEI and CRT, when indicated [23].

STAGE C: HEART FAILURE

BACKGROUND

Stage C heart failure (HF) is defined as the presence of structural heart disease with prior or current symptoms of HF [29].

CHALLENGES

Despite the availability of imaging and biomarkers, the history and physical examination remain the key components and first steps in the diagnosis of asymptomatic, symptomatic compensated stage C HF. The **first challenge** is how to make the diagnosis of HF in patients with or even without multiple active co-morbidities (e.g., severe COPD or fluid overload from chronic renal failure, or in the very obese patients). Once the diagnosis is made, the **second challenge** is to maintain the stable status of chronic systolic dysfunction (stage C) and to prevent its deterioration into acute decompensated heart failure (ADHF). The **third challenge** is that current therapies are only modestly effective in returning patients to their previous baseline despite providing acute improvement in the signs and symptoms of ADHF.

STRATEGIC MAPPING

In the management of patients with stage C HF, the **first step** is to confirm the diagnosis, the fluid status, and the extent of right and left HF. The **second step** is to identify the high risk patients by matching their risk profile based on published literature (profiling) and then to search for their high-risk predicting factors. Because of acute changes or frequent relapses, advanced testing including cardiopulmonary stress testing and invasive hemodynamic measurement and monitoring should be performed. Once the diagnosis of HF is confirmed, the **third step** is to give generic guideline directed medical therapy (GDMT). The goals of the treatment plan at this stage consist of (1) improving symptoms; (2) managing destabilizing factors; (3) reducing hospital readmission; and (4) reducing mortality.

HIGH-RISK MARKERS

According to the current literature, the markers which identify the high risk for developing severe HF include advanced age, diabetes mellitus, overweight, very low body weight (low muscle mass), AF or chronic kidney disease (CKD).

HIGH-RISK PREDICTORS

These are advanced age, re-admission more than twice during the last 1 year, anemia, CKD, AF, pulmonary hypertension, hyponatremia [30].

INVESTIGATIONS

Symptoms to look for

In the history interview of a patient with stable stage C HF, the usual question is about shortness of breath (SOB). The presence of SOB is proof of fluid overload in the lungs. Further questioning will focus on the symptoms due to fluid overload in the liver, stomach, abdominal wall, and leg. The questions involving symptoms from left HF causing low cardiac output are about fatigue, confusion, or lack of energy. Other questions are focused on a low sodium diet, fluid restriction, and chest pain to rule out CAD or pulmonary HTN.

CLINICAL PEARLS
How to know whether patients adhere to a low sodium diet and fluid restriction The question to check whether the patient has asymptomatic fluid overload is nocturia. Normally, a middle-aged person needs to wake up once at night to go to the bathroom to urinate (none at a younger age). If a patient needs to wake up more than once to urinate, then the fluid intake for that day is more than enough.

In order to check whether the patient maintains a low sodium diet at home, then the question is: When you go out for dinner at a restaurant, do the foods taste too salty? If the answer is yes, then the patient does maintain a low sodium diet at home. If the answer is no, then the patient may not be adhering to a strict low sodium diet at home. The reason is that restaurants may frequently use extra salt to make the food taste better.

Signs to look for

In the physical examination of a patient with stable stage C HF, the focus is on detecting fluid overload. Usually inspection of the legs shows ankle edema, then auscultation of the lungs may reveal rales in the two bases and at the end, and inspection of the neck should be carried out to ascertain the level of jugular venous distension. However, fluid accumulation does not start from the legs.

 CLINICAL PEARLS
Where to check the fluid in patients with compensated HF The first place where the HF patient begins to accumulate fluid is in the abdominal wall. This layer of tissue in the abdominal wall is hard when squeezed. The patient could sense that the abdomen feels heavier or bigger. Once the abdomen accumulates more than 5 liters of fluid, then edema begins to show at the ankle. The fluid in the abdominal wall, in the abdominal cavity, or in the legs is in the extravascular compartment. Next it is important to check the fluid in the liver, spleen, right ventricle (JVD), and lungs. This fluid is in the intravascular compartment.

This distinction between intra- versus extravascular fluid overload is very important because this information will help to predict the progress of treatment and length of hospitalization. The best example of patient with extravascular compartment fluid overload is the patient with endstage renal disease on hemodialysis (HD) and normal cardiac function. If the patient misses one day of HD, the patient will come to the hospital with extravascular fluid overload (no hepatomegaly, no JVD, no rales in lungs). As soon as the patient has HD, the patient improves right away. This is patient has extravascular fluid overload and no HF.

In contrast, for patients with intravascular fluid overload (hepatomegaly, JVD, rales in lungs) with or without extravascular compartment fluid overload, the treatment takes longer and the prognosis is poorer.

SMART TESTING

All patients would have had a basic work-up including an electrocardiogram (EKG), echocardiography, and a stress test during stage A or B HF. Now these patients become symptomatic and their diseases progresses into stage C. This is the time they need advanced testing, if clinically indicated. The selection of these advanced diagnostic tests depends on the level of certainty of evidence regarding risks and benefits, how these risks and benefits compare with potential alternatives, and what the comparative cost or cost-effectiveness of the diagnostic test would be.

Cardiopulmonary stress testing Cardiopulmonary stress (CPX) testing has been shown to have significant predictive value in HF. Peak VO_2 <14 mL/kg/min (<12 mL/kg/min on beta-blocker) has traditionally defined patients at high risk of adverse events and poor prognosis [30], however, other markers have been shown to have predictive power including VE/VCO_2 slope >34 [31] and in obese patients lean peak VO_2 <19 mL/kg/min [32]. Declining CPX parameters are an early marker of disease progression and should prompt referral for evaluation for advanced options in appropriate patients.

Invasive hemodynamic measurements Routine use of pulmonary artery catheterization in normotensive patients with adequate response to diuresis is not recommended. However when clinical assessment is insufficient to determine intracardiac filling pressures, invasive hemodynamic measurements should be performed (ACC/AHA Class 1C) [1]. In patients with recurrent hospitalizations, intolerant to guideline directed medical therapy (GDMT) or significant functional decline, invasive hemodynamic measurements can provide necessary information to guide future therapy. Significantly reduced cardiac output with elevated filling pressures may prompt use of IV inotropes and begin the evaluation for advanced options. In patients being considered for mechanical circulatory support or cardiac transplantation, complete right heart catheterization should be performed including assessment of pulmonary vascular resistance.

MANAGEMENT

The treatment of HF implies the use of guideline directed medical therapy (GDMT) which is listed in Table 6.11. The patient should have a long and comprehensive discussion with the clinician about the treatment plan.

Angiotensin converting enzyme inhibitor

ACEI should be given as early as possible at the first office visit or during the index hospitalization. In the absence of significant renal dysfunction, ACEI should be initiated at low doses with gradual titration to achieve

Table 6.11 Guideline directed medical therapy for heart failure [1]

HF therapy	Recommendation class/Level of evidence
Angiotensin converting enzymes inhibitors	All patients with a reduced EF to prevent HF (Class I, LOE A).
Beta-blockers	Patients with a history of MI and reduced EF (class I, LOE B).
	All patients with a reduced EF to prevent HF (class I, LOE C).
Mineralocorticoid receptor antagonists	Patients with NYHA class II–IV and who have LVEF <35% (Class I, LOE A).
	Post-MI patients who have LVEF ≤40% who develop symptoms of HF or who have a history of diabetes mellitus (Class I, LOE B).
Diuretics	Patients with fluid retention (Class I, LOE C).
Hydralazine/dinitrate isosorbide	African Americans with NYHA class III–IV HFrEF already optimal therapy with ACE-I and BB (Class I, LOE A).
	Patients with current or prior symptomatic HFrEF in whom an ACE-I or ARB cannot be used owing to drug intolerance, hypotension, or renal insufficiency (Class IIa, LOE B).
Angiotensin receptor blockers	Patients with HFrEF with current or prior symptoms who are ACE-I intolerant (Class I, LOE A)
Digoxin	Patients with HFrEF (Class IIa, LOE B).

Adapted from ACC/AHA HF guidelines [1]. ACEI = angiotensin converting enzyme inhibitor; ARB = angiotensin receptor blocker; BB = beta-blockers; EF = ejection fraction; HF = Heart failure; HFpEF = Heart failure with preserved ejection fraction; LVEF = left ventricular ejection fraction; LOE = level of evidence; MI = myocardial infarction; NYHA = New York Heart Association.

doses equivalent to those in RCTs. If hypotension is present, holding beta-blockers (BB) and ACEI/ARB may be beneficial to allow for adequate diuresis and ensure target organ perfusion. Current data support a class effect with ACEI; however, preference should be given to a long-acting ACEI to increase compliance and ensure consistent neurohormonal blockade. Some cautions should be used when considering initiation of ACEI in patients with hyponatremia, as there are concerns for hypotension.

For patients that are unable to tolerate an ACEI (due to cough, hypotension, and renal dysfunction) ARBs have been shown to be well-tolerated and to reduce CV risk as indicated in the results of the pooled data from the Candesartan in Heart Failure: Assessment of Reduction in Mortality and Morbidity (CHARM)-Added and CHARM-Alternative trials, see below [33].

EVIDENCE-BASED MEDICINE
CHARM Low-Left Ventricular Ejection Fraction
Trials Pooled data from the CHARM-Added and CHARM-Alternative randomized placebo controlled trials in patients with New York Heart Association (NYHA) functional class (FC) II–IV HF and reduced EF ($\leq$40%) was analyzed for the composite outcome of CV death and HF hospitalization, with all-cause mortality as the secondary endpoint. The primary endpoint occurred in 36% of the candesartan group and 41% of the placebo group (HR: 0.82, $P < 0.001$); all-cause mortality was also significantly reduced with candesartan (HR: 0.88, $P = 0.018$). Overall, candesartan reduced all-cause mortality, HF admissions, and CV death in patients with reduced EF when added to GDMT or when used in place of ACEI [34].

New standard of care: Neprilysin inhibition and ARB

Neprilysin, a neutral endopeptidase, degrades several endogenous vasoactive peptides, including natriuretic peptides, bradykinin, and adrenomedullin. Inhibition of neprilysin increases the levels of these substances, countering the neurohormonal overactivation that contributes to vasoconstriction, sodium retention, and maladaptive remodeling. In the past, the combined inhibition of ACEI and neprilysin was associated with serious angioedema. In the Prospective comparison of ARNI with ACEI to Determine Impact on. Global Mortality and morbidity in Heart Failure (PARADIGM-HF) trial, LCZ696, which consists of the neprilysin inhibitor sacubitril (AHU377) and the ARB valsartan, was designed to minimize the risk of serious angioedema [35].

EVIDENCE-BASED MEDICINE
The PARADIGM-HF Trial 8442 patients with NYHA FC II, III, or IV HF and an EF of 40% or less were randomly assigned to receive either LCZ696 (at a dose of 200 mg twice daily) or enalapril (at a dose of 10 mg twice daily), in addition to recommended therapy. The results showed that 17%

patients receiving LCZ696 and 19.8% patients receiving enalapril died (hazard ratio for death from any cause, 0.84; 95% CI, 0.76 to 0.93; $P < 0.001$); of these patients, 13.3% and 16.5%, respectively, died from CV causes (hazard ratio, 0.80; 95% CI, 0.71 to 0.89; $P < 0.001$).

As compared with enalapril, LCZ696 also reduced the risk of hospitalization for HF by 21% ($P < 0.001$) and decreased the symptoms and physical limitations of HF ($P = 0.001$). The LCZ696 group had higher proportions of patients with hypotension and non-serious angioedema but lower proportions with renal impairment, hyperkalemia, and cough than the enalapril group. The conclusion is that LCZ696 was superior to enalapril in reducing the risks of death and of hospitalization for HF and became the new standard of care in future guidelines [35].

Beta-blockers

Beta-blockers have been shown to reduce morbidity and mortality in all patients with HF, including those already on ACEI [25]. Unlike ACEI, there is no evidence of a class effect with BB. Only carvedilol [36], sustained-release metoprolol (succinate) [37], and bisoprolol [38] have been shown to have favorable effects on survival and disease progression by RCTs. One study, the *Carvedilol Or Metoprolol European (COMET) trial* showed superiority of carvedilol when compared to short acting metoprolol tartrate [39]. A meta-analysis of 15 placebo controlled trials (nine using carvedilol and six using metoprolol of which four used the short-acting form and two used an extended-release drug), suggested that carvedilol may produce a greater improvement in LVEF [40].

As with ACEI, doses should start low and be titrated to achieve doses similar to those in RCTs. BB can be started early, in the absence of contraindications such as hypotension or symptomatic bradycardia. Caution should be used when starting BB in patients that have required inotropic therapy during their index hospitalization and in newly diagnosed HF.

Aldosterone antagonists

For patients with NYHA Class II–IV HF symptoms already on GDMT (BB, ACEI, diuretics), the addition of mineralocorticoid receptor antagonists (MRA) have been shown to improve survival and reduce HF related hospitalizations. The ACC/AHA guidelines recommend MRA therapy (spironolactone, eplerenone) in patients with EF ≤35% in the absence of contraindications [1]. Aldosterone blockade should also be considered in symptomatic patients with LVEF ≤ 40% if fibrosis should be prevented, after recent myocardial infarction (MI) according to the results of the Eplerenone in Mild Patients Hospitalization and Survival Study in HF (EMPHASIS-HF) trial [41].

CLINICAL PEARLS
How to give an aldosterone antagonist When adding an aldosterone antagonist, selection of a starting dose should be based on the glomerular filtration rate (GFR); if the GFR is >50 mL/min/1.73 m [2] spironolactone can be started at 12.5 mg–25 mg daily, and for eplerenone 25 mg daily should be used. When the GFR is <30 mL/min/m [2] doses should be 12.5 mg every other day and 25 mg every other day, respectively. Supplemental potassium should be discontinued and close monitoring of renal function and serum potassium level at 3 days, 1 week, and then monthly for at least the first 3 months, should be done. Extra caution should be used in the elderly with relatively low muscle mass [1]. Spironolactone (non-selective aldosterone antagonist) carries the risk of painful gynecomastia in male patients, which may require switching to the more expensive agent eplerenone (selective antagonist) [1].

Vasodilators (hydralazine and nitrates)

These should be considered in patients intolerant to ACEIs or ARBs due to renal function or hyperkalemia or in patients with persistent symptoms in spite of treatment with renin angiotensin aldosterone antagonists and BB, particularly in African Americans.

The addition of hydralazine-isosorbide dinitrate to African Americans with NYHA FC II-IV HF already on optimal medical therapy is recommended to reduce morbidity and mortality [1,42]. It is also a Class IIa recommendation for African Americans with Stage C HF who are intolerant of ACEI/ARB therapy. Hydralazine and isosorbide-dinitrate should be initiated at low doses (37.5/20 mg, one tablet three times daily) and titrated to a goal of two tablets three times daily as tolerated. The high incidence of side-effects (headache, gastrointestinal disturbance, and dizziness) has limited adherence to this drug.

Digoxin for atrial fibrillation

In patients with mild to moderate HF, digoxin has been shown to improve symptoms, exercise tolerance, and reduce rates of hospitalization, but had no effect on mortality. In patients with severe systolic HF with persistence of symptoms despite maximal therapy with ACEIs, BB, and diuretics, digoxin has been shown to reduce symptoms and decrease hospitalizations. Digoxin is best used for heart rate control in the setting of atrial fibrillation combined with HF [1]. A recent study showed that digoxin could be detrimental to patients with AF.

Long-acting nitrates

Long-acting nitrates are commonly prescribed to enhance activity tolerance in patients with HFpEF. However, in a multicenter, double-blind, crossover study, 110 patients with HFpEF were randomly assigned to a regimen of isosorbide mononitrate (from 30 mg to 60 mg to 120 mg once daily) or placebo. The results showed that in the group receiving the 120-mg dose of isosorbide mononitrate, as compared with the placebo group, there was a non-significant trend toward lower daily activity (-381 accelerometer units; 95% confidence interval [CI], -780 to 17; $P = 0.06$) and a significant decrease in hours of activity per day (-0.30 hours; 95% CI, -0.55 to -0.05; $P = 0.02$). During all dose regimens, activity in the isosorbide mononitrate group was lower than that in the placebo group (-439 accelerometer units; 95% CI, -792 to -86; $P = 0.02$). Activity levels decreased progressively and significantly with increased doses of isosorbide mononitrate (but not placebo). There were no significant between-group differences in the 6-minute walk distance, quality-of-life scores, or NT-proBNP levels. Therefore, patients with HFpEF who received isosorbide mononitrate were less active and did not have better quality of life or submaximal exercise capacity than did patients who received the placebo. With these results, the addition of long-acting nitrates may not be beneficial for patients with HFpEF [43].

Device therapy

Approximately one-third of those with HF will develop a prolonged QRS (>120 ms), typically with a LBBB pattern and subsequent ventricular dyssynchrony. The ventricular dys-synchrony places the already taxed ventricle at a mechanical disadvantage by increasing LV end diastolic dimension (LVEDD), delaying opening and closure of the aortic valve, delaying opening of the mitral valve, and may worsen functional mitral regurgitation. Cardiac resynchronization therapy (CRT) was developed to correct this hemodynamic disadvantage through biventricular pacing and simultaneous activation of both ventricles. The Comparison of Medical Therapy, Pacing, and Defibrillation in Heart Failure (COMPANION) and Cardiac Resynchronization in Heart Failure (CARE-HF) trials demonstrated the

CRT survival benefit, reduction in mitral regurgitation, increased EF, and improved symptoms in patients with NYHA FC III-IV HF [44, 45].

Recently, the Resynchronization Defibrillation for Ambulatory Heart Failure (RAFT) trial showed both a morbidity and mortality benefit from CRT-D in patients with NYHA FC II-III symptoms when compared to an implantable cardiac defibrillator (ICD) alone [46].

EVIDENCE-BASED MEDICINE

The RAFT Trial The RAFT trial randomized 1798 patients with NYHA FC II-III HF, EF ≤30% and QRS duration ≥120 ms or paced QRS ≥200 ms to either ICD alone or CRT-D. The primary outcome of the study was death from any cause or HF hospitalization. CRT-D therapy resulted in a significant reduction in mortality of 29% vs. 35% in ICD-alone (HR: 75, $P = 0.003$), and HF hospitalizations of 19.5% versus 26% (HR: 68, $P < 0.001$). However, CRT-D was associated with significantly higher adverse events compared with ICD alone (118 vs. 61, respectively, $P < 0.001$) [46].

These trials confirmed the benefits of CRT for patients with LVEF <35%, sinus rhythm, and LBBB with QRS > 150 ms and NYHA Class III and IV symptoms [1].

Revascularization for heart failure patients

One of the most common causes of LV dysfunction is CAD. It could be manifested as localized wall motion abnormalities on echocardiography. Patients with LV dysfunction have higher mortality during coronary artery bypass surgery (CABG), therefore, there is a need to assess myocardial viability (stunned or hibernated myocardium) in order to select the patients who would survive and benefit from CABG.

Iron for anemia

What are the benefits and safety of long-term intravenous (i.v.) iron therapy in iron-deficient patients with HF? In the CONFIRM-HF trial, 304 ambulatory symptomatic HF patients with LVEF ≤45%, elevated BNP, and iron deficiency (ferritin <100 ng/ml or 100–300 ng/mL if transferrin saturation <20%) were given i.v. iron, as ferric carboxymaltose (FCM, $n = 152$) or placebo (saline, $n = 152$) for 52 weeks. There was no difference in mortality; however, there was an improvement in the 6-minute walk test

(6MWT) (baseline to week 24) and the rate of hospitalization for worsening HF [47].

ACTION POINTS

1 For the stage A HF patient: The main message is to change lifestyle and undergo treatment of risk factors in order to prevent ventricular remodeling.

2 For the asymptomatic stage B and C HF patient: The main treatments of stage B asymptomatic HF patients with abnormal structural changes place emphasis primarily on prevention with healthy lifestyle change (low salt, low cholesterol diet, fluid restriction, exercise, control of HTN and DM, medications such as BB and ACEI).

3 The new medication neprilysin inhibition with ARB should be given to the stage C patient.

4 Revascularization is indicated if there is large area of reversible ischemia.

5 Avoidance of all precipitating or aggravating factors is very important to prevent any clinical deterioration. BNP can help to identify the sicker patients and monitor their optimal response to treatment. ICD implantation is indicated if the EF is still <30% after a few months of GDMT (including BB and ACEI).

6 CRT may help to prevent HF.

7 Medications or the seven measures to prevent HF or reverse the structural abnormality (LVH or dilation) are to be pursued aggressively.

REFERENCES

1. Hunt SA, Abraham WT, Chin MH, et al. 2009 focused update incorporated into the ACC/AHA 2005 Guidelines for the Diagnosis and Management of Heart Failure in Adults: a report of the American College of Cardiology Foundation/American Heart Association Task Force on Practice Guidelines: developed in collaboration with the International Society for Heart and Lung Transplantation. *Circulation.* 2009;119:e391.

2. Mehta PA, Cowie MR. Gender and heart failure: A population perspective. *Heart.* 2006;92(Suppl 3):iii14–iii18.

3. Matsushita K, Blecker S, Pazin-Filho A, et al. The association of hemoglobin a1c with incident heart failure among people without diabetes: the atherosclerosis risk in communities study. *Diabetes.* 2010 Aug;59(8):2020.

4. Newman AB, Gottdiener JS, McBurnie MA, et al. Associations of subclinical cardiovascular disease with frailty. *J Gerontol A Biol Sci Med Sci.* 2001;56(3): M158–M166.

5. Mathew ST, Gottdiener JS, Kitzman D, et al. Congestive heart failure in the elderly: the Cardiovascular Health Study. *Am J Geriatr Cardiol.* 2004 Mar–Apr; 13(2):61–68.

6. Kenchaiah S, Narula J, Vasan RS. Risk factors for heart failure. *Med Clin North Am.* 2004;88:1145–1172.

7. Gardin JM, Siscovick D, Anton-Culver H, et al. Sex, age, and disease affect echocardiographic left ventricular mass and systolic function in the free-living elderly: the Cardiovascular Health Study. *Circulation.* 1995;91:1739–1748.

8. Piepoli M, Coats AJS. Chronic heart failure: a multisystem syndrome. *Eur Heart J.* 1996;17:1777–1778.

9. Fried LP, Borhani NO, Enright P, Furberg CD, Gardin JM, Kronmal RA, Kuller LH, Manolio TA, Mittelmark MB, Newman A, et al. The Cardiovascular Health Study: design and rationale. *Ann Epidemiol.* 1991 Feb;1(3):263–267.

10. The SOLVD Investigators. Effect of enalapril on mortality and the development of heart failure in asymptomatic patients with reduced left ventricular ejection fractions. *N Engl J Med.* 1992;3:327.

11. Pfeffer MA, Braunwald E, Moyé LA, et al. Effect of captopril on mortality and morbidity in patients with left ventricular dysfunction after myocardial infarction. Results of the survival and ventricular enlargement trial. *The SAVE Investigators. N Engl J Med.* 1992;327:669.

12. Ezekowitz J, McAlister FA, Humphries KH, et al. The association among renal insufficiency, pharmacotherapy, and outcomes in 6,427 patients with heart failure and coronary artery disease. *J Am Coll Cardiol.* 2004;44:1587.

13. Packer M, Bristow MR, Cohn JN, et al. The effect of carvedilol on morbidity and mortality in patients with chronic heart failure. U.S. Carvedilol Heart Failure Study Group. *N Engl J Med.* 1996;334:1349–1355.

14. Hjalmarson A, Goldstein S, Fagerberg B, et al. Effects of controlled-release metoprolol on total mortality, hospitalizations, and well-being in patients with heart failure: The Metoprolol CR/XL Randomized Intervention Trial in congestive heart failure (MERIT-HF). MERIT-HF Study Group. *JAMA.* 2000;283(10):1295–1302.

15. Effect of ramipril on mortality and morbidity of survivors of acute myocardial infarction with clinical evidence of heart failure. The Acute Infarction Ramipril Efficacy (AIRE) Study Investigators. *Lancet.* 1993 Oct 2;342(8875):821–828.

16. Køber L, Torp-Pedersen C, Carlsen JE, Bagger H, Eliasen P, Lyngborg K, Videbaek J, Cole DS, Auclert L, Pauly NC. A clinical trial of the angiotensin-converting-enzyme inhibitor trandolapril in patients with left ventricular dysfunction after myocardial infarction. Trandolapril Cardiac Evaluation (TRACE) Study Group. *N Engl J Med.* 1995 Dec 21;333(25):1670–1676.

17. Effect of metoprolol CR/XL in chronic heart failure: Metoprolol CR/XL Randomised Intervention Trial in Congestive Heart Failure (MERIT-HF). *Lancet.* 1999 Jun 12;353(9169):2001–2007.

18. McKelvie RS, Yusuf S, Pericak D, Avezum A, Burns RJ, Probstfield J, Tsuyuki RT, White M, Rouleau J, Latini R, Maggioni A, Young J, Pogue J. Comparison

of candesartan, enalapril, and their combination in congestive heart failure: randomized evaluation of strategies for left ventricular dysfunction (RESOLVD) pilot study. The RESOLVD Pilot Study Investigators. *Circulation*. 1999 Sep 7;100(10):1056–1064.

19. Pitt B, Poole-Wilson PA, Segal R, et al. On behalf of the ELITE II Investigators. Effect of losartan compared with captopril on mortality in patients with symptomatic heart failure: randomised trial – the Losartan Heart Failure Survival Study ELITE II. *Lancet*. 2000;255:1582–1587.

20. McMurray JJ, Ostergren J, Swedberg K, Granger CB, Held P, Michelson EL, Olofsson B, Yusuf S, Pfeffer MA; CHARM Investigators and Committees. Effects of candesartan in patients with chronic heart failure and reduced left-ventricular systolic function taking angiotensin-converting-enzyme inhibitors: the CHARM-Added trial. *Lancet*. 2003 Sep 6;362(9386):767–771.

21. Turakhia MP, Santangeli P, Winkelmayer WC, et al. Increased mortality associated with digoxin in contemporary patients with atrial fibrillation findings from the TREAT-AF Study. *J Am Coll Cardiol*. 2014;64(7):660–668.

22. Lai C, Sun D, Cen R, et al. Impact of long-term burden of excessive adiposity and elevated blood pressure from childhood on adulthood left ventricular remodeling patterns: The Bogalusa Heart Study. *J Am Coll Cardiol*. 2014;64(15):1580–1587.

23. Folsom AR, Shah AM, Lutsey PL. American Heart Association's Life's Simple 7: Avoiding Heart Failure and Preserving Cardiac Structure and Function. *Am J Med*. 2015 Sep;128(9):970–976.e2. doi: 10.1016/j.amjmed.2015.03.027. Epub 2015 Apr 20.

24. deFilippi CR, de Lemos JA, Tkaczuk AT, et al. Physical activity, change in biomarkers of myocardial stress and injury, and subsequent heart failure risk in older adults. *J Am Coll Cardiol*. 2012;60(24):2539–2547.

25. O'Connor CM, Whellan DJ, Lee KL. Efficacy and safety of exercise training in patients with chronic heart failure: HF-ACTION randomized controlled trial. *JAMA*. 2009;301:1439–1450.

26. Piepoli MF, Davos C, Francis DP, Coats AJ. Exercise training meta-analysis of trials in patients with chronic heart failure (ExTraMATCH). *BMJ*. 2004;328: 189.

27. O'Connor CM, Whellan DJ, and the HF-ACTION Investigators. Efficacy and safety of exercise training in patients with chronic heart failure: HF-ACTION randomized controlled trial. *JAMA*. 2009;301(14):1439–1450.

28. Agha G, Loucks E, Tinker L, et al. Healthy Lifestyle and Decreasing Risk of Heart Failure in Women: The Women's Health Initiative Observational Study. *J Am Coll Cardiol*. 2014;64(17):1777–1785.

29. Goldenberg I, Kutyifa V, Klein H, et al. Survival with cardiac-resynchronization therapy in mild heart failure. *N Engl J Med*. 2014;370:1694–1701.

30. Bettari L, Fiuzat M, Shaw LK, et al. Hyponatremia and long-term outcomes in chronic heart failure – an observational study from the Duke Databank for Cardiovascular Diseases. *J Card Fail*. 2012;18(1):74–81.

31. Mancini DM, Eisen H, Kussmaul W, Mull R, et al. Value of peak exercise oxygen consumption for optimal timing of cardiac transplantation in ambulatory patients with heart failure. *Circulation*. 1991;83:778–786.

32. Arena R, Myers J, Aslam SS, Varughese EB, Peberdy MA, et al. Peak VO_2 and VE/VCO_2 slope in patients with heart failure: a prognostic comparison. *Am Heart J.* 2004;147:354–360.

33. Osman AF, Mehra MR, Lavie CJ, Nunez E, Milani RV. The incremental prognostic importance of body fat adjusted peak oxygen consumption in chronic heart failure. *J Am Coll Cardiol.* 2000;36:2126–2131.

34. Young JB, Dunlap ME, Pfeffer MA et al. Mortality and morbidity reduction with candesartan in patients with chronic systolic heart failure and left systolic dysfunction. *Circulation.* 2004;110:2618–2626.

35. McMurray JJV, Packer M, Desai AS, et al. Angiotensin–neprilysin inhibition versus enalapril in heart failure. *N Engl J Med.* 2014 Sep 11;371(11):993–1004.

36. Dargie HJ, et al. Effect of carvedilol on outcome after myocardial infarction in patients with left-ventricular dysfunction: the CAPRICORN randomized trial: the CAPRICORN investigators. *Lancet.* 2001;357:1385–1390.

37. MERIT-HF Study Group. Effect of metoprolol CR/XL in chronic heart failure: Metoprolol randomized Intervention Trial in Congestive Heart failure (MERIT-HF). *Lancet.* 1999:353:2001–2007.

38. CIBIS-II Investigators and Committee. The cardiac insufficiency bisoprolol study II (CIBIS-II): a randomized control trial. *Lancet.* 1999;353:9–13.

39. Remme WJ, Torp-Pedersen C, Cleland JF, et al. Carvedilol protects better against vascular events than metoprolol in heart failure: Results from COMET. *J Am Coll Cardiol.* 2007;49(9):963–971.

40. Packer M, Antonopoulos GV, Berlin JA, et al. Comparative effects of carvedilol and metoprolol on left ventricular ejection fraction in heart failure: results of a meta-analysis. *Am Heart J.* 2001;141:899.

41. Zannad F, McMurray JJ, Krum H, et al. Eplerenone in patients with systolic heart failure and mild symptoms. *N Engl J Med.* 2011;364:11–21.

42. Cohn JN, Johnson G, Ziesche S, et al. A comparison of enalapril with hydralazine-isosorbidedinitrate in the treatment of chronic congestive heart failure. *N Engl J Med.* 1991;325:303–310.

43. Redfield M, Anstrom KJ, et al. for the NHLBI Heart Failure Clinical Research Network. Isosorbide mononitrate in heart failure with preserved ejection fraction. *N Engl J Med* 2015;373:2314–2324. DOI: 10.1056/NEJMoa1510774.

44. Cleland JG, Daubert JC, Erdman E, et al. The effect of cardiac resynchronization on morbidity and mortality in heart failure. *N Engl J Med* 2005;352:1539–1549.

45. Bristow MR, Saxon LA, Boehmer J, for the COMPANION Investigators. The Comparison of Medical Therapy, Pacing and Defibrillation in Heart Failure Cardiac Resynchronization therapy with or without an implantable defibrillator in advanced chronic heart failure. *N Engl J Med.* 2004;350:2140–2150.

46. Tang A, Wells GA, Talajic M, Malcolm AO, et al. Cardiac resynchronization therapy for mild-to-moderate heart failure. *N Engl J Med.* 2010;363:2385–2395.

47. Ponikowski P, van Veldhuisen DJ, Comin-Colet J, et al., on behalf of the CONFIRM-HF Investigators. Beneficial effects of long-term intravenous iron therapy with ferric carboxymaltose in patients with symptomatic heart failure and iron deficiency. *Eur Heart J.* 2014 Aug 31. pii: ehu385.

CHAPTER 7

Acute Decompensated and Chronic Stage D Heart Failure

Patrick Campbell, Selim R. Krim, Thach Nguyen, Marvin Eng, Yidong Wei, Hau Van Tran and Hector Ventura

Management of Complex Cardiovascular Problems, Fourth Edition. Edited by Thach N. Nguyen, Dayi Hu, Shao Liang Chen, Moo Hyun Kim and Cindy L. Grines.
© 2016 John Wiley & Sons, Ltd. Published 2016 by John Wiley & Sons, Ltd.

NEW UNDERSTANDINGS

Conventional understandings define acute decompensated heart failure (ADHF) as the sudden or gradual onset of the signs or symptoms of heart failure (HF) requiring unplanned office visits, emergency room visits, or hospitalization. In this real world practice book, ADHF is understood as being composed of two contradictory sets of findings:

1 Fluid overload in the venous system, mainly the two vital venous compartment (pulmonary and hepatic).

2 Low perfusion in three other arterial compartments, mainly cerebral (causing dizziness or change of mental status), renal (causing renal failure) and distal peripheral arterial system (causing fatigue or exercise intolerance).

ADHF is diagnosed when the fluid storage capacity of the pulmonary arterial and venous system is exceeded, leading to shortness of breath (SOB) and subsequent exudation of plasma into the alveoli causing respiratory distress.

STRATEGIC MAPPING

For patients with ADHF, **the first step** is to confirm the diagnosis of severe fluid overload in the right heart system with or without hypoperfusion in the arterial system. **The second step** is to treat pulmonary fluid overload (impending pulmonary edema) and underlying problems which destabilize the recently compensated HF. While the SOB and respiratory distress are being reversed, the patient should receive guideline directed medical therapy (GDMT) for HF with angiotensin converting enzyme inhibitors (ACEI), angiotensin receptor blockers (ARB), angiotensin receptor neprilysin inhibitors (ARNI) or beta-blockers (BB). Implantable cardioverter defibrillator (ICD) and chronic resynchronization therapy (CRT) (if qualified) can be implanted once the patient stabilizes and is on optimal medical therapy.

HIGH-RISK MARKERS

Respiratory difficulty and distress

The patient with ADHF may have SOB, and its severity should be practically evaluated when the patient needs use of accessory muscles to breathe. Without appropriate treatment, the patient will go into respiratory failure requiring urgent intubation and artificial ventilation.

Hypotension

The patient with ADHF may be profiled based on systolic blood pressure (BP) at presentation: high, normal, and low BP. The sickest one is the patient with hypotension. In contrast, most of the patients with normal or high BP have a preserved left ventricular ejection fraction (LV EF), respond

Table 7.1 Predictors of high risk or advanced HF by decreasing order of severity

1. Frequent (≥2) hospitalizations or ED visits for HF in the past year
2. Frequent systolic blood pressure <90 mmHg
3. Progressive decline in serum sodium
4. Progressive deterioration in renal function (e.g., rise in BUN and creatinine)
5. Intolerance to ACEI due to hypotension and/or worsening renal function
6. Intolerance to beta-blockers due to worsening HF or hypotension
7. Persistent dyspnea on dressing or bathing, requiring rest
8. Frequent ICD shocks
9. Weight loss without other cause (e.g., cardiac cachexia)

HF: Heart failure; ED: Emergency department; BUN: blood urea nitrogen; ACEI: angiotensin converting enzyme inhibitor; ICD: implantable cardioverter defibrillator.

rapidly to therapy, and have low in-hospital mortality. The reason is that an elevated BP indicates the presence of adequate contractile reserve and suggests that abnormal vasoconstriction and volume expansion are the main culprits of ADHF [1].

HIGH-RISK PREDICTORS

At the first encounter of a patient admitted because of ADHF, according to the Acute Decompensated Heart Failure National (ADHERE) *Registry* BUN ≥43 mg/dL was the single strongest predictor of mortality and that patients with BUN ≥43 mg/dL combined with SBP <115 mmHg and serum creatinine ≥2.75 mg/dL had the highest mortality risk [2]. Other predicting factors signaling high risk or advanced HF are listed in Table 7.1.

INVESTIGATIONS

As the patient arrives with SOB, a quick screening to identify patients who require urgent or emergent care, and subsequent hospitalization is of utmost importance in order to prevent respiratory failure and unplanned intubation.

Symptoms to look for

The main symptom of ADHF is shortness of breath (SOB). The patients may have worsening SOB which becomes intolerable, and progresses to impending respiratory crisis. The second symptom signaling the utmost severity of ADHF is the change of mental status. The patient can become obtunded due to lack of oxygen, either from of low oxygen saturation from impaired respiratory function or due to low cerebral perfusion caused by hypotension. Can the patient with ADHF present with the symptom of chest pain?

CLINICAL PEARLS
How to differentiate chest pain from CAD versus chest pain from pulmonary hypertension secondary to COPD For patients with pulmonary hypertension (HTN) secondary to chronic obstructive pulmonary disease (COPD), the patient would have SOB when exercising and as the patient continues to exercise, the SOB becomes worse and then chest heaviness follows. This is the classic scenario for chest pain caused by pulmonary HTN secondary to lung disease. However, this patient may have concomitant CAD as they become older. At that time, angina pain from CAD may occur before or at the same time as SOB from COPD, and not after severe SOB from COPD.

Signs to look for

The signs belong to two mechanisms causing ADHF (overload in the venous system and low perfusion in the arterial system). The signs of venous fluid overload are in the lungs (rales), elevated jugular venous distention (JVD), liver congestion and enlargement. When fluid overload in the lungs become severe, causing pulmonary edema, the patient will develop the signs of respiratory distress (increased respiratory rate, need to use accessory muscles to breathe, diffuse sweating, complaining of being exhausted, etc). The sternomastoid muscle in the neck is shown to contract prominently when the patient needs to use the whole chest to inspire. The signs of low perfusion include low blood pressure and mental obtundation.

CLINICAL PEARLS
Causes of hypotension in ADHF The reduced BP in the patient with ADHF may be related to poor LV systolic dysfunction. However, careful clinical evaluation

is necessary to exclude volume depletion, especially in the setting of beta-blockade or endstage HF where the expected compensatory reflex increase in heart rate is blunted. Orthostatic hypotension is also due to multiple anti-hypertensives, sodium and fluid restriction, autonomic dysfunction, and advancing age. Volume depletion is not uncommonly seen in advanced HF patients who adhere to a strict low sodium diet while on strong diuretics. Restrictive cardiomyopathy and right HF with pulmonary HTN may also limit the LV stroke volume and result in low cardiac output syndrome and low BP [1].

Signs and symptoms requiring immediate action

The problems which need to be solved urgently and are the compelling reasons requiring inpatient management or monitoring as listed in Table 7.2.

Table 7.2 Signs and symptoms that should prompt admission

Recommend hospitalization	Consider hospitalization
Hypotension	Evidence of worsening congestion
	Increased liver function tests suggesting hepatic congestion
	Weight gain
Declining renal function	Electrolyte disturbances
Change in mental status	Co-morbid conditions that can worsen heart failure
	Pneumonia
	Pulmonary embolism
	Diabetes
	Stroke or transient ischemic attack
Dyspnea at rest	Frequent defibrillators discharges
Arrhythmia	Newly diagnosed heart failure with signs and symptoms of congestion
Atrial fibrillation	
Ventricular tachycardia	
Acute coronary syndromes	

Adapted from HFSA Guidelines, *J Card Fail.* 2010. Source: Lindenfeld et al. 2010. Reproduced with permissions from Elsevier [28].

CLINICAL PEARLS
Which is the first sign predicting the appearance of acute decompensated heart failure? The first sign predicting ADHF is the unexplained elevation of the International Ratio (INR). Due to congestion of the liver, coumadin cannot be metabolized as usual, so the INR becomes higher. This is the earliest sign predicting the imminent appearance of ADHF, even if the patient is totally asymptomatic.

SMART TESTING

Besides the history and physical examination, B-type natriuretic peptide (BNP) level can be used to support a diagnosis of HF. However this biomarker can also be elevated due to a range of cardiac and non-cardiac causes, such as AF, pulmonary embolism or chronic obstructive pulmonary disease (COPD) and severe pneumonia. Renal function with blood urea nitrogen (BUN) and creatinine level should be measured at baseline because the selection and intensity of treatment for HF depend on these levels. Na and K level should be measured as they can be depleted with diuretics and cause significant arrhythmia. Can troponin level be elevated in patients with ADHF mimicking acute coronary syndrome?

CLINICAL PEARLS
Can diastolic heart failure precipitate and mimic acute coronary syndrome? On many occasions, patients come with mild ADHF (mild to moderate SOB) and early signs of mild overload in the pulmonary vascular system (minimal rales in the lungs and mild liver congestion, no frank JVD). However these patients have positive troponin and the EKG shows prominent T wave inversion in multiple leads, suggesting acute coronary syndrome (Figure 7.1). The coronary angiogram shows no lesion. The left ventricular end diastolic pressure is high and the coronary perfusion pressure is below 20 mmHg. Therefore the patient lacks perfusion due to high LVEDP and low diastolic aortic pressure, even if the coronary arteries are clean. This problem is recognized more frequently now (Figures 7.2 and 7.3).

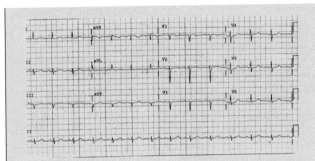

Figure 7.1 EKG before the index emergency room visit.

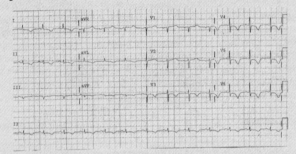

Figure 7.2 EKG on the index visit (diffuse T waves inversion in all leads V1-V6, I and AvL).

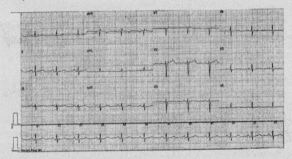

Figure 7.3 EKG 3 months later (The T waves changes reversed to normal upright).

DIAGNOSES

Once all the information is collected from the medical history, physical examination and testing, a diagnosis of whether the patient has ADHF needs to be made. In the real world practice, for the purpose of reimbursement, the conventional diagnoses could be coded as acute on chronic systolic HF, chronic systolic HF, etc. However, for the purpose of treatment of ADHF patients in the hospital, one of the lead editors of this book (TN) uses the pathologic diagnoses which need to be corrected: right heart failure causing fluid overload, live congestion, and hypotension causing hypoperfusion. These different diagnoses are listed in Table 7.3.

CLINICAL PEARLS
How to differentiate moderate versus severe HF Using the concept of differentiating the diagnosis of HF to right and left HF, and the fluid overload from intravascular and extravascular compartments, clinicians may separate patients with poor or good prognosis. If the patient has rales in the lungs, jugular venous distention (JVD), liver enlargement, and liver congestion (painful to gentle percussion on the right upper quadrant), this patient has fluid overload in the intravascular compartment. The storage capacity of the pulmonary vascular system is exceeded. In contrast, if the patient has ONLY fluid overload in the abdominal wall, ascites, and edema in the legs or thighs, then this patient has fluid overload in the extravascular compartment while the pulmonary vascular system is not compromised.

The patients with intravascular fluid overload are sicker, and respond quickly with diuretics because the diuretics remove the fluid from the entire blood without a direct effect on the extravascular fluid of the body. However these patients need a higher dose of diuretics and their length of hospital stay is longer. On the other hand, patients with only mild intravascular fluid overload and prominent extravascular fluid overload, present with less severe symptoms (less SOB), respond slowly to treatment at the initial stage, but improve more quickly and the length of stay is shorter. In these patients, it will take longer to absorb the extravascular fluid into the intravascular compartment before the fluid is expelled by the kidneys.

Table 7.3 Diagnoses of heart failure

---

1. **Pathological diagnosis**
   a Dilated versus non-dilated cardiomyopathy
   b Reduced versus preserved ejection fraction
   c Systolic dominant versus diastolic dominant dysfunction
2. **Fluid status**
   d **Fluid status**
      i.   Overload
      ii. Euvolemic status
      iii. Hypovolemic status
   e **Intravascular fluid overload**
      i.   Jugular venous distension
      ii. Liver congestion
      iii. Spleen congestion
      iv. Pulmonary congestion
   f **Extravascular fluid overload**
      i.   Abdominal wall edema
      ii. Ascites
      iii. Scrotal edema
      iv. Leg edema
      v.   Pre-sacral edema
      vi. Dependent areas in the upper extremities (back of arm, elbow)
3. **Right versus left heart failure**
   g **Left heart failure without low cardiac output**
      i.   Normal blood pressure during acute decompensated heart failure
   h **Right heart failure**
      i.   Shortness of breath is predominant symptom
      ii. Edema is predominant sign
   i **Left heart failure with low cardiac output**
      i.   Fatigue is predominant symptom
      ii. Confusion
      iii. Sleepiness
      iv. Cold hands and feet

MANAGEMENT

Strategic mapping

The **first treatment** of ADHF is to relieve the fluid overload in the pulmonary vascular system. It could be done with IV diuretics and if the problem is not corrected quickly enough or the patient is still symptomatic, an IV vasodilator such as nitroglycerin would be helpful to lower preload and relieve pulmonary congestion. Once the urgent problem is treated, the precipitating factors need to be treated or reversed. Then GDMT should be implemented. Right on the day of admission or the next day, patient management should be programmed to include cardiac rehabilitation. Discharge planning should be started on the second day of admission if the expected day of discharge is the 3rd or 4th day of hospitalization.

Intravenous diuretics   Intravenous (IV) diuretics can be given as a bolus, and safely initiated at doses up to 2.5 times their current outpatient oral dose. The question of high versus standard dose diuretics in ADHF was studied in the Diuretic Optimization Strategies Evaluation (DOSE) trial. The low-dose strategy involved total daily IV doses of furosemide equivalent to prior oral dose, while the high-dose strategy was 2.5 times the oral dose. The result showed that the high-dose strategy did result in greater fluid removal and change in weight compared to the low-dose strategy [3].

After initiation of IV diuresis, careful hemodynamic monitoring and frequent clinical assessment are required. Assessment of volume status should occur at least once a day including evaluation of rales in the lungs, jugular venous distention, abdominal wall edema, hepatomegaly, ascites, peripheral edema (dependent areas in the lower extremities, upper extremities, and pre-sacral area), and daily weight. Re-evaluation of symptoms aids in guiding continued management and should focus on the symptoms that prompted hospital admission (dyspnea, orthopnea, nocturnal cough, altered mental status, and fatigue). As BNP is high in decompensated HF, could the level of BNP guide treatment of the patient with ADHF? The ACCF/AHA recommendations on diuretics for hospitalized patients with HF are summarized in Table 7.4 [1].

CRITICAL THINKING
N-terminal pro B type natriuretic peptide
level IS NOT ACCURATE in guiding diuretic therapy
Clinicians often struggle with accurate assessment of volume status, effectiveness of diuretic therapy, and determining timing of discharge after IV diuresis. The Trial of Intensified vs. Standard Medical Therapy in Elderly Patients With Congestive Heart Failure (TIME-CHF) trial compared biomarker guided (N-terminal pro BNP) with symptom-guided management for the treatment of ADHF. The study demonstrated that NT-BNP guided therapy was not superior to symptom-guided therapy. Routine use of BNP targets does not reduce readmissions or improve quality of life. Clinicians should tailor HF therapy and intensity of diuretic therapy based on symptoms in order to achieve the New York Heart Association (NYHA) functional class II prior to discharge [4].

Table 7.4 ACCF/AHA Diuretics recommendations for hospitalized patients with heart failure

RECOMMENDATION	COR	LOE
Diuretics		
HF patients hospitalized with fluid overload should be treated with IV diuretics	I	B
HF patients receiving loop diuretic therapy should receive an initial parenteral dose greater than or equal to their chronic oral daily dose; dose should then be serially adjusted	I	B
Serum electrolytes, urea nitrogen, and creatinine should be measured during the titration of HF medications, including diuretics	I	C
When diuresis is inadequate, it is reasonable to (A) give higher doses of IV loop diuretics or (B) add a second diuretic (e.g., thiazide)	IIa	B
Low-dose dopamine infusion may be considered with loop diuretics to improve diuresis	IIb	B

COR: class of recommendation; HF: heart failure; LOE: level of evidence. Adapted from Reference [1].

While IV diuresis is pursued, careful monitoring of renal function and electrolytes is required to ensure adequate electrolyte replacement and to adjust diuretic dosing as necessary. If large volume diuresis occurs, more frequent laboratory evaluation of renal function and electrolytes may be required. However, in many patients, after a few days on diuretics, the diuresis decreases. Why?

CLINICAL PEARLS
How to overcome diuretic resistance Often, especially in the critically ill or patients on chronic loop diuretics, conventional doses of loop diuretics do not result in an optimal response. This is referred as 'diuretic resistance'. There are currently three suggested mechanisms: (1) Rebound sodium retention, when the sodium absorption blockade in the loop of Henle results in increased sodium reabsorption in the distal nephron; (2) Post-diuretic effect: when the effect of the diuretic begins to wane, there is a compensatory rebound and increase in

sodium retention by the kidney; and (3) 'Braking phenomenon' – decreased efficacy of diuretics after successive diuretic use which has been reported to decrease as much as 40% after 3 days of treatment [5]. It is likely that diuretic resistance is due to a combination of these mechanisms. Treatment strategies to overcome diuretic resistance include: stricter salt restriction; addition of a second agent, typically a thiazide-type diuretic, to loop diuretics; or continuous IV infusions of diuretics [5].

For patients who fail to respond adequately to IV diuresis, the current ACC/AHA and Heart Failure Society of America (HFSA) guidelines recommend considering the addition of an IV vasodilator (nitroglycerin/nitroprusside or nesiritide) [Class IIB, Level of evidence: B] [1].

IV vasodilator The goal of IV vasodilators is to relieve dyspnea in normotensive or hypertensive patients hospitalized with acute HF [1], because these patients have increased systec arterial vasoconstriction which impairs the forward-pumping ability of the LV.

High-dose IV nitroglycerin This promptly alleviates symptoms of congestion, reduces the need for mechanical ventilation, and reduces the rate of admission to the intensive care unit (ICU) [7]. IV NTG is started at 20 mcg/min and titrated upwards in a stepwise fashion with 10–50 mcg/min increments. The endpoints are: improvements of symptoms; development of drug-related side-effects; change in systolic blood pressure; or a maximum dose of 200–500 mcg/min. The side-effects of nitroglycerin are worsening hypoxia or pulmonary edema due to ventilation–perfusion mismatch caused by vasodilation of the non-aerated alveoli.

Nesiritide The early studies of nesiritide demonstrated improvement in symptoms, acute hemodynamics, weight loss, urine output, renin-angiotensinogen aldosterone system (RAAS) activation, and decreased diuretic use without significant neurohormonal stimulation [7, 8]. However there was greater risk of arrhythmia and hypotension. Therefore, in select patients with adequate BP, when there is intolerance to nitroglycerin or nitroprusside and significant congestion unresponsive to IV diuresis alone, nesiritide could be considered to improve congestion and acutely reduce symptoms in the early admission period.

Nitroprusside   Few studies have evaluated sodium nitroprusside (SNP) in patients with acute HF. One retrospective, non-randomized study of patients hospitalized with advanced, low-output HF found that the use of SNP improved hemodynamic measurements without worsening renal function or the need for higher rates of inotropic support. Due to the risks of excessive hypotension, thiocyanate toxicity, and methemoglobinemia, treatment with SNP requires invasive blood pressure monitoring and careful titration by highly trained nursing staff in the intensive care setting [9].

Treatment of precipitating factors   After stabilizing the patient from respiratory difficulty or distress with diuretics, then the clinician should evaluate and treat possible precipitating events because these events destabilize the precarious balance between fluid intake and output. The common conditions which precipitate ADHF are listed in Table 7.5.

Once the urgent period passes, then the clinician would review the treatment plan and be sure that the patient receives optimal GDMT. The medications include angiotensin converting enzyme inhibitors (ACEI), or angiotensin receptor blockers (ARB), angiotensin receptor neprilysin inhibitors (ARNI) or beta-blockers (BB). Initiation of beta-blocker therapy at a low dose is recommended after the optimization of volume status and discontinuation of IV agents.

Table 7.5 Common precipitating factors

1. Non-adherence to GDMT, diet, fluid and/or sodium restriction.
2. Accelerated or uncontrolled hypertension.
3. Arrhythmia (atrial fibrillation most commonly).
4. Acute myocardial infarction.
5. Concurrent infection (pneumonia, viral illness).
6. Medications – addition of negative inotropes (calcium channel blockers, beta-blockers).
7. Medications – that increase sodium retention (steroids, non-steroidal anti-inflammatory drugs, thiazolidinediones).
8. Pulmonary embolism.
9. Excessive ETOH or illicit drug use.
10. Endocrinological co-morbidities – diabetes mellitus, hypo/hyperthyroidism.
11. Acute cardiovascular disease – valvular disease, aortic dissection, myopericarditis, endocarditis.

GDMT: Guideline-Determined Medical Therapy.

Physical activities   Although bed rest is recommended during the acute phase of hospitalization to improve diuresis, early ambulation with physical therapy should begin within the first 24 hours of admission.

Renal failure   Approximately 30% of patients who are hospitalized with HF experience worsening renal function during hospitalization. Declining renal function can also complicate management as many medications could worsen renal failure or increase the risk of medication toxicity. In the setting of acute renal failure during hospitalization, diuretics should be reduced or discontinued. If the renal function continues to decline, reducing or holding the dose of ACEI or ARB may be necessary. The track record of negative renal protection trials demonstrates the complexity of acute HF management and highlights the need for new renal-specific therapies to improve decongestion and preserve renal function [10].

Hyponatremia   In patients admitted with severe hypervolemic hyponatremia who are at risk of or having active cognitive deficits, all other possible causes of hyponatremia (the syndrome of inappropriate antidiuretic hormone [SIADH], hypothyroidism, or hypoaldosteronism) should be ruled out. Then fluid restriction is the first treatment. If the hyponatremia still persists, arginine vasopressin (AVP) antagonists (conivaptan and tolvaptan) may be used. Even AVP corrects the serum sodium and may improve diuresis; there was no mortality benefit. During AVP antagonist administration, liberalization of sodium restriction, frequent assessment of serum sodium, and discontinuation of therapy once serum sodium is >135 mg/dL are important. Long-term use is not recommended. Overly rapid correction of hyponatremia may cause osmotic demyelination and this is why tolvaptan therapy should be initiated only in a hospital where serum sodium can be closely monitored [11, 12].

Non-invasive ventilation   Patients with acute pulmonary edema or a pending hypertensive crisis can benefit from non-invasive ventilation strategies, including continuous positive airway pressure (CPAP) and bi-level positive airway pressure (BiPAP).

FOCUS CARE: THE REALLY SICK PATIENTS

Some patients are sicker and progressing towards endstage or refractory HF (Stage D). In these patients, there is a need to evaluate potential complicating co-morbidities (uncontrolled diabetes, ischemic heart disease, or COPD), reassessment of medical therapy, and assessment of patient and care-giver understanding. Once exacerbating factors have been eliminated, focus should shift to identification of those patients that may be progressing to endstage HF and who may require other advanced HF options (Table 7.6).

Table 7.6 Evaluation of advanced heart failure patients

1. Clinical assessment of heart failure (physical exam, history).
2. Review complicating comorbidities.
3. Assess adherence to Guideline-Determined Medical Therapy.
4. Evaluate for possible cardiac ischemia.
5. Evaluate for arrhythmia.
6. Assess lifestyle (older patients living alone, sodium intake, caregiver understanding).
7. Assess for barriers to adherence.
8. Assess for progression to end-stage/refractory heart failure.

SYSTEM-BASED PRACTICE: DISCHARGE

Strategic mapping

Once the patient's HF has been stabilized and medical therapy has achieved appropriate resolution of symptoms, planning for discharge should begin. The discharge planning process requires a thorough review including laboratory results, GDMT, exercise tolerance, and level of patient's education of HF. A multidisciplinary team should coordinate discharge preparation efforts including social workers, HF nurses, pharmacists, hospitalists, and consultants. Education must include the patient, caregivers, and other family members and focus on lifestyle changes including sodium restriction, fluid restriction, monitoring of daily weight, and a graded exercise program or referral to a cardiac rehabilitation program. Patients and caregivers should be educated on signs and symptoms of HF exacerbation, and what to do if symptoms worsen, compliance with outpatient testing and office visits during the early follow-up (vulnerable period) and thereafter. These plans for follow-up should be scheduled and discussed in detail with the patient and caregivers. There are three problems to be solved before discharging a patient: polypharmacy, dietary compliance instruction and readmission prevention measures.

Polypharmacy According to the GDMT guidelines, the patient should be treated with ACEI or ARB, BB, or ARNI. However, as medical therapy for HF has progressed, the list of drugs that improve symptoms and reduce mortality grew. In patients with Stage D HF the list of medications can become daunting, reaching 10 or more medications (BB, ACEI, diuretic, hydralazine-isosorbide dinitrate, mineralo-receptor antagonist, ASA, anticoagulants, digoxin, and statins). This list does not include medications seen in patients with other common co-morbid conditions (chronic obstructive lung disease (COPD), DM, or arthritis). This is why in these patients with HF, polypharmacy reduces adherence to medical regimens, increases risk of drug-interactions, and increases the risk of side-effects. This problem should be addressed when coordinating MDGT and done at least 2 days before discharge so the patient's medication could be adjusted and side-effects monitored before discharge.

Dietary compliance counseling Patients and caregivers are often aware of the dietary restrictions, but are unclear on the sodium content of many foods. Often, patients are simply unwilling to adhere to the required sodium and fluid restrictions. As patients age, they often become forgetful and medication intake can be missed or delayed. The patients and care-givers should be educated about a low sodium diet, low cholesterol diet, fluid restriction (<64 ounces a day), weight gain (2.2 pound is equal to 1 liters of fluid retained), etc.

Metrics on the day of discharge On the day of discharge providers should ensure that patients have met goals and an appropriate checklist is completed (Table 7.7) [13].

Proactive readmission prevention measures The metrics which had the biggest impact on the day the patient is being discharged home are listed in Table 7.8 [14].

Table 7.7 Heart failure discharge checklist

1. Guideline-Determined Medical Therapy has been reviewed and has been stable for 24 hours.
2. Potential exacerbating/confounding co-morbidities have been addressed.
3. Exercise tolerance has returned to New York Heart Association Class II.
4. Volume status has been optimized.
5. Education has been provided.
6. Clinic follow-up has been scheduled.

Table 7.8 **Metrics on discharge day with biggest impact**

1. **Medication management post-discharge:** Is the patient familiar and competent with his or her medications?
2. **Early follow-up:** Does the patient have a follow-up visit scheduled within a week of discharge and is she or he able to get there?
3. **Symptom management:** Does the patient fully comprehend the signs and symptoms of early fluid overload that require medical attention and whom to contact if they occur?

SYSTEM-BASED PRACTICE: EARLY AND RECURRENT READMISSION

Scope of the problem

Readmission for HF occurs in approximately 50% of patients within 6 months of discharge, and approximately 24% occur within the first 30 days [15]. Nearly one half to two-thirds of the readmissions appear to be triggered by potentially remediable factors, including poor discharge planning, non-adherence to recommendations regarding diet and medical treatment, inadequate follow-up, poor social supports, and delays in seeking medical attention [16]. There is increasing interest in restructuring the care of ambulatory HF patients to reduce fragmentation, enhance patient self-efficacy, and improve cost-effectiveness, quality, and clinical outcomes while smoothing the transition from hospital to home [16]. This section is a summary of reference [16].

Conventional transitional care interventions

Interventions are designed to stabilize the patients in the vulnerable period, during transitioning from hospital setting to home care. Efforts at HF disease management typically take the form of nursing-intensive interventions focused on ensuring the delivery of guideline-based medical therapy (therapeutic modification); enhancing patient self-efficacy through education regarding adherence and self-management (education); and regular surveillance for early signs of clinical deterioration (monitoring) [16]. Home visits are defined as visits by clinicians, such as nurses or pharmacists, who educate, reinforce self-care instructions, perform physical examinations, or provide other care (e.g. physical therapy or medication reconciliation). Structured telephone support is defined as monitoring, education, or self-care management (or various combinations) using simple telephone technology after discharge in a structured format

---

Table 7.9 Questions for the home monitoring program

1. What is the best approach to operationalizing the concept of home monitoring for heart failure patients?

2. What are the standards in the structure of the home monitoring program for heart failure disease management interventions?

3. What is the intensity and duration of the home monitoring program?

4. Who are the target populations?

5. Which are the core components of these multidimensional, multidisciplinary home monitoring interventions essential to improvement in clinical outcomes?

(e.g., series of scheduled calls with a specific goal, structured questioning, or use of decision-support software) [16]. Using data from 18 prospective randomized trials with a mean observation period of 8 months, Phillips et al. [17] identified a 25% reduction in the rates of all-cause hospital readmission (relative risk 0.75, 95% confidence interval [CI], 0.65–0.88) and a statistically non-significant trend toward reduced mortality (relative risk 0.87; 95% CI, 0.73–1.03). The questions for the home monitoring program to succeed are listed in Table 7.9.

The key components

In the meta-analysis by Phillips et al. [17] the intensity of post-discharge surveillance was not a major determinant of benefit, with comparable outcomes observed in those receiving a single post-discharge home visit, more frequent home visits with or without frequent telephone follow-up, and extended home care services. The data collectively suggest that the real benefits of HF disease management may be related not to the intensity of home monitoring after discharge, but to improvements in patient adherence to instructions regarding diet, weight control, and medications and greater use of evidenced-based medical therapies, including BB, ACEI, and spironolactone [18]. The consistent message appears to be that in patients with HF who are well-managed with evidence-based medical therapy, there is limited incremental impact of intensive home monitoring on clinical outcomes [16].

Problems with telemonitoring

Data from trials of implantable hemodynamic monitors suggest that weight gain is a relatively poor surrogate for intracardiac filling pressures and may be inadequate to recognize impending decompensation in sufficient time to intervene to prevent hospitalization. Because changes in filling pressures are often apparent several weeks before symptoms worsen, it seems tautological that more frequent, and even automated, home monitoring should facilitate disease management by allowing providers to intervene early to prevent HF decompensation, largely by adjusting doses of diuretics [16]. This lack of efficacy may be fed in part by excessive reliance on remote monitoring of weights and symptoms, which are likely insensitive and late markers of incipient HF decompensation [16].

With studies from remote follow-up of implantable cardiac defibrillators and cardiac resynchronization therapy devices, changes in certain routinely monitored parameters, such as the percentage of ventricular pacing, presence of arrhythmia, activity levels, and mean heart rates at rest or during exertion, or heart rate variability, did not help clinicians to better anticipate impending decompensation. The only randomized prospective trial conducted to date (Diagnostic Outcome Trial in Heart Failure [DOT-HF]), treatment guided by routine monitoring of intrathoracic impedance did not improve clinical outcomes and actually increased the likelihood of HF hospitalizations [18].

Implantable hemodynamic monitors

In The CardioMEMS Heart Sensor Allows Monitoring of Pressure to Improve Outcomes in NYHA Class III Heart Failure Patients (CHAMPION) trial [19], 550 patients with HF (independent of ejection fraction), NYHA class III symptoms, and a prior hospitalization for HF received a wireless implantable pulmonary artery pressure sensor (CardioMEMS; CardioMEMS, Inc., Atlanta, GA) and were randomized to treatment with or without the assistance of sensor data. At 6 months, management guided by the pressure sensor was associated with a statistically significant 30% reduction in the primary endpoint of HF hospitalizations (event rate, 0.31 versus 0.44; hazard ratio 0.70, 95% CI, 0.60–0.84, $P < 0.0001$), with a low rate of system-related complications (1.4%). These results were seen despite high background use of evidence-based medical therapies in the population as a whole (78% treated with ACEI or ARB, 91% with BB, and 42% with an aldosterone antagonist) and may have been related to the marked increase in the number of adjustments to HF medications by physicians who had access to the sensor data (2468; mean 9.1 adjustments per patient) relative to those without access to the data (1061; 3.8 per patient) [19]. These data suggest that for selected patients with advanced HF symptoms, continuous monitoring of intracardiac pressures may provide a reliable signal both for early detection of deterioration and for tracking effectiveness of early intervention that can facilitate improvements in clinical outcomes.

Personalized and hi-tech medicine

Tailoring the optimal disease management intervention for a given patient may require consideration of several factors, including the severity of disease, the setting in which care is being delivered (including the geographic distance between patients and their providers), and the patient's capacity for self-management, as well as the specific metrics that are being used to evaluate efficacy. Telemonitoring approaches, although apparently ineffective for high-risk populations with advanced HF or recent HF hospitalization, may yet be suitable for patients at lower risk who still require intermittent surveillance [20]. Higher-risk patients may require more intensive clinic-based follow-up, perhaps facilitated in selected cases by implantable hemodynamic monitors, either as stand-alone devices or as integrated modifications to implantable defibrillators and cardiac resynchronization devices. Leveraging technology to promote greater self-efficacy for patients may also be important [21]. Mobile phone applications can be designed to enhance patient adherence to dietary recommendations and medical treatment. Next-generation remote monitoring approaches already suggest the potential to more efficiently close the HF management loop by enabling HF patients to self-adjust diuretic dosing according to daily intracardiac pressure measurements without the routine need for remote supervision, much as diabetic patients self-adjust insulin dosing on the basis of readouts from home glucose monitors. Realizing the promise of disease management to improve patient outcomes requires creativity and a comprehensive, multidimensional approach. The telephone and a digital scale are simply not enough [16].

In summary, the success of home monitoring as an adjunct to HF care depends on the fundamental assumption that routine surveillance of HF symptoms and physiological data will facilitate early detection of clinical deterioration and direct corrective intervention to avert adverse clinical outcomes. An effective strategy must therefore accomplish several goals [16] (Table 7.10).

ADVANCED (STAGE D) HEART FAILURE

Management

Despite the pharmacologic progress made in the last three decades and the improvement in survival of HF patients, many patients reach an advanced stage. Early signs and symptoms suggesting advanced stage of HF are summarized in Table 7.3. With regard to treatment, current options for patients with refractory HF include cardiac transplant, mechanical circulatory support (MCS), and palliative measures [1].

Table 7.10 Needs for a successful program

1. Data collection must help to accurately anticipate decompensation with sufficient lead time to permit intervention.
2. Data must be transmitted efficiently in a format that is easily interpretable and enables timely intervention.
3. Personnel receiving the data must be qualified to interpret the data and respond appropriately.
4. Patient must receive and implement the treatment recommendation.
5. System must provide timely feedback to confirm resolution of the perturbation or indicate the need for further intervention.
6. Failure or delay in execution of any of these steps may fatally disrupt the feedback loop, preventing even an effective intervention from improving outcomes in practice.

Inotrope therapy

Positive inotropic agents are most commonly used in the setting of cardiogenic shock and in ADHF with evidence of pulmonary congestion and signs of hypoperfusion. **Dobutamine** (a β-adrenergic agonist) is recommended for treatment of patients with low cardiac output and reduced blood pressure. Concomitant use of β-blockers with dobutamine may attenuate the benefit of either agent [22]. **Milrinone** (a phosphodiesterase inhibitor), is preferred over dobutamine in patients without hypotension but with low cardiac output and symptoms of hypoperfusion. Milrinone acts by inhibiting the phosphodiesterase enzyme which is an enzyme that breaks down cyclic adenosine monophosphate (cAMP) resulting in a net increase in cAMP levels which in turn results in the ionotropic effects. Thus the effects of milrinone are independent of beta adrenergic receptors. Hence, β-blocker usage is not contraindicated with milrinone. However, concerns have been raised with the use of these agents, particularly in the long term and on a continuous basis, due to increased arrhythmia and mortality [23]. Therefore long-term continuous or intermittent infusion of inotropes is only recommended as a bridge to heart transplantation or for palliation of symptoms in patients with refractory HF who are not eligible for a more definitive therapy such as heart transplantation or mechanical circulatory support.

Ultrafiltration

Ultrafiltration may be an effective approach to alleviating congestion symptoms in patients with acute HF [1]. In the UNLOAD trial (Ultrafiltration vs. Intravenous Diuretics for Patients Hospitalized for Acute

Table 7.11 ACCF/AHA recommendations for ultrafiltration and IV inotropes for hospitalized patients with heart failure

Ultrafiltration	COR	LOE
Ultrafiltration may be considered for patients with obvious volume overload	IIb	B
Ultrafiltration may be considered for patients with refractory congestion	IIb	C
IV Inotropes		
Inotropic agents may be considered as temporary support for patients with cardiogenic shock who are awaiting definitive therapy or the resolution of acute precipitating problems	I	C
Inotropic agents may be considered as bridge therapy in patients with stage D HF who are refractory to standard medical and device therapy and are awaiting MCS or heart transplantation	IIa	B
Inotropic agents may be considered as short-term therapy for patients with severe systolic dysfunction, low BP, and significantly depressed cardiac output	IIb	B
Inotropic agents may be considered as palliative therapy in patients with stage D HF who are refractory to standard medical and device therapy and not eligible for MCS or heart transplantation	IIb	B

COR: Class of recommendation; HF: heart failure LOE: level of evidence; MCS: mechanical circulatory support. Adapted from Reference [1].

Decompensated Congestive Heart Failure), ultrafiltration was associated with greater fluid volume loss, sodium removal, and weight loss as compared with IV diuretic therapy. No significant improvement in dyspnea was observed. A reduction in 90-day hospital readmissions in patients with acute HF was also noted, although this finding was based on a small number of events [24]. The 2013 ACCF/AHA guidelines recommend considering ultrafiltration for patients with obvious volume overload and those with congestion refractory to standard medical therapy [1]. (Table 7.11).

Mechanical circulatory support

Owing to a limited number of available organ donors each year (2500 cardiac transplant/year in the United States), mechanical circulatory support is increasingly used in patients with advanced HF either as bridge to transplantation (BTT) or permanent therapy, otherwise known as

---

Table 7.12 Indications for left ventricular assist devices

1. Bridge to transplantation strategy in patients who are in cardiogenic shock and too sick to wait or who have temporary contraindications for transplant.
2. As a permanent therapy or so called 'destination therapy' for patients considered ineligible for cardiac transplantation,
3. As a bridge to myocardial recovery such as in patients with acute myocarditis where recovery is expected.
4. As bridge-to-decision or bridge-to-bridge, it is used for those patients who present with severe shock or following cardiac arrest and are supported with a temporary support ventricular assist devices to see if they become candidates for a long-term support device.

'destination therapy' (DT). Today, two continuous flow devices 'Thoratec HM II' and 'Heartware HVAD' (COMPANY AND CITY) are commonly used in the US. While the Heartware device is only approved for BTT strategy, the HM II remains the only device approved for BTT and DT. These second (HM II) and third generation devices (HVAD, Heartware) are smaller in size, offer greater durability, and lower risk of infection and device failure when compared to earlier generation pulsatile flow devices. The indications of LVAD are listed in Table 7.12.

EVIDENCE-BASED MEDICINE
The new magnetically levitated left ventricular assist system In the single-arm, prospective, multicenter HM3 CE Mark study, a full magnetically levitated left ventricular assist system (LVAD) showed favorable safety and efficacy outcomes in patients with The HeartMate 3 LV assist system (St. Jude Medical) was designed to provide enhanced hemocompatibility and long-term support for patients with advanced HF. The system is placed within the pericardium with the inflow conduit inserted into the left ventricle and the outflow graft secured to the ascending aorta. The fully magnetically levitated rotor has large blood-flow paths (0.5 mm along the side and 1 mm above and below the rotor) to reduce shear forces. At 6 months, 88% of patients continued on support, 4% received transplants and 8% died. The 6-month survival rate was 92%, which was higher than the 88% INTERMACS performance goal (HR = 0.34; P = .0093). The

HeartMate 3 reduced mortality risk by 66%, which was lower than the Seattle Heart Failure Model-predicted survival of 78% ($P = .0093$). NYHA classification ($P < .0001$), 6-minute walk test ($P < .0001$) and quality-of-life scores ($P < .0001$) also showed improvement within the 6-month period [25].

Heart transplantation

Heart transplantation remains the treatment of choice for patients with HF refractory to medical therapy. Data from the registry of the International Society for Heart and Lung Transplant (ISHLT) showed that, patient survival at 1 and 3 years for patients that received cardiac transplantation, was approximately 85 and 79%, respectively [27]. Moreover, among patients who survived the first year, the median survival was up to 14 years. Right heart catheterization and cardiopulmonary exercise stress (CPX) test are crucial tools to determine the need for cardiac transplant. A cardiac index value of less than 2.5 L/min/m2 suggests advanced disease. Similarly, a reduced maximal oxygen consumption of less than 12 mL/kg/1 /min (or <14 mL/Kg/min for patients using beta blockers) signifies advanced HF stage and warrants evaluation for cardiac transplant. The indications for cardiac transplant are listed in Table 7.13.

End of life care and palliative therapy

Palliative measures including inotropes should be considered and offered to patients with advanced HF, who do not qualify for either cardiac

Table 7.13 Indications for cardiac transplant

1. Cardiogenic shock requiring either continuous intravenous inotropic support or MCS with an intra-aortic balloon pump counterpulsation device or MCS.
2. Persistent NYHA class IV congestive HF symptoms refractory to maximal medical therapy (LVEF<20%; peak VO_2 <12 mL/kg/min).
3. Intractable or severe anginal symptoms in patients with coronary artery disease not amenable to percutaneous or surgical revascularization.
4. Intractable life-threatening arrhythmias unresponsive to medical therapy, catheter ablation, and/or implantation of intracardiac defibrillator [27].

MCS: Mechanical Circulatory Support; NYHA = New York Heart Association; HF = heart failure; LVEF = left ventricular ejection fraction.

transplantation or mechanical circulatory support and are unresponsive to medical therapy. Hospice care at home, hospital, or at specialized centers may be considered for patients with NYHA Class IV symptoms with life expectancy of 6 months or less and with refractory HF. Hospices generally provide oral medications and symptomatic management. Some hospices may provide complex treatments such as intravenous inotropes or continuous positive airway pressure (CPAP). Continued participation of the clinician and meticulous management of fluid status is essential to maximize quality of life even after the patient enrolls in a hospice [28].

ACTION POINTS

1 **New definition:** In this book, ADHF is understood as being composed of two contradictory sets of findings: (1) Fluid overload in the venous system, mainly the two vital venous compartment (pulmonary and hepatic); and (2) Low perfusion in three other arterial compartments, mainly cerebral (causing dizziness or change of mental status), renal (causing renal failure) and distal peripheral arterial system (causing fatigue or exercise intolerance). ADHF is diagnosed when the fluid storage capacity of the pulmonary arterial and venous system is exceeded, leading to shortness of breath (SOB) and subsequent exudation of plasma into the alveoli causing respiratory distress.

2 **Guideline-directed management:** Once the patients with ADHF are stabilized, they should receive guideline-directed medical therapy for HF with angiotensin converting enzyme inhibitors, angiotensin receptor blockers, angiotensin receptor neprilysin inhibitors or beta-blockers.

3 **New observation: Diastolic heart failure can precipitate and mimic acute coronary syndrome:** On many occasions, patients came with mild ADHF (mild to moderate SOB and early signs of mild overload in the pulmonary vascular system (minimal rales in the lungs and mild liver congestion, no frank JVD). However these patients had troponin positive and EKG showed prominent T wave inversion in multiple leads, suggesting acute coronary syndrome. Coronary angiogram showed no lesion. The left ventricular end diastolic pressure was high and the coronary perfusion pressure was below 20 mmHg. Therefore the patient lacked perfusion due to high LVEDP and low diastolic aortic pressure; even the coronary arteries were clean.

4 Which are the metrics on discharge day with biggest impact on preventing of readmission? There are three:

1 **Medication management post-discharge:** Is the patient familiar and competent with his or her medications?

2 **Early follow-up:** Does the patient have a follow-up visit scheduled within a week of discharge and is she or he able to get there?

3 **Symptom management:** Does the patient fully comprehend the signs and symptoms of early fluid overload that require medical attention and whom to contact if they occur?

5 Key components for success in home monitoring: The intensity of post-discharge surveillance was not a major determinant of benefit, with comparable outcomes observed in those receiving a single post-discharge home visit, more frequent home visits with or without frequent telephone follow-up, and extended home care services. The data collectively suggest that the real benefits of HF disease management may be related not to the intensity of home monitoring after discharge, but to improvements in patient adherence to instructions regarding diet, weight control, and medications and greater use of evidenced-based medical therapies, including BB, ACEI, and spironolactone. The consistent message appears to be that in patients with HF who are well-managed with evidence-based medical therapy, there is limited incremental impact of intensive home monitoring on clinical outcomes.

REFERENCES

1. Yancy CW, Jessup M, Bozkurt B, Butler J, et al. 2013 ACCF/AHA Guideline for the Management of Heart Failure: Executive Summary: A Report of the American College of Cardiology Foundation/American Heart Association Task Force on Practice Guidelines. *Circulation.* 2013;128:1810–1852.

2. Peterson PN, Rumsfeld JS, Liang L, et al. A validated risk score for in-hospital mortality in patients with heart failure from the American Heart Association get with the guidelines program. *Circ Cardiovasc Qual Outcomes.* 2010;3(1): 25–32.

3. Felker MG, Lee KL, Bull DA, et al. Diuretic strategies in patients with acute decompensated heart failure. *N Engl J Med.* 2011;364(9):797–805.

4. Pfisterer M, Buser P, Rickli H, et al. BNP-Guided vs Symptom-Guided Medical Therapy. The Trial of Intensified vs Standard Medical Therapy in Elderly Patients With Congestive Heart Failure (TIME-CHF) Randomized Trial. *JAMA.* 2009;301(4):383–392.

5. Wilcox CS, Mitch WE, Kelly RA, et al. Response of the kidney to furosemide: effects of salt intake and renal compensation. *J Lab Clin Med.* 1983;102:450–458.

6. Levy P, Compton S, Welch R, et al. Treatment of severe decompensated heart failure with high-dose intravenous nitroglycerin: a feasibility and outcome analysis. *Ann Emerg Med.* 2007;50(2):144–152.

7. Colucci WS, Elkayam U, Horton DP, et al. Intravenous neseritide, a natriuretic peptide, in the treatment of decompensated congestive heart failure. *Nesteritide Study Group. N Eng J Med.* 2000;343:246–253.

8. VMAC Committee. Intravenous nesiritide vs. nitroglycerine for treatment of decompensated congestive heart failure: a randomized controlled trial. *JAMA.* 2002;287:1531–40.

9. Mullens W, Abrahams Z, Francis GS, et al. Sodium nitroprusside for advanced low-output heart failure. *J Am Coll Cardiol.* 2008;52(3):200–207.

10. Ronco C, Haapio M, House AA. Cardiorenal syndrome. *JACC.* 2008:52:1527–1539.

11. Konstam MA, Gheorghiade M, Burnett JC, Jr., et al. Effects of oral tolvaptan in patients hospitalized for worsening heart failure: the EVEREST Outcome Trial. *JAMA.* 2007;297(12):1319–1331.

12. Gheorghiade M, Niazi I, Ouyang J, et al. Vasopressin V2-receptor blockade with tolvaptan in patients with chronic heart failure: Results from a double-blind, randomized trial. *Circulation.* 2003;107:2690–2696.

13. Writing Committee Members, Bonow RO, Ganiats TG, Beam CT, et al. ACCF/AHA/AMA-PCPI 2011 Performance Measures for Adults With Heart Failure: A Report of the American College of Cardiology Foundation/American Heart Association Task Force on Performance Measures and the American Medical Association-Physician Consortium for Performance Improvement. *Circulation.* 2012;125:2382–2401.

14. http://blog.cardiosource.org/post/overcoming-challenges-to-reduce-readmissions/

15. Krumholz HM, Merril AR, Schone EM, et al. Patterns of hospital performance in acute myocardial infarction and heart failure 30-day mortality and readmissions. *Circ Cardiovasc Qual Outcomes.* 2009;2:407–413.

16. Desai AS. Home monitoring heart failure care does not improve patient outcomes looking beyond telephone-based disease management. *Circulation.* 2012;125:828–836.

17. Phillips CO, Wright SM, Kern DE, et al. Comprehensive discharge planning with postdischarge support for older patients with congestive heart failure: a meta-analysis. *JAMA.* 2004;291:1358–1367.

18. Konstam MA, Konstam V. Heart failure disease management: a sustainable energy source for the health care engine. *J Am Coll Cardiol.* 2010;56:379–381.

19. Abraham W, Adamson P, Bourge R et al., for the CHAMPION Trial Study Group. Wireless pulmonary artery haemodynamic monitoring in chronic heart failure: a randomised controlled trial. *Lancet.* 2011 377:658–666.

20. Hernandez AF, Greiner MA, Fonarow GC, et al. Relationship between early physician follow-up and 30-day readmission among Medicare beneficiaries hospitalized for heart failure. *JAMA.* 2010;303:1716–1722.

21. Ritzema J, Troughton R, et al. Physician-directed patient self-management of left atrial pressure in advanced chronic heart failure. *Circulation.* 2010; 121:1086–1095.

22. Abraham W. Response *Circulation.* 2012;125:837.

23. Cuffe MS, Califf RM, Adams KF, et al. Short-term intravenous milrinone for acute exacerbation of chronic heart failure: A randomized controlled trial. *JAMA.* 2002;287:1541–1547.

24. Rose EA, Gelijns AC, Moskowitz AJ, Heitjan DF, Stevenson LW, Dembitsky W, et al. Long-term use of a left ventricular assist device for end-stage heart failure. *N Engl J Med.* 2001;345:1435–1443.

25. Netuka I, Sood P, Pya Y, et al. Fully Magnetically Levitated Left Ventricular Assist System for Treating Advanced HF A Multicenter Study. *J Am Coll Cardiol.* 2015;66:257–989.

26. Mehra M, Kobashigawa J, Starling R, et al. Listing criteria for heart transplantation: International Society for Heart and Lung Transplantation guidelines for the care of transplant candidates – 2006. *J Heart Lung Transplant.* 2006;25:1024–1042.

27. Goodlin SJ, Hauptman PJ, Arnold R, Grady K, Hershberger RE, Kutner J, et al. Consensus statement: Palliative and supportive care in advanced heart failure. *J Card Fail.* 2004;10:200–209.

28. Lindenfeld J, Albert NM, Boehmer JP, et al. HFSA 2010 Comprehensive Heart Failure Practice Guideline. *J Card Fail.* 2010;16:e1–194 (table 2).

CHAPTER 8

Atrial Fibrillation

Mihail Gabriel Chelu, Ali Oto, Tuan D. Nguyen, Phan Dinh Phong, Tung Mai, Thomas Bump and Rajasekhar Nekkanti

Management of Complex Cardiovascular Problems, Fourth Edition. Edited by Thach N. Nguyen, Dayi Hu, Shao Liang Chen, Moo Hyun Kim and Cindy L. Grines.
© 2016 John Wiley & Sons, Ltd. Published 2016 by John Wiley & Sons, Ltd.

BACKGROUND

Atrial fibrillation (AF) is a cardiac arrhythmia that is characterized by the following on an ECG or rhythm strip [1]:

1 Irregular RR intervals in the absence of complete AV block and some level of heart block or digoxin toxicity.

2 No distinct P waves on the surface ECG except in coarse AF with some atrial activity which can be confused with flutter.

3 An atrial cycle length (when P waves are visible) that is variable and <200 milliseconds.

AF can be classified as paroxysmal, persistent, and longstanding persistent AF based on its duration [1]. Recurrent AF is defined as having at least two episodes of AF. Paroxysmal AF is defined as AF with spontaneous termination within 7 days. Persistent AF is defined as AF lasting more than 7 days and requiring some means to terminate it. Longstanding persistent AF is defined as continuous AF lasting more than 12 months. 'Permanent' AF implies a decision has been made not to restore or maintain sinus rhythm by any means, pharmacological or electrical cardioversion, or catheter or surgical ablation. If the decision has been made to restore sinus rhythm, AF should be reclassified.

CHALLENGES

The **first challenge** is in the diagnosis and differential diagnosis of AF. Several supraventricular arrhythmias may present with rapid irregular RR intervals that can mimic AF: frequent atrial ectopy, multifocal atrial tachycardia, atrial tachycardias with variable atrioventricular (AV) block, atrial flutter with variable AV block, atrioventricular nodal reentrant tachycardia with block in the lower common pathway, and dual antegrade atrioventricular nodal conduction [1, 2].

The **second challenge is** that there are many possible risk factors for AF identified in the medical literature, however they are not necessarily related to the development but the risk of thromboembolic events (Table 8.1). While many of these factors can be potentially corrected, there were no data showing that their correction resulted in AF prevention or cure. That is because they are not necessarily causally related. One of the examples is that statins have not been proven to be useful in prevention of AF in post-coronary artery bypass graft surgery (CABG) patients [1]. In two particular clinical situations, the American College of Cardiology/American heart Association/Heart rhythm Society (ACC/AHA/HRS) guidelines suggest angiotensin converting enzyme inhibitors (ACEI) or angiotensin-receptor blocker (ARB) for primary prevention of new-onset

Table 8.1 Selected risk factors for development of AF

Risk factors
Age
Hypertension
Diabetes mellitus
Coronary artery disease
Myocardial infarction
Heart failure
Valvular heart disease
Cardiothoracic surgery
Obstructive sleep apnea
Obesity
Exercise
Alcohol
Smoking
Hyperthyroidism
Family history
Genetic variants

AF in patients with HF with reduced left ventricular ejection fraction (LVEF) or in the setting of hypertension [1].

The **third challenge** is in the management of AF. Only some patients respond to medications which convert AF to sinus rhythm or to maintain the sinus rhythm after successful cardioversion. For patients with AF, the only intervention proven so far to reduce mortality is oral anticoagulation for prevention of stroke [3]. The **fourth challenge** is that in the use of oral anticoagulants, there is a need to discuss with patients about the risk-benefit ratio of medication and the fact that not all patients require anticoagulation.

STRATEGIC MAPPING

The initial evaluation involves a comprehensive history and physical examination and its goals are listed in Table 8.2.

For patients with symptomatic AF, sinus rhythm restoration improves their quality of life and exercise capacity (Figure 8.1). This depends on whether AF really is causing the symptoms. Strategies aimed at restoration and maintenance of sinus rhythm include pharmacologic or electric cardioversion, class IC and III anti-arrhythmic drugs (AAD) and catheter-based ablation or any of its combinations. Sinus rhythm restoration and maintenance should be undertaken only after exclusion

---

Table 8.2 Goals of the history and physical examination

---

1. Confirm the diagnosis and assess the burden of AF.
2. Determine its possible causes and in particular potentially reversible factors (e.g. hyperthyroidism, after thoracic surgery).
3. Identification of risk factors for development of AF.
4. Risk stratification for thromboembolic risk.
5. Assess the impact on cardiovascular (CV) (including worsening heart failure (HF) or other systems.

---

of left atrial appendage (LAA) thrombus and/or adequate anticoagulation according to their stroke risk.

For asymptomatic patients, it is important to determine that they are indeed asymptomatic and that they are not at risk for thromboembolic events. Not all patients who have asymptomatic AF benefit from a rate control strategy, particularly younger individuals. For a 20-year-old patient who has AF, maintenance of AF is not a good strategy, even if symptoms are minimal. When the rate is difficult to be controlled with

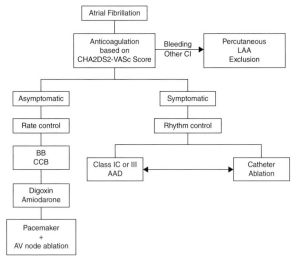

Figure 8.1 Strategy for management of atrial fibrillation. (CI: contraindication; LAA: left atrial appendage; BB: beta-blocker; CCB: non-dihydropyridine receptor calcium channel blockers; AAD: anti-arrhythmic drugs.

medical therapy and in particular in patients with tachycardia induced cardiomyopathy, AV node ablation and permanent pacemaker implant should be considered (Figure 8.1). Catheter-based ablation is superior to AAD for paroxysmal, persistent, or longstanding persistent AF.

Stroke prevention

As the only intervention proved so far to reduce mortality in patients with AF is oral anticoagulation for prevention of stroke [3], it is therefore critical to anticoagulate any patient according with their stroke risk (CHA2DS2-VASc score) (Figure 8.1). The choice between warfarin and novel oral anticoagulants (NOAC) (dabigatran, rivaroxaban, apixaban, edoxaban) should be made according to each patient's individual benefits (lowest rate of ischemic stroke), risks (lowest rate of bleeding) and co-morbidities (valvular heart disease, renal function, etc.). Patients with bleeding from oral anticoagulants and other conditions that preclude their use may benefit from percutaneous LAA occlusion as one closure device (the Watchman, Boston Scientific, Mapple Grove, MN has recently been approved by the Federal Drug Administration [FDA]). However there is an important caveat: not all strokes come from the LAA. Surgical or hybrid AF ablation should be offered to symptomatic patients undergoing surgery for other compelling indications. LAA ligation should be considered at the time of surgery to minimize thromboembolic risk.

HIGH-RISK MARKERS

1 **Highly symptomatic AF:** Patients with highly symptomatic AF should be treated aggressively with a rhythm restoration strategy to minimize the rate of recurrent hospitalizations.
2 **Persistent, uncontrolled rapid ventricular rate:** Patients with a persistent, uncontrolled rapid ventricular rate should be followed up closely for decline of left ventricular (LV) ejection fraction (EF) due to tachycardia induced cardiomyopathy. More than that, rate control should be undertaken to prevent cardiomyopathy from happening in the first place.
3 **Prior transient ischemic attack (TIA)/cerebro-vascular accident (CVA), vascular disease, diabetes mellitus (DM), and female gender:** These factors appear to confer the highest risk for further thromboembolic events in patients with AF and therefore particular attention should be paid in anticoagulating these subsets of patients.

   Patients with **side-effects or contraindications to antiarrhythmic or oral anticoagulants** drugs have high morbidity and mortality rates.

4 **Syncope:** Patients presenting with syncope and AF should be thoroughly investigated for sinus node dysfunction and pauses and a pacemaker implant should be considered whenever appropriate.

HIGH-RISK PREDICTORS

1 **Increased age** is associated with higher risk of stroke. The severity of stroke in AF patients tends to be more severe than in patients without AF [4]. **Left ventricular function** may be affected by fast ventricular rate, irregularity, loss of atrial contraction, and increased filling pressures. AF is associated with three times increase in risk of HF.

2 **Predictors of mortality:** The independent predictors of mortality were: age, chronic kidney disease, AF as primary presentation, prior transient ischemic attack (TIA), chronic obstructive pulmonary disease (COPD), malignancy, minor bleeding, and diuretic use while statin use appeared to be predictive of a lower mortality rate [5].

INVESTIGATIONS

Symptoms to look for

The symptoms of AF may range from no symptoms to palpitations, dyspnea, hypotension, dizziness/lightheadedness, syncope, decreased exercise capacity, and fatigue. Sometimes the first manifestation of AF is a due to thromboembolic event resulting in sensory or motor deficit.

Signs to look for

Confirm AF with the irregular irregularity of the rhythm of the apical beat or of the radial pulse. Need to check for sign of fluid overload, past cerebrovascular accident (CVA), past history of coronary artery disease (CAD), peripheral artery disease (PAD), carotid bruit, abdominal bruit, chronic kidney disease.

SMART TESTING

The selection of a diagnostic test depends on the level of certainty of evidence regarding risks and benefits, how these risks and benefits compare with potential alternatives, and what the comparative cost or cost-effectiveness of the diagnostic test would be.

For patients with AF, in addition to the EKG, pacemaker, implantable cardioverter defibrillator (ICD), and implantable loop recorders (ILR) have become valuable tools in diagnosing, quantification of AF burden, and evaluation of efficacy of different interventions for AF rate and rhythm control.

 CLINICAL PEARLS
The best way to confirm paroxysmal atrial fibrillation if strongly suspected In the Cryptogenic Stroke and Underlying AF (CRYSTAL AF) trial, paroxysmal atrial fibrillation (PAF) was detected by an ILR in 9% of patients at 6 months and more than 12% of patients at 12 months compared with 1.4% and 2% of patients, respectively, who were monitored by conventional methods [6].

An echocardiogram provides useful information about LVEF, valvular disease, and atrial size. Transesophageal echocardiography (TEE) plays a central role in the management of AF, particularly when sinus rhythm is contemplated, and LAA thrombus presence needs to be excluded to reduce the risk of thromboembolism during or after cardioversion (Table 8.3).

Table 8.3 Evaluation of patients with atrial fibrillation

History
Pattern (paroxysmal, persistent, longstanding persistent, or permanent)
  symptoms
  prior treatment
  Determination of its cause
  Review of associated cardiac and extracardiac disease
  Identify potentially reversible risk factors
  Assess thromboembolic risk
  Family history

Physical exam
  Signs suggesting AF: irregular pulse, irregular jugular venous pulsations, and variation in the intensity of the first heart sound
  Signs suggestive of valvular heart disease

ECG
  Diagnosis
  Atrial enlargement on sinus rhythm electrocardiogram
  Left ventricular hypertrophy
  Accessory pathway
  Identify evidence of coronary artery disease

Chest X-ray
  Cardiac size
  Identify pulmonary disease

(continued)

Table 8.3 (*Continued*)

Blood chemistry
Blood count
Serum electrolytes
Renal function
Liver function
Thyroid function

Transthoracic echocardiography
Assess left ventricular function
Identify underlying structural heart disease
Measure atrial size

Transesophageal echocardiography
Identify left atrial thrombi and guide timing of cardioversion
Identify high risk features for thrombus formation
Identify underlying structural heart disease

Holter monitor/Event monitor/Implantable loop recorder
Diagnose and evaluate of AF burden
Assess ventricular rate

Treadmill test
Identify coronary artery disease
Diagnose exercise induced AF
Assess ventricular rate during exercise

Electrophysiology study
Identify and ablate supraventricular tachycardias triggering AF
Ablation of atrial flutter
Ablation of AF

ACUTE MANAGEMENT

The management of AF includes prevention of thromboembolic events, selection of rhythm control or rate control, pharmacological or invasive conversion, and ablation. These options should be discussed in details with patients and family. A well-informed patient should ask about treatment options and question the success, failure or complication of the proposed treatment.

Strategic mapping

The three goals in the acute management of AF are: [1] symptom control; [2] restoration of adequate cardiac function; and [3] prevention of thromboembolic events. The urgency and type of intervention are dictated by the severity of hemodynamic compromise. Different strategies can be undertaken including rate or rhythm control. Duration of AF as well as anticoagulation status of the patient should be taken into consideration when rhythm control strategy is selected. If the patient is hemodynamically unstable and AF is believed to play a major role in the instability, emergent cardioversion should be performed urgently.

Stroke prevention   Unfractionated heparin (UFH) and low molecular weight heparin (LMWH) are usually initiated in the acute setting. Vitamin K antagonist (VKA) may be initiated concomitantly as it takes a few days to reach a target International Normalized Ratio (INR) of 2–3. Novel anticoagulants (NOAC) have a quick onset of action and have become a very good alternative to VKA in appropriate patients.

Acute rate control   Intravenous beta-blockers (esmolol, propranolol, and metoprolol) and non-dihydropyridine receptor calcium channel blockers (CCB) (verapamil and diltiazem) are effective in reducing the heart rate in the acute setting. Beta-blockers block the sympathetic tone while non-dihydropyridine receptor CCB have a direct effect on slowing AV nodal conduction through the blockade of L-type calcium channels. Oral formulations of these medications may be used in the acute setting if the heart rate does not require rapid decrease. Suggested dosages of these agents are listed in Table 8.4.

 CLINICAL PEARLS
How to select medications for acute rate control of atrial fibrillation Non-dihydropyridine receptor calcium channel blockers (CCB) (e.g. intravenous cardiazem) are the first drug of choice if the blood pressure is stable. Non-dihydropyridine receptor CCB should not be used in patient with decompensated HF as this may lead to further decompensation due to their inotropic negative effects. **Beta-blockers** and non-dihydropyridine receptor CCB are contraindicated in AF with antegrade conduction over an accessory pathway (Wolff-Parkinson-White syndrome) as the AV nodal conduction slowing would favor ventricular activation over the accessory pathway and would a trigger rapid ventricular response. In patients with severe structural disease, intravenous **digoxin and amiodarone** may also be used; however they are less effective and

Table 8.4 Drugs for acute and chronic rate control in atrial fibrillation

Drug	Route/dose	Comments
Beta-blockers		
Metoprolol	IV 2.5–5.0 mg bolus over 2 min; up to 3 doses (tartrate)	Bradycardia
	Oral 25–100 mg twice daily (tartrate)	Heart block
		Hypotension
	Oral 50–400 mg once daily (succinate)	Depression
		Fatigue
		Erectile dysfunction
Atenolol	Oral 25–100 mg once daily	
Esmolol	IV 500 mcg/kg bolus over 1 min, then 50–300 mcg/kg/min	
Propranolol	IV 1 mg over 1 min, up to 3 doses at 2 min intervals	
	10-40 mg three to four times daily	
Nadolol	Oral 10–240 mg daily	
Carvedilol	Oral 3.125–25 mg every 12 hours	
Bisoprolol	Oral 2.5–10 mg once daily	
Calcium channel blockers		
Verapamil	IV (0.07–0.15 mg/kg) bolus over 2 min, may give an additional 10.0 mg after 30 min if no response, then 0.005 mg/kg/min infusion	Bradycardia
		Heart block
		Hypotension
		Depression
	Oral 180–480 mg once daily (extended release)	Fatigue
		Inotrope negative – do not use in heart failure
Diltiazem	IV 0.25 mg/kg bolus over 2 min, then 5–15 mg/h	
	Oral 120–360 mg once daily (extended release)	
Digitalis glycoside		
Digitalis	IV 0.25 mg with repeat dosing to a maximum of 1.5 mg over 24 hours	Control heart rate at rest
		Contraindicated in renal failure
	Oral 0.125–0.25 mg once daily	
Class III anti-arrhythmic		
Amiodarone	IV 150 mg over 10 min, then 1 mg/min for 6 hours, then 0.5 mg/min for 18 hours	Hypotension
		bradycardia
		phlebitis (when used intravenously)
	Oral 100–200 mg once daily	Second line due to side-effects

have a delayed effect. There are data suggesting that digoxin increases risk. The onset of action of digoxin is after an hour with a peak at 6 hours. Amiodarone has an onset of action after several hours.

If patients develop bradycardia upon receiving the medication to control the HR, withholding the medications may suffice. If the patient becomes symptomatic, a temporary pacemaker wire may be needed. Sometimes, when there is hemodynamic compromise, emergent cardioversion may be required.

Acute rhythm control   Frequently, the AF episodes terminate themselves spontaneously. However, in patients with hemodynamic compromise despite rate control or when rhythm control strategy is pursued, pharmacologic or direct current cardioversion (DCCV) may be used. Although less effective than DCCV, pharmacologic cardioversion has the advantage of not requiring sedation. In either case, measures to avoid a thromboembolic event should be implemented.

CLINICAL PEARLS
Anticoagulation for pharmacologic or electrical cardioversion If duration of AF is <48 hours, start anticoagulation and proceed with cardioversion (UFH or LMWH). If the duration of AF is >48 hours or unknown, a trans-esophageal echocardiography (TEE) should be performed to exclude LAA thrombus prior to cardioversion and proceed to cardioversion only in the absence of detectable thrombus. Alternatively, patients should be anticoagulated with VKA in therapeutic range for at least 3 weeks before attempting cardioversion if TEE is not desired. NOACs appear safe for cardioversion but are not currently Federal Drug Agency (FDA) approved for cardioversion (see discussion below).

Direct current cardioversion   DCCV represents the delivery of an electrical shock synchronized with the QRS complex. Appropriate anticoagulation should be employed around the time of cardioversion to minimize the risk of thromboembolic events. DCCV is not a completely benign procedure and there are associated potential risks: thromboembolism, sedation-related complications, ventricular tachycardia and fibrillation, bradyarrhythmias, skin burns or irritation from electrodes, muscle soreness, and device function alterations.

 CLINICAL PEARLS
Tips for a successful direct current cardioversion
Before proceeding with elective cardioversion, digoxin toxicity or severe hypokalemia should be excluded and electrolyte imbalances should be corrected. If DCCV fails after multiple attempts with the electrodes in anterolateral position, the electrodes could be repositioned on the antero-posterior axis (front and back). An initial high energy shock is more effective and may reduce the number of shocks required and duration of sedation. Anti-arrhythmic drugs could be administered early to facilitate electrical cardioversion or if the initial shocks fails.

Pharmacologic cardioversion A number of class IC and III anti-arrhythmic drugs are effective in restoring sinus rhythm or facilitate restoration by cardioversion. They are listed in Table 8.5.

Ibutilide has a success rate of sinus conversion in approximatively 50% and pretreatment improves the efficacy of electrical cardioversion [7–9]. The major risk is QT prolongation and subsequent ensuing of polymorphic VT/torsades de pointes in up to 3–4% of patients. The later may be mitigated by preadministration of high doses of intravenous magnesium sulfate [10]. Therefore, pharmacologic cardioversion should be performed in a monitored setting for up to 4 hours after administration and with connected defibrillator pads on and resuscitative equipment in the room. Ibutilide should be avoided in patients with hypokalemia, prolonged QT, and with LVEF <30% [7]. Intravenous **amiodarone** may be used for cardioversion of AF, but the effect may be delayed [11,12].

Dofetilide is moderately effective in cardioversion of AF to sinus rhythm [13]. The main side-effect is QT prolongation and consequent proarrhythmia. Dofetilide is initiated in the hospital setting so the QT interval could be monitored for the first five doses. Dosage is based on creatinine clearance and corrected QT duration. Every prescriber should complete an educational program and register the Tikosyn® (dofetilide) prescriber certification form with Pfizer prior to prescribing dofetilide.

Table 8.5 Drugs for pharmacologic cardioversion of atrial fibrillation

Drug	Route/dose	Potential side-effects	Monitor
Class IC anti-arrhythmic			
Flecainide	Oral 200–300 mg once	Hypotension Atrial flutter with 1:1 AV conduction Ventricular proarrhythmia Avoid in patients with CAD and significant structural heart disease	Blood pressure Heart rate
Propafenone	Oral 450–600 mg once	Hypotension Atrial flutter with 1:1 AV conduction Ventricular proarrhythmia Avoid in patients with CAD and significant structural heart disease	Blood pressure Heart rate
Class III anti-arrhythmic			
Ibutilide	IV 1 mg over 10 minutes; may repeat 1 mg once if necessary (weight <60 kg use 0.01 mg/kg)	Hypotension QT prolongation Torsades de pointes	Blood pressure QT interval Electrolytes
Amiodarone	IV 150 mg over 10 min, then 1 mg/min for 6 hours, then 0.5 mg/min for 18 hours	Hypotension Bradycardia Phlebitis	Blood pressure Heart rate
Dofetilide	CrCl (mL/min) Oral >60: 500 mcg BID 40–60: 250 mcg BID 20–40: 125 mcg BID <20: not recommended	QT prolongation Torsades de pointes; Adjust dose for renal function, body size, and age	QT interval Rhythm Electrolytes Renal function Drug interactions

AV: atrioventricular; CAD: coronary artery disease; CrCl: creatinine clearance.

'Pill-in-the-pocket' strategy The class IC AADs (**flecainide or propafenone**) may be used in a single dose 'pill-in-the-pocket' strategy to restore sinus rhythm in patients with symptomatic and infrequent episodes of AF at the onset of an episode [14, 15]. The single dose should be preceded by at least 30 minutes dose of beta-blocker or non-dihydropyridine CCB to prevent atrial flutter with rapid 1:1 ventricular response. This approach can be taken in an unmonitored outpatient setting after an initial trial in the inpatient setting to ensure there is no proarrhythmic response or bradycardia due to sinus or AV node dysfunction.

Prevention of thromboembolic events For patient with AF, it is paramount to determine the risk of stroke in each patient and anticoagulate patients at high risk. The current guidelines recommend using the CHA2DS2-VASc score for risk stratification (Table 8.6) [16].

A score of 2 or greater is an indication for anticoagulation while for a score of 0, aspirin or no anticoagulation are options with a preference for the later due to risk of bleeding from aspirin. For a score of 1 the indications are not as clearly defined (may use aspirin or oral anticoagulants). A discussion with the patient should be undertaken to determine the best strategy. The results of a study by Chao et al. when the score = 1 is presented below.

Table 8.6 **CHA2DS2-VASc score for stroke risk stratification**

CHA2DS2-VASc acronym	Points	Score	Adjusted stroke rate (%/year)
Congestive heart failure	1	0	0%
Hypertension	1	1	1.3%
Age ≥75 years	2	2	2.2%
Diabetes mellitus	1	3	3.2%
Stroke/TIA/TE	2	4	4.0%
Vascular disease (prior MI, PAD, or aortic plaque)	1	5	6.7%
Age 65–74 years	1	6	9.8%
Sex category (female)	1	7	9.6%
		8	6.7%
		9	15.2%

TIA: transient ischemic attack; TE: thromboembolism; MI: myocardial infarction; PAD: peripheral arterial disease.

CRITICAL THINKING
Risk of stroke when CHA2DS2-VASc score = 1 In a review of data of 12,935 males with a CHA2DS2-VASc score of 1 and 7900 females with a CHA2DS2-VASc score of 2 who were not receiving anti-platelet or anticoagulant drugs, the risk of ischemic stroke and the impact of different component risk factors were investigated. The results showed that among 12,935 male AF patients with a CHA2DS2-VASc score of 1, 1858 patients (14.4%) experienced ischemic stroke during the follow-up of 5.2 ± 4.3 years, with an annual stroke rate of 2.75%. The risk of ischemic stroke ranged from 1.96%/year for AF patients with vascular disease to 3.50%/year for those aged 65–74 years. For AF females with a CHA2DS2-VASc score of 2, 14.9% of them experienced ischemic stroke with an annual stroke rate of 2.55%. The risk of ischemic stroke increased from 1.91%/year for patients with HTN to 3.34%/year for those aged 65–74 years.

One statistical caveat: In this review, the patients aged >74 were excluded because they had CHA2DS2-VASc score = or >2. Therefore, the conclusion of this study could only apply to patients younger than 75.

In real world practice, oral anticoagulants should be considered for AF patients with one additional stroke risk factor (i.e. CHA2DS2-VASc score of 1 (males) or 2 (females)) given their high risk of ischemic stroke [17].

CLINICAL PEARLS
Anticoagulants for Asian patients Because of the high rate of stroke and intra-cranial bleeding, the Japanese guidelines give optional treatments with oral anticoagulants for patients with CHA2DS-VASc = 1 at age 65–74 or if there is vascular disease [18].

Predicting the bleeding risk   Although the CHA2DS2-VASc score calculation is great for predicting the risk of stroke, it was not accurate in predicting the risk of bleeding so the **HAS-BLED scoring system** was designed to predict the bleeding risks (Table 8.7). A score ≥3 is considered a high risk for bleeding [19].

The HAS-BLED score per se should not be used to exclude patients from antithrombotic therapy; rather, it indicates caution, requests efforts to

Table 8.7 HAS-BLED Risk Score

Letter	Clinical parameter	Points
H	Hypertension (systolic blood pressure >160 mmHg)	1
A	Abnormal renal or liver function (1 point each)	1 or 2
S	Stroke	1
B	Bleeding	1
L	Labile INRs	1
E	Elderly age (>65 years)	1
D	Drugs or alcohol (1 point each)	1 or 2

correct the potentially reversible risk factors for bleeding, and encourages a regular review of the patients following the initiation of antithrombotic therapy [20].

Once the patient has indications for treatment, the available antithrombotic agents are listed in Table 8.8. UFH and LMWH are typically used in the acute setting and for bridging before and after procedures that require OAC drugs discontinuation.

Aspirin does not reduce the risk of stroke; even aspirin plus clopidogrel is superior to aspirin alone in patients with AF who were unsuitable for oral anticoagulation and who had ≥1 stroke risk factor. However, warfarin was superior to the combination of aspirin and clopidogrel [21]. Three new anticoagulants recently approved by the FDA include direct thrombin inhibitor (dabigatran) and factor Xa inhibitors (rivoraxaban and apixaban). Their beneficial effects were evidenced in the RE-LY, ROCKET-AF and ARISTOTLE trials [22–24].

CLINICAL PEARLS
Discriminative selection of NOACs and warfarin
Among all four NOACs, all decreased stroke compared to warfarin; however, apixaban decreased the most (37%). Apixaban and edoxaban had lowest rate of major bleeding (0.63%). Rivaroxaban also has a good safety profile, but the incidence of major bleeding is similar, but not inferior, to that of warfarin [25]. However this information is from historical data, not head-to-head comparisons. The types of bleeding seen with NOACs are less serious than of warfarin. There is less intracranial hemorrhage with NOACs (0.2% to 0.35%) or 2 or 3 out of 1000 patients. Significant bleeding is very unusual [26]. Edoxaban and

rivaroxaban also have the advantage of once-daily dosage while the other two have BID dosage. These more frequent dosages may affect a patient's compliance which ultimately affects the efficacy of treatment in the real world, independent of the conclusions from clinical trials [27].

Anticoagulants for cardioversion   Warfarin was the standard of care drug for cardioversion. None of the NOACs are FDA approved for cardioversion. However, subgroup analyses of all three NOACs support

Table 8.8 Antithrombotic and anticoagulants for stroke prevention

Drug	Route/dose	Comments
Heparin products		
UFH	IV Bolus of 50–100 units/kg (maximum: 4000 units), then 12 units/kg/hour (maximum: 1000 units/hour) as continuous infusion. Check aPTT every 4–6 hours; adjust to target of 50–70 seconds.	May cause skin necrosis May lead to HIT
LMWH	SQ 1 mg/kg every 12 hours	Not approved for use in patient on dialysis May lead to HIT Use with caution in elderly and low weight patients Does not clearly defined in obese patients
Antiplatelets		
Aspirin	Oral 81–325 mg once daily	Avoid use in severe liver disease
Clopidogrel	Oral 75 mg once daily	Usually in combination with aspirin
Vitamin K antagonists		
Warfarin	Oral dose adjustment based on INR	Multiple food interactions Multiple drug interactions

(continued)

Table 8.8 (*Continued*)

Drug	Route/dose	Comments
Direct thrombin inhibitors		
Dabigatran	Oral 150 mg every 12 hours Oral 75 mg every 12 hours if CrCl 15 mL/min–30 mL/min	Intestinal absorption reduced in patients taking PPIs Increased risk of bleeding in patients taking verapamil, amiodarone, quinidine, ketoconazole Not approved for CrCl <15 mL/minute or patients on dialysis Premature discontinuation increases the risk of thrombotic events
Factor Xa inhibitors		
Rivoraxaban	Oral 20 mg once daily Oral 15 mg once daily if CrCl 30 mL/min–49 mL/min	Take with food Not approved for CrCl <15 mL/minute or patients on dialysis Avoid use in moderate-to-severe hepatic impairment Not approved for prosthetic heart valves or significant rheumatic heart disease Premature discontinuation increases the risk of thrombotic events
Apixaban	Oral 5 mg every 12 hours Oral 2.5 mg every 12 hours (Patients ≥2 of the following conditions: ≥80 years of age, weight ≤60 kg, or a serum creatinine level ≥1.5 mg/dL)	Not approved for CrCl <25 mL/minute or patients on dyalisis Not approved for prosthetic heart valves or significant rheumatic heart disease Avoid use in severe hepatic impairment Premature discontinuation increases the risk of thrombotic events

UFH: unfractionated heparin; HIT: Heparin induced thrombocytopenia; LMWH: low molecular weight heparin; INR: international normalized ratio; PPI: proton pump inhibitor; CrCl: creatinine clearance.

Table 8.9 Efficacy and risk of NOACs

RELY	Dabigatran	Dabigatran	Warfarin
Stroke	1.5	1.11	1.69
Major bleeding	2.7	3.1	3.4
ROCKET AF	**Rivaroxaban**	**Warfarin**	**P**
Stroke	1.7	2.4	
Major bleeding	3.6	3.4	
ARISTOTLE	**Apixaban**	**Warfarin**	**P**
Stroke	1.27	1.6	
Major bleeding	4.07	6.01	
ENGAGE TIMI 48	**Edoxaban**	**Edoxaban**	**Warfarin**
Stroke	1.57	1.8	
Major bleeding	2.75	3.43	

their safety in patients receiving long-term anticoagulation (>3 weeks) around the time of cardioversion.

CHRONIC MANAGEMENT

Strategic mapping

The four goals in long term management of AF are:

1 Symptom control.

2 Stroke prevention.

3 Prevention of tachycardia induced cardiomyopathy.

4 Reduction in hospitalizations.

The strategy for chronic management of AF is largely dictated by symptoms. Patients that have minimal or no symptoms due to AF may be managed with a rate control strategy; however for young patients or due to patient's preference, or intolerance (inconvenience with drugs or anticoagulants) the patients should explore the option of rhythm control. For patients that are highly symptomatic, a strategy aimed at restoring and maintaining sinus rhythm should be used.

Rate control by medications The first line and most frequent medications are beta-blockers followed by non-dihydropyridine receptor calcium channel blockers (verapamil and diltiazem). Oral BB and non-dihydropyridine receptor calcium channel blockers are effective in reducing the heart rate in an outpatient setting. Digoxin is effective only in reducing the resting heart rate and should be reserved for patients that have concomitant reduced LVEF due to additional mild positive inotropic effect. Amiodarone is used as a second line agent for rate control due to its side-effects and interaction with other medications. Patients on amiodarone should be monitored periodically for side-effects. Both digoxin and amiodarone can be used in combination with BBs and CCBs.

Invasive rate control with AV node ablation and pacemaker
Patients with difficult medical rate control may benefit from pacemaker implant and AV node ablation [28]. This allows regularization of the ventricular rate and therefore no rate control medications are needed. However, continuation of oral anticoagulation is necessary according with the CHA2DS2-VASc score. This strategy should be in particular reserved for tachycardia-induced cardiomyopathy or elderly patients that are refractory to medical rate control as this leads to lifelong pacemaker dependency. Whenever possible, AV node ablation should be performed 4–6 weeks after pacemaker implant to ensure proper function of the pacemaker and proper healing without infection. Pacemaker malfunction, lead dislodgement, and/or infection can lead to catastrophic consequences. The initial rate of the pacemaker should be set at 90–100 bpm and then gradually decreased because sudden decrease after AV node ablation was reported to be associated with sudden cardiac death due to torsades de pointes or VF [29]. Finally, since RV pacing may lead to depression of LVEF, biventricular pacing should be considered in any patient with LVEF<50%, or an upgrade to biventricular pacing should be considered whenever there is a decline in LVEF [30].

Long-term rhythm control   Three strategies are employed to achieve long-term rhythm control: anti-arrhythmic drugs, catheter-based ablation, and surgical or hybrid ablation.

Anti-arrhythmic drugs (AAA) for maintenance of sinus rhythm
AADs are used to restore and maintain sinus rhythm (Table 8.10) and as a consequence, to reduce symptoms and hospitalizations. AADs have modest efficacy in maintaining sinus rhythm and drug-induced proarrhythmia or extra-cardiac side-effects are frequent. Therefore, safety rather than efficacy considerations should primarily guide the choice of an AAD and they should not be used in asymptomatic patients. Clinically, anti-arrhythmic drugs may only reduce the frequency and severity of AF episodes. Drugs should be tailored to individual patients and if one agent fails it is acceptable to use another one. The most effective drugs are class IC and III anti-arrhythmics but other classes may be used in select patients depending on suspected AF mechanism and co-morbidities (Table 8.10).

Table 8.10 Drugs for maintenance of sinus rhythm

Drug	Route/dose	Potential side-effects	Monitor
Class IA anti-arrhythmic			
Disopyramide	Oral 100–200 mg once every 6 hours (immediate release) 200–400 mg once every 12 hours (extended release)	QT prolongation HF Prostatism Glaucoma	QT interval LVEF
Quinidine	Oral 324–648 mg once every 8 hours	QT prolongation Diarrhea	QT interval
Class IC anti-arrhythmic			
Flecainide	Oral 50–200 mg once every 12 hours	Hypotension Atrial flutter with 1:1 AV conduction Ventricular proarrhythmia Avoid in patients with CAD and significant structural heart disease	Blood pressure Heart rate QRS duration at peak heart rate
Propafenone	Oral 150–300 mg once every 8 hours (immediate release) 225–425 mg once every 12 hours (extended release)	Hypotension Atrial flutter with 1:1 AV conduction Ventricular proarrhythmia Avoid in patients with CAD and significant structural heart disease	Blood pressure Heart rate QRS duration at peak heart rate
Class III anti-arrhythmic			
Amiodarone	Oral 600–800 mg daily in divided doses to a total load of up to 10 g, then 200 mg daily as maintenance	Pulmonary Gastrointestinal Thyroid (hypo- and hyperthyroidism) Neurologic Skin Cardiac Genitourinary	TSH LFTs CXR PFTs Ophthalmologic exam
Dronaderone	Oral 400 mg once every 12 hours	Bradycardia Heart failure Long-standing persistent AF/flutter Liver disease Prolonged QT interval	LFTs QT interval ECG LVEF
Sotalol	Oral 40–160 mg once every 12 hours	Bradycardia QT prolongation	QT interval Renal function

(continued)

Table 8.10 *(Continued)*

Drug	Route/dose	Potential side-effects	Monitor
Dofetilide	CrCl (ml/min) >60 500 mcg BID 40–60 250 mcg BID 20–40 125 mcg BID <20 not recommended	QT prolongation Torsades de pointes; adjust dose for renal function, body size, and age	QT interval Rhythm Electrolytes Renal function Drug interactions

AV: Atrioventricular; CAD: coronary artery disease; CXR: Chest X-ray; EKG: electro-cardiogram; LFTs: Liver function tests; LVEF: Left ventricular ejection fraction; PFTs: pulmonary function tests; TSH: Thyroid stimulating hormone.

Class Ia AAD have a very limited use for rhythm control. Disopyramide is a sodium channel blocker with potent anticholinergic effect. Disopyramide was shown to reduce AF recurrence after electrical cardioversion [31], and may be useful in AF that occurs in the setting of high vagal tone ('vagally mediated AF'), such as sleep, and in hypertrophic cardiomyopathy associated with dynamic outflow tract obstruction [34] due to its negative inotropic effects. It should be avoided in structural heart disease.

CLINICAL PEARLS
Discriminating selection of anti-arrhythmic drugs for maintenance of sinus rhythm

Flecainide and propafenone are effective in restoring and maintaining sinus rhythm [32]. They should not be used in patients with structural heart disease or CAD. QRS duration should be monitored at peak heart rate as widening QRS complex at peak heart rate of more than 25% compared to baseline may increase the risk of proarrhythmia.

Amiodarone has blocking effects on multiple ion channels. Amiodarone is the most effective anti-arrhythmic drug for maintenance of sinus rhythm in patients with paroxysmal or persistent AF but also has the most side-effects [33]. Patients on amiodarone should be inquired at each visit about side-effects (hypothyroidism, pulmonary (dyspnea, cough, or pleuritic chest pain; new interstitial or alveolar infiltrate), etc and should be carefully monitored. Dronedarone is a structural analogue to amiodarone. It lacks the iodine moieties, and therefore has fewer side-effects than amiodarone, but is also less efficacious [34]. It is contraindicated in HF.

Sotalol is a potassium channel and beta-blocker that has moderate effectiveness in maintaining sinus rhythm [1]. Sotalol prolongs the QT interval and this should be monitored. It is renally cleared and should be used with caution or avoided in patients with CKD or unstable renal function.

Dofetilide is a potassium channel blocker that is moderately effective in maintaining sinus rhythm. Dofetilide is initiated in the patient and QT should be monitored, as excessive prolongation may lead to torsades de pointes.

INVASIVE MANAGEMENT

Catheter ablation Catheter ablation of AF is indicated for select patients that have symptomatic AF. Catheter ablation of AF was shown in numerous studies to be superior to anti-arrhythmic drugs. There is a substantial body of literature defining the safety and efficacy of catheter ablation of AF. Therefore, the 2012 Heart Rhythm Society/European Heart Rhythm Association/European Cardiac Arrhythmia Society (HRS/EHRA/ECAS) Expert Consensus Statement on Catheter and Surgical Ablation of Atrial Fibrillation no longer requires refractoriness or intolerance to at least one Class 1 or 3 anti-arrhythmic medication as a primary indication of catheter ablation for patients with symptomatic AF [35]. The approach to catheter-based ablation of AF depends on the duration of AF (paroxysmal, persistent, longstanding persistent) and other variables (atrial size, LVEF, etc.).

Ablation of pulmonary veins Ablation of paroxysmal AF is predicated on the presence of a trigger. The presence of a trigger was substantiated by the landmark observation by Haissaguerre and colleagues that AF is often initiated by a focal source originating from the pulmonary veins (PVs) and that ablation of that focal trigger can eliminate AF [36]. The anatomical substrate for the PV trigger is constituted by myocardial muscle fibers that extend 1 to 3 cm from the left atrium (LA) into all the PVs [37–39]. Isolation of the trigger by creating a lesion encircling the PV constitutes the basis for the catheter-based ablation of AF [44]. Two modalities are employed for paroxysmal AF ablation: point by point radiofrequency (RF) ablation or circumferential lesions with the cryoballoon. Cryoballoon ablation appears to be as effective as RF ablation for paroxysmal AF ablation [40].

In a meta-analysis by Parker et al. the efficacy and effectiveness of catheter ablation versus AAD showed that AF reduced the recurrence of atrial arrhythmias by 71% (RR 0.29, 95% CI 0.20–0.41, $P < 0.00001$, with random effects model) at one year. There were 23.2% patients in AF ablation group and 76.6% patients in the control group that had recurrence of atrial tachyarrhythmia. There were fewer complications and adverse events reported in the ablation group compared with the control group (RR 0.72, 95% CI 0.40–1.30, $P = 0.28$, with a random effects model) [41].

Typically, AF is a progressive disease. Progression from paroxysmal AF to persistent and longstanding persistent AF is accompanied by multiple changes at molecular, cellular, and atrial level. Therefore, the strategy for persistent and longstanding persistent AF ablation involves more extensive ablation and results are lower than for paroxysmal AF. If a catheter ablation is determined to be the best strategy for a particular patient, it is recommended that the patient be referred to an electrophysiologist early in the disease process to obtain optimal results.

Surgical MAZE ablation   The basis for more extensive ablation in persistent and longstanding persistent AF is the multiple random propagating wavelets theory. This is based on the hypothesis that AF is due to multiple independent wavelets occurring simultaneously and propagating randomly throughout the left and right atria [42]. AF maintenance requires a minimum number of wavelets occurring at the same. For this to happen, slowed conduction, shortened refractory periods, and increased atrial mass are necessary. These factors contribute to AF maintenance by enhancing spatial dispersion of refractoriness which promotes heterogeneous conduction delay and block. This theory has led to the development of the surgical Maze procedure [43, 44]. The lesion set of the surgical Maze procedure is aimed at reducing the critical excitable mass of atrial tissue that can support the minimal number of circulating wavelets necessary to maintain AF. Subsequently, some of the surgical Maze procedure lesions were adopted in various iterations in catheter-based ablation of persistent and longstanding persistent AF ablation. There is no good agreement in the EP community on the optimal strategy for persistent and longstanding persistent AF ablation.

Catheter-based ablation of AF is associated with important risks of major complications (4.5%): 1.3% rate of cardiac tamponade, 0.94% rate of stroke or TIA, a 0.04% rate of atrial-esophageal fistula, and a 0.15% rate of death [45–48]. The indications for ablation are listed in Table 8.11.

Table 8.11 Indications for catheter based and surgical ablation of AF

Class I

AF catheter ablation is useful for symptomatic paroxysmal AF refractory or intolerant to at least 1 class I or III anti-arrhythmic medication when a rhythm control strategy is desired.

Class IIa

AF **catheter ablation** is reasonable for selected patients with symptomatic persistent AF refractory or intolerant to at least 1 class I or III anti-arrhythmic medication.

In patients with recurrent symptomatic paroxysmal AF, **catheter ablation** is a reasonable initial rhythm control strategy prior to therapeutic trials of anti-arrhythmic drug therapy, after weighing risks and outcomes of drug and ablation therapy.

An AF **surgical ablation** procedure is reasonable for selected patients with AF undergoing cardiac surgery for other indications.

Class IIb

AF **catheter ablation** may be considered for symptomatic longstanding (>12 months) persistent AF refractory or intolerant to at least 1 class I or III anti-arrhythmic medication, when a rhythm control strategy is desired.

AF **catheter ablation** may be considered prior to initiation of anti-arrhythmic drug therapy with a class I or III anti-arrhythmic medication for symptomatic persistent AF, when a rhythm control strategy is desired.

A stand-alone AF **surgical ablation** procedure may be reasonable for selected patients with highly symptomatic AF not well-managed with other approaches.

Class III: Harm

AF catheter ablation should not be performed in patients who cannot be treated with anticoagulant therapy during and following the procedure.

AF catheter ablation to restore sinus rhythm should not be performed with the sole intent of obviating the need for anticoagulation.

MANAGEMENT OF COMPLEX PROBLEMS OR HIGH-RISK PATIENT SUBSETS

Selection of NOACs for patients with high risk of bleeding   As all anticoagulants carry a risk of bleeding so the risk of stroke should be balanced against the risk of bleeding. This is why the selection of an antithrombotic agent needs to take in consideration of clinical factors, clinician's, patient's preference and cost. Warfarin has a delayed onset of action, has numerous interactions with other medications and food, and requires repeated INR testing. However, it is very inexpensive, there is an agent for reversal, and compliance can be verified. The NOACs have rapid onset/offset of action, have more predictable pharmacology, fewer drug interactions, less major bleeding, and do not require monitoring. They are significantly more expensive, and compliance is. There is no evidence to recommend one agent over another because the NOACs have never been compared in head-to-head trials difficult to monitor. Reversal agents of NOACs are now available.

Anticoagulants for patients with chronic kidney disease   Warfarin is the drug of choice for patients with severe CKD and ESRD patients on HD. None of the NOAC is approved for severe CKD or patients on HD.

Dose reduction for patients with high risk of bleeding   In the Effective aNticoaGulation with factor x: A next GEneration in Atrial Fibrillation (ENGAGE AF-TIMI 48) trial, a strategy of 50% dose reduction was used for patients who met 1 of 3 specified criteria: creatinine clearance of 30 to 50 mg/dL, weight ≤60 kg, and patients who were on potent P-glycoprotein inhibitors. The result of this dose reduction allowed for the preservation of efficacy (lowest rate of ischemic stroke) and enhancement of the safety profile (lowest rate of bleeding, mainly intra-cranial bleeding). The study randomized patients to warfarin, a higher dose of edoxaban, or a lower dose of edoxaban [49]. Dabigatran was FDA approved at a dose of 75 mg twice daily for those with low CrCl (15 mL/min to 30 mL/min) based on entirely on pharmacological modeling. Rivaroxaban dose should be reduced to 15 mg once daily for a CrCl between 15 mL/min–50 mL/min. Apixaban dose should be reduced to 2.5 mg twice daily for patients with ≥2 of the following conditions: ≥80 years of age, weight ≤60 kg, or a serum creatinine level ≥1.5 mg/dL

Treatment of bleeding caused by NOACs   Because of their relatively short half-lives, withholding the medication and providing supportive care is generally sufficient to ensure adequate hemostasis in cases of mild to moderate bleeding. For patients who have a life-threatening bleeding (intracranial or GI, etc.) or requiring urgent surgery, there are three options:

1 Prothrombin complex concentrates.

2 Hemodialysis.

3 Reversal agents.

Prothrombin complex concentrates   Administer 75 to 80 units/kg of activated prothrombin complex concentrate (aPCC) which contain significant amounts of clotting factors, including Factors II, VII, IX, and X. However, more studies are needed to clearly define the role of PCCs since the use of these agents can be complicated by thrombosis. Fresh frozen plasma has not been shown to be effective at reversing the effects of NOACs [50].

Hemodialysis   For patients with severe bleeding on long-term dabigatran, hemodialysis could remove 40% to 60% of dabigatran during a 4-hour session because dabigatran is 80% renally cleared [51]. In contrast, rivaroxaban and apixaban are both highly protein bound, so they cannot be removed by hemodialysis.

Reversal agents for NOACs   Idarucizumab (Praxbind by Boehringer Ingelheim Pharmaceuticals Inc Ridgefield CT) is a reversal agent recently approved for patients taking Pradaxa (Boehringer Ingelheim Pharmaceuticals Inc Ridgefield CT) in emergency or life-threatening situations when bleeding could not be controlled. Praxbind is given intravenously and its effect lasts for at least 24 hours. The anticoagulant effect of Pradaxa was fully reversed in 89% of patients within four hours of receiving Praxbind. The most common side-effects of Prabind are low potassium (hypokalemia), confusion, constipation, fever and pneumonia. Reversing the effect of Pradaxa exposes patients to the risk of blood clots and stroke from their underlying disease (such as atrial fibrillation). Patients should resume their anticoagulant therapy as soon as medically appropriate [52].

Risk of bleeding with triple therapy: NOACs and P2Y12 inhibitors after DES   There are two ways to solve the problems of increased bleeding with NOACS and P2Y12 inhibitors:

1 Remove ASA as in the WOEST trial [53]. The results showed less bleeding.

2 Shorten to 6 weeks triple therapy instead of 6 months as in the Triple Therapy in Patients on Oral Anticoagulation After Drug Eluting Stent Implantation (ISAR-TRIPLE) trial [54].

In this randomized, open-label trial, 614 patients receiving OAC and ASA who underwent DES implantation were randomized to either 6-week clopidogrel therapy ($n = 307$) or 6-month clopidogrel therapy ($n = 307$). The primary endpoint was a composite of death, myocardial infarction (MI), definite stent thrombosis, stroke, or Thrombolysis In Myocardial Infarction (TIMI) major bleeding at 9 months. The results showed that the primary endpoint occurred in 30 patients (9.8%) in the 6-week group compared with 27 patients (8.8%) in the 6-month group (hazard ratio [HR]: 1.14; 95% CI: 0.68 to 1.91; $P = 0.63$). There were no significant differences for the secondary combined ischemic endpoint of cardiac death, MI, definite stent thrombosis, and ischemic stroke (12 [4.0%] vs. 13 [4.3%]; HR: 0.93; 95% CI: 0.43 to 2.05; $P = 0.87$) or the secondary bleeding endpoint of TIMI major bleeding (16 [5.3%] vs. 12 [4.0%]; HR: 1.35; 95% CI: 0.64 to 2.84; $P = 0.44$). So the conclusion is that six weeks of triple therapy was not superior to 6 months with respect to net clinical outcomes. These results suggest that physicians should weigh the trade-off between ischemic and bleeding risk when choosing the shorter or longer duration of triple therapy [54].

Dabigatran in patients with DAPT   In a post-hoc analysis from the RE-LY trial [55] concomitant antiplatelet therapy (single or double) did not affect the relative advantages of dabigatran in comparison with warfarin, but led to a significant increase in the overall risk of major bleeding when combined with any treatment arm. The risk appeared to increase by 50% when a single antiplatelet agent was combined with either warfarin or dabigatran, and it was doubled with DAPT. However, the lowest absolute risks were noted for patients receiving dabigatran 110 mg twice daily.

For **apixaban and rivaroxaban**, data on the association with DAPT derive from randomized clinical trials in the setting of ACS/PCI: for apixaban, the dosage used for these patients in the APPRAISE-2 trial was the same used in AF trials (5 mg twice daily) [56] while for rivaroxaban, the dosage was 2- to 4-fold lower (2.5 to 5.0 mg twice daily vs. 15 to 20 mg once daily).

Ticagrelor and prasugrel instead of clopidogrel are now the preferred choices, on top of aspirin alone, in patients with ACS. There are insufficient data about any of these drugs in the setting of a combination therapy with aspirin and an OAC or with an OAC alone.

The role of NOACs in the management of patients requiring DAPT will be likely clarified after the availability of data from four upcoming large-scale randomized clinical trials testing multiple antithrombotic regimens: RE-DUAL PCI for dabigatran (NCT02164864, enrolling), PIONEER AF-PCI for rivaroxaban (NCT01830543, enrolling), EVOLVE AF-PCI for edoxaban (announced), and AUGUSTUS for apixaban (announced) [57].

NOACs in patient receiving NSAID   In the RE-LY trial, the use of non-steroidal anti-inflammatory drugs was linked to increased bleeding risk and a higher rate of hospitalizations. Patients with AF who used NSAIDs reaped similar relative benefits as non-users with dabigatran (Pradaxa, Boehringer Ingelheim) vs. warfarin. The mortality ($P = .2109$), intracranial hemorrhage ($P = .3631$) and MI ($P = .6674$) rates were similar between groups; NSAID users demonstrated greater risk for major bleeding ($P < .0001$), particularly major gastrointestinal bleeding ($P = .0004$), as well as life-threatening bleeding ($P = .0103$) and any bleeding ($P < .0001$). Additionally, NSAID users were hospitalized more frequently ($P < .0001$). Further, the lowest absolute numbers for any bleeds were observed with DE 110 mg [58].

Left atrial appendage occlusion in AF   The meta-analysis from the WATCHMAN Left Atrial Appendage Closure (LAAC) Device for Embolic PROTECTion in Patients with Atrial Fibrillation (PROTECT) AF and Prospective Randomized Evaluation of the WATCHMAN™ LAA Closure Device in Patients With Atrial Fibrillation Versus Long Term Warfarin Therapy (PREVAIL) randomized controlled trials compared left atrial appendage (LAA) closure vs. warfarin for the prevention of stroke, systemic embolism and CV death (2406 patients). The mean follow-up duration was 2.69 years. Closure with the Watchman device (Boston Scientific, Marlborough, MA) yielded 0.15 hemorrhagic strokes per 100 patient-years vs. 0.96 per 100 patient-years with warfarin (HR = 0.22; $P = .004$). CV or unexplained mortality also was significantly lower in the LAA closure group (1.1 vs. 2.3 events per 100 person-years; HR = 0.48; $P = .006$), as was non-procedural bleeding (6% vs. 11.3%; HR = 0.51; $P = .006$). Rates of all-cause mortality or systemic embolism were 1.75 per 100 person-years in the LAA closure group vs. 1.87 per 100 person-years in the warfarin group, (HR = 1.02; 95% CI, 0.62–1.7). Patients treated with the device experienced 1.6 ischemic strokes per 100 person-years, whereas warfarin was associated with 0.9 ischemic strokes per 100 person-years (HR = 1.95; $P = .05$) [59].

Another percutaneous epicardial LAA closure device (Lariat snare device; SentreHEART, Inc, Palo Alto, California), which does not require the placement of intracardiac hardware, was shown to be effective in closing the LAA [31]. This device is FDA approved for soft tissue closure and is used off label for stroke prevention in AF. Preliminary data in small studies suggests efficacy in stroke prevention at the expenses of high complication rate [60]. Surgical LAA occlusion should be considered in any AF patient at the time of cardiac surgery for other indications.

ACTION POINTS

1 AF tends to be a chronic condition. Progression from paroxysmal to persistent AF and to longstanding persistent makes intervention aimed at restoring sinus rhythm less efficient. Early intervention and perhaps early referral to an electrophysiologist should be considered to ensure maximum success of interventions for rhythm control restoration.

2 The goals of care are: decrease mortality, minimize thromboembolic risk, control of symptoms, improve quality of life and exercise capacity, prevent hospitalizations, and prevent tachycardia-induced cardiomyopathy.

3 Significant advances have been made in the past decade, particularly with regards to oral anticoagulation, devices for left atrial appendage closure, catheter and surgical ablation, and device therapy, but there are still areas that need to be addressed by future therapies, devices, and clinical trials.

REFERENCES

1. January CT, Wann LS, Alpert JS, Calkins H, Cleveland JC, Jr., Cigarroa JE, et al. 2014 AHA/ACC/HRS Guideline for the Management of Patients With Atrial Fibrillation: A Report of the American College of Cardiology/American Heart Association Task Force on Practice Guidelines and the Heart Rhythm Society. *J Am Coll Cardiol.* 2014.

2. European Heart Rhythm A, European Association for Cardio-Thoracic S, Camm AJ, Kirchhof P, Lip GY, Schotten U, et al. Guidelines for the management of atrial fibrillation: the Task Force for the Management of Atrial Fibrillation of the European Society of Cardiology (ESC). *Eur Heart J.* 2010;31(19):2369–429.

3. Hylek EM, Go AS, Chang Y, Jensvold NG, Henault LE, Selby JV, et al. Effect of intensity of oral anticoagulation on stroke severity and mortality in atrial fibrillation. *N Engl J Med.* 2003;349(11):1019–1026.

4. Wolf PA, Abbott RD, Kannel WB. Atrial fibrillation: a major contributor to stroke in the elderly. *The Framingham Study. Arch Intern Med.* 1987;147(9):1561–1564.

5. Lip GY, Laroche C, Ioachim PM, Rasmussen LH, Vitali-Serdoz L, Petrescu L, et al. Prognosis and treatment of atrial fibrillation patients by European cardiologists: One Year Follow-up of the EURObservational Research Programme-Atrial Fibrillation General Registry Pilot Phase (EORP-AF Pilot registry). *Eur Heart J.* 2014.

6. Sanna T, Diener HC, Passman RS, et al; CRYSTAL AF Investigators. Cryptogenic stroke and underlying atrial fibrillation. *N Engl J Med.* 2014;370:2478–2486.

7. Murray KT. Ibutilide. *Circulation.* 1998;97(5):493–497.

8. Oral H, Souza JJ, Michaud GF, Knight BP, Goyal R, Strickberger SA, et al. Facilitating transthoracic cardioversion of atrial fibrillation with ibutilide pretreatment. *N Engl J Med.* 1999;340(24):1849–54.

9. Ellenbogen KA, Clemo HF, Stambler BS, Wood MA, VanderLugt JT. Efficacy of ibutilide for termination of atrial fibrillation and flutter. *Am J Cardiol.* 1996;78(8A):42–45.

10. Patsilinakos S, Christou A, Kafkas N, Nikolaou N, Antonatos D, Katsanos S, et al. Effect of high doses of magnesium on converting ibutilide to a safe and more effective agent. *Am J Cardiol.* 2010;106(5):673–676.

11. Khan IA, Mehta NJ, Gowda RM. Amiodarone for pharmacological cardioversion of recent-onset atrial fibrillation. *Int J Cardiol.* 2003;89(2–3):239–248.

12. Letelier LM, Udol K, Ena J, Weaver B, Guyatt GH. Effectiveness of amiodarone for conversion of atrial fibrillation to sinus rhythm: a meta-analysis. *Arch Intern Med.* 2003;163(7):777–785.

13. Singh S, Zoble RG, Yellen L, Brodsky MA, Feld GK, Berk M, et al. Efficacy and safety of oral dofetilide in converting to and maintaining sinus rhythm in patients with chronic atrial fibrillation or atrial flutter: the symptomatic atrial fibrillation investigative research on dofetilide (SAFIRE-D) study. *Circulation.* 2000;102(19):2385–2390.

14. Alboni P, Botto GL, Baldi N, Luzi M, Russo V, Gianfranchi L, et al. Outpatient treatment of recent-onset atrial fibrillation with the 'pill-in-the-pocket' approach. *N Engl J Med.* 2004;351(23):2384–2391.

15. Khan IA. Single oral loading dose of propafenone for pharmacological cardioversion of recent-onset atrial fibrillation. *J Am Coll Cardiol.* 2001;37(2):542–547.

16. Lip GY, Nieuwlaat R, Pisters R, Lane DA, Crijns HJ. Refining clinical risk stratification for predicting stroke and thromboembolism in atrial fibrillation using a novel risk factor-based approach: the euro heart survey on atrial fibrillation. *Chest.* 2010 Feb;137(2):263–272.

17. Presented at the ESC 2014 by Chao TF, Liu CJ, Lip G, Shih-Ann Chen

18. Japanese Circulation Society Joint Working Group. Guidelines for Pharmacotherapy of Atrial Fibrillation (JCS 2013). *Circ J.* 2014;78(8):1997–2021. Epub 2014 Jun 26.

19. Pisters R, Lane DA, Nieuwlaat R, et al. A novel user-friendly score (has-bled) to assess 1-year risk of major bleeding in patients with atrial fibrillation: The Euro Heart Survey. *Chest.* 2010;138(5):1093–1100.

20. Camm AJ, Lip GY, De Caterina R, et al. 2012 Focused update of the ESC Guidelines for the management of atrial fibrillation: an update of the 2010 ESC Guidelines for the management of atrial fibrillation. Developed with the special contribution of the European Heart Rhythm Association. *Eur Heart J.* 2012;33:2719–2747.

21. Investigators AWGotA, Connolly S, Pogue J, Hart R, Pfeffer M, Hohnloser S, et al. Clopidogrel plus aspirin versus oral anticoagulation for atrial fibrillation in the Atrial fibrillation Clopidogrel Trial with Irbesartan for prevention

of Vascular Events (ACTIVE W): a randomised controlled trial. *Lancet.* 2006;367(9526):1903–1912.

22. Connolly SJ, Eikelboom J, Joyner C, Diener HC, Hart R, Golitsyn S, et al. Apixaban in patients with atrial fibrillation. *N Engl J Med.* 2011;364(9):806–817.

23. Connolly SJ, Ezekowitz MD, Yusuf S, Eikelboom J, Oldgren J, Parekh A, et al. Dabigatran versus warfarin in patients with atrial fibrillation. *N Engl J Med.* 2009;361(12):1139–1151.

24. Patel MR, Mahaffey KW, Garg J, Pan G, Singer DE, Hacke W, et al. Rivaroxaban versus warfarin in nonvalvular atrial fibrillation. *N Engl J Med.* 2011;365(10):883–891.

25. Sharma M, Cornelius VR, Patel JP, Davies JG, Molokhia M. Efficacy and harms of direct oral anticoagulants in the elderly for stroke prevention in atrial fibrillation and secondary prevention of venous thromboembolism: systematic review and meta-analysis. *Circulation.* 2015;132:194–204.

26. Graham DJ, Reichman ME, Wernecke M, et al. Cardiovascular, bleeding, and mortality risks in elderly Medicare patients treated with dabigatran or warfarin for nonvalvular atrial fibrillation. *Circulation.* 2015;131:157–164.

27. Giugliano R, Ruff C, Braunwald C. and the Effective Anticoagulation with Factor Xa Next Generation in Atrial Fibrillation–Thrombolysis in Myocardial Infarction 48 (ENGAGE AF-TIMI 48) Edoxaban versus Warfarin in Patients with Atrial Fibrillation. *N Engl J Med.* 2013;369:2093–2104.

28. Wood MA, Brown-Mahoney C, Kay GN, Ellenbogen KA. Clinical outcomes after ablation and pacing therapy for atrial fibrillation : a meta-analysis. *Circulation.* 2000;101(10):1138–1144.

29. Geelen P, Brugada J, Andries E, Brugada P. Ventricular fibrillation and sudden death after radiofrequency catheter ablation of the atrioventricular junction. *Pacing Clin Electrophysiol.* 1997;20(2 Pt 1):343–348.

30. Curtis AB, Worley SJ, Adamson PB, Chung ES, Niazi I, Sherfesee L, et al. Biventricular pacing for atrioventricular block and systolic dysfunction. *N Engl J Med.* 2013;368(17):1585–93.

31. Karlson BW, Torstensson I, Abjorn C, Jansson SO, Peterson LE. Disopyramide in the maintenance of sinus rhythm after electroconversion of atrial fibrillation. A placebo-controlled one-year follow-up study. *Eur Heart J.* 1988;9(3):284–290.

32. Aliot E, Capucci A, Crijns HJ, Goette A, Tamargo J. Twenty-five years in the making: flecainide is safe and effective for the management of atrial fibrillation. *Europace.* 2011;13(2):161–173.

33. Singh BN, Singh SN, Reda DJ, Tang XC, Lopez B, Harris CL, et al. Amiodarone versus sotalol for atrial fibrillation. *N Engl J Med.* 2005;352(18):1861–1872.

34. Piccini JP, Hasselblad V, Peterson ED, Washam JB, Califf RM, Kong DF. Comparative efficacy of dronedarone and amiodarone for the maintenance of sinus rhythm in patients with atrial fibrillation. *J Am Coll Cardiol.* 2009;54(12):1089–1095.

35. Calkins H, Kuck KH, Cappato R, Brugada J, Camm AJ, Chen SA, et al. 2012 HRS/EHRA/ECAS expert consensus statement on catheter and surgical ablation of atrial fibrillation: recommendations for patient selection, procedural techniques, patient management and follow-up, definitions, endpoints, and research trial design: a report of the Heart Rhythm

Society (HRS) Task Force on Catheter and Surgical Ablation of Atrial Fibrillation. Developed in partnership with the European Heart Rhythm Association (EHRA), a registered branch of the European Society of Cardiology (ESC) and the European Cardiac Arrhythmia Society (ECAS); and in collaboration with the American College of Cardiology (ACC), American Heart Association (AHA), the Asia Pacific Heart Rhythm Society (APHRS), and the Society of Thoracic Surgeons (STS). Endorsed by the governing bodies of the American College of Cardiology Foundation, the American Heart Association, the European Cardiac Arrhythmia Society, the European Heart Rhythm Association, the Society of Thoracic Surgeons, the Asia Pacific Heart Rhythm Society, and the Heart Rhythm Society. *Heart Rhythm.* 2012;9(4):632–696 e21.

36. Haissaguerre M, Jais P, Shah DC, Takahashi A, Hocini M, Quiniou G, et al. Spontaneous initiation of atrial fibrillation by ectopic beats originating in the pulmonary veins. *N Engl J Med.* 1998;339(10):659–666.
37. Nathan H, Eliakim M. The junction between the left atrium and the pulmonary veins. An anatomic study of human hearts. *Circulation.* 1966;34(3):412–422.
38. Ho SY, Sanchez-Quintana D, Cabrera JA, Anderson RH. Anatomy of the left atrium: implications for radiofrequency ablation of atrial fibrillation. *J Cardiovasc Electrophysiol.* 1999;10(11):1525–1533.
39. Weiss C, Gocht A, Willems S, Hoffmann M, Risius T, Meinertz T. Impact of the distribution and structure of myocardium in the pulmonary veins for radiofrequency ablation of atrial fibrillation. *Pacing Clin Electrophysiol.* 2002;25(9):1352–1356.
40. Pappone C, Rosanio S, Oreto G, Tocchi M, Gugliotta F, Vicedomini G, et al. Circumferential radiofrequency ablation of pulmonary vein ostia: A new anatomic approach for curing atrial fibrillation. *Circulation.* 2000;102(21):2619–2628.
41. Packer DL, Kowal RC, Wheelan KR, Irwin JM, Champagne J, Guerra PG, et al. Cryoballoon ablation of pulmonary veins for paroxysmal atrial fibrillation: first results of the North American Arctic Front (STOP AF) pivotal trial. *J Am Coll Cardiol.* 2013;61(16):1713–1723.
42. Moe GW. On the multiple wavelet hypothesis of atrial fibrillation. *Arch Int Pharmacodyn.* 1964;140:183–188.
43. Cox JL. The surgical treatment of atrial fibrillation. IV. Surgical technique. *J Thorac Cardiovasc Surg.* 1991;101(4):584–592.
44. Cox JL, Canavan TE, Schuessler RB, Cain ME, Lindsay BD, Stone C, et al. The surgical treatment of atrial fibrillation. II. Intraoperative electrophysiologic mapping and description of the electrophysiologic basis of atrial flutter and atrial fibrillation. *J Thorac Cardiovasc Surg.* 1991;101(3):406–426.
45. Cox JL, Schuessler RB, Boineau JP. The surgical treatment of atrial fibrillation. I. Summary of the current concepts of the mechanisms of atrial flutter and atrial fibrillation. *J Thorac Cardiovasc Surg.* 1991;101(3):402–405.
46. Cox JL, Schuessler RB, D'Agostino HJ, Jr., Stone CM, Chang BC, Cain ME, et al. The surgical treatment of atrial fibrillation. III. Development of a definitive surgical procedure. *J Thorac Cardiovasc Surg.* 1991;101(4):569–583.
47. Cappato R, Calkins H, Chen SA, Davies W, Iesaka Y, Kalman J, et al. Updated worldwide survey on the methods, efficacy, and safety of catheter ablation for human atrial fibrillation. *Circ Arrhythm Electrophysiol.* 2010;3(1):32–38.

48. Damiano RJ, Jr., Schwartz FH, Bailey MS, Maniar HS, Munfakh NA, Moon MR, et al. The Cox maze IV procedure: predictors of late recurrence. *J Thorac Cardiovasc Surg.* 2011;141(1):113–121.

49. Cuff CT, Giugliano RP, Antman EM, et al. Evaluation of the novel factor Xa inhibitor edoxaban compared with warfarin in patients with atrial fibrillation: design and rationale for the Effective aNticoaGulation with factor xA next GEneration in Atrial Fibrillation-Thrombolysis In Myocardial Infarction study 48 (ENGAGE AF-TIMI 48). *Am Heart J.* 2010;160:635–641.

50. Babilonia K, Trujillo T. The role of prothrombin complex concentrates in reversal of target specific anticoagulants. *Thromb J.* 2014;12:8.

51. http://www.medscape.org/viewarticle/852477_transcript

52. Pollack C, Reilly P, Eikelboom J, et al. Idarucizumab for Dabigatran Reversal. *N Engl J Med.* 2015;373:511–520.

53. Dewilde WJ, Oirbans T, Verheugt FW, et al. Use of clopidogrel with or without aspirin in patients taking oral anticoagulant therapy and undergoing percutaneous coronary intervention: an open-label, randomised, controlled trial. *Lancet.* 2013;381:1107–1115.

54. Fiedler KA, Maeng M, Mehilli J, et al. Duration of Triple Therapy in Patients Requiring Oral Anticoagulation After Drug-Eluting Stent ImplantationThe ISAR-TRIPLE Trial *J Am Coll Cardiol.* 2015;65(16):1619–1629. doi:10.1016/j.jacc.2015.02.050

55. Dans AL, Connolly SJ, Wallentin L, et al. Concomitant use of antiplatelet therapy with dabigatran or warfarin in the Randomized Evaluation of Long-Term Anticoagulation Therapy (RE-LY) trial. *Circulation.* 2013;127:634–640.

56. Alexander JH, Lopes RD, James S, et al. Apixaban with antiplatelet therapy after acute coronary syndrome. *N Engl J Med.* 2011;365:699–708.

57. Capodanno D, Lip GY, Windecker S, et al. Triple antithrombotic therapy in atrial fibrillation patients with acute coronary syndromes or undergoing percutaneous coronary intervention or transcatheter aortic valve replacement. *EuroIntervention.* 2015;10:1015–1021.

58. Ezekowtiz M. Clinical outcomes of atrial fibrillation patients receiving NSAIDs in the RE-LY trial. Presented at: European Society of Cardiology Congress; September 1, 2015; London, England.

59. Reddy VY, Doshi SK, Sievert H, Buchbinder M, Neuzil P, Huber K, et al. Percutaneous left atrial appendage closure for stroke prophylaxis in patients with atrial fibrillation: 2.3-Year Follow-up of the PROTECT AF (Watchman Left Atrial Appendage System for Embolic Protection in Patients with Atrial Fibrillation) Trial. *Circulation.* 2013;127(6):720–729.

60. Sievert H, Rasekh A, Bartus K, et al. Left atrial appendage ligation in nonvalvular atrial fibrillation patients at high risk for embolic events with ineligibility for oral anticoagulation: Initial report of clinical outcomes. *JACC Clin Electrophysiol* 2015;Nov 25:[Epub ahead of print]. See more at: www.acc.org/latest-in-cardiology/journal-scans/2015/11/25/12/32/left-atrial-appendage-ligation-in-nonvalvular-atrial-fibrillation?WT.mc_ev=EmailOpen&w_pub=JScan151203&w_nav=JScan#sthash.LgrtGQG3.dpuf

CHAPTER 9
Ventricular Tachycardia

Sorin Lazar, Bao V. Ho, Phillip Tran, Pham Nhu Hung, Thomas Bump and Evgeny Shlyakhto

Management of Complex Cardiovascular Problems, Fourth Edition. Edited by Thach N. Nguyen, Dayi Hu, Shao Liang Chen, Moo Hyun Kim and Cindy L. Grines.
© 2016 John Wiley & Sons, Ltd. Published 2016 by John Wiley & Sons, Ltd.

BACKGROUND

Ventricular tachycardia (VT) is an arrhythmia that originates in ventricular muscle and/or the ventricular specialized conduction system. It is a wide complex tachycardia (WCT) that presents with wide QRS complexes (usually at least or longer than 120 ms) and a rate greater than 100 bpm. The QRS complexes during tachycardia are uniform in morphology in the case of monomorphic VT, and are of varying morphologies in the case of polymorphic VT. Episodes of VT that terminate spontaneously within 30 seconds of their onset and are not hemodynamically compromising are non-sustained VT (NSVT). The term sustained VT is applied to episodes of VT that last longer than 30 seconds or require therapy for termination because of hemodynamic collapse. Ventricular fibrillation (VF) is a ventricular tachyarrhythmia in which there are no distinct QRS complexes on the surface electrocardiogram (ECG).

CHALLENGES

The **first challenge** is to be sure that a patient with WCT has VT and not a condition that mimics VT. The **second challenge** is to identify the cause of VT using a cost-effective diagnostic approach. Then the **third challenge** is to select and deliver successfully the most appropriate therapy for terminating VT and preventing its recurrences.

STRATEGIC MAPPING

First, when a WCT or VF causes cardiac arrest or severe hemodynamic compromise, immediate resuscitation is required. Second, sustained VT needs to be terminated or incessant VT to be suppressed. Once the patient is stable, identify and correct contributing factors such as ischemia, electrolyte disturbances, or drug toxicity and prevent recurrence of VT and/or sudden cardiac death (SCD). Specific syndromes of VT, if present, must be accurately identified.

The treatment options in the management of VT include antiarrhythmic drugs, electrical therapy (cardioversion, defibrillation and antitachycardia pacing) delivered by external or implanted devices, ablative therapy (catheter-based or surgical), coronary revascularization with or without aneurysmectomy, and even heart transplantation. Frequently, a combination of these therapeutic options is required to manage successfully a patient with VT.

HIGH-RISK PROFILING

A patient who has had a cardiac arrest or syncope from VT is at high risk for an adverse outcome if no completely reversible cause of VT can be identified. On the other hand, patients with idiopathic monomorphic VT arising from the right or left ventricular outflow tracts, or the fascicular region of the left ventricle (LV), or the mitral annular region, are at low risk for syncope, cardiac arrest, or arrhythmic death. Therefore, in order to risk-profile a particular patient, the physician must attempt to identify exactly which type of VT is present. Also, the nature of co-existing cardiac diseases must be assessed accurately.

HIGH-RISK PREDICTORS

The discovery that a patient has VT should lead to an investigation into whether the patient has coronary artery disease (CAD), left ventricular (LV) systolic dysfunction, inherited arrhythmia syndrome, or structural heart disease. A high risk of death is found in patients with VT and certain types of structural heart disease listed in Table 9.1.

Electrophysiological studies (see below) can be used for risk stratification in patients with prior myocardial infarction (MI), asymptomatic nonsustained VT, and LV ejection fraction less than or equal to 40%. High risk of lethal VT or ventricular fibrillation (VF) is indicated when a clinically relevant, hemodynamically significant sustained VT is induced.

Table 9.1 List of structural heart disease with high risk of VT [1]

1. Ischemia or severe LV systolic dysfunction.
2. Hypertrophic cardiomyopathy (HCM) and at least one risk factor (prior cardiac arrest, spontaneous sustained or non-sustained VT, family history of SCD, LV thickness greater than or equal to 30 mm, and an abnormal blood pressure response to exercise).
3. Arrhythmogenic dysplasia with evidence of extensive right ventricular (RV) disease or LV involvement.
4. Non-compaction of the LV.
5. Cardiac sarcoidosis.
6. Giant cell myocarditis.
7. Chagas disease.
8. Familial cardiomyopathy associated with sudden cardiac death.

Symptoms to look for

Symptoms produced by VT depend on the rate of tachycardia, the severity of underlying heart disease, and on whether the patient is upright or supine. At faster rates, especially in patients with structural heart disease, symptoms may vary from palpitations, dyspnea, dizziness, or syncope to severe hemodynamic instability and cardiac arrest. At slower rates, VT often does not cause significant hemodynamic compromise and the patient may be relatively asymptomatic. If the episode is prolonged, though, even an initially asymptomatic patient can gradually develop tachycardia-mediated cardiomyopathy with congestive heart failure (HF).

Patients with the Brugada syndrome (BrS) or type 3 long QT syndrome (LQTS3) tend to have their symptoms (such as cardiac arrest or agonal nocturnal breathing) at night while sleeping. Patients with type 1 long QT syndrome (LQT1) or catecholaminergic polymorphic VT (CPVT) tend to have arrhythmias during exercise or emotional stress. Patients with type 2 long QT syndrome (LQT2) tend to have arrhythmias following sudden loud noises.

Signs to look for

If a patient is examined during an episode of VT, the examiner must immediately assess the hemodynamic and neurologic state of the patient, including measuring of vital signs and level of consciousness. There are no specific signs of VT: other types of arrhythmia such as supraventricular tachycardia (SVT), atrial flutter, or atrial fibrillation (AF) can have exactly the same effect on vital signs and neurologic function as VT. The physical examination of a patient with VT should also search for signs of underlying diseases such as cardiomyopathies, valvular disease, drug toxicity, and metabolic disorders.

SMART TESTING

Strategic mapping VT presents in a variety of ways. It can be the rhythm that is recorded when a patient presents with a cardiac arrest or with palpitations. It can be detected by inpatient telemetric monitoring or by outpatient ambulatory monitoring. It can be provoked during a stress test or during an electrophysiological study (EPS). It can appear as an event that has been recorded by a pacemaker, an implantable cardioverter/defibrillator (ICD), or an implantable loop monitor (ILM). The recording of VT may be in the form of a 12-lead ECG; a single or multichannel surface electrocardiographic rhythm strip; or intracardiac ECG obtained by electrode catheters during an electrophysiologic study (EPS) or by pacing leads of an implantable device.

So, the tests needed from the patients with VT include a 12-lead ECG which should be obtained during WCT, as long as the patient is hemodynamically stable and doesn't need immediate cardioversion before the ECG can be obtained [12]. Then blood tests are done to screen for electrolyte abnormalities and drug toxicity, etc. Next is cardiac imaging such as echocardiography or cardiac magnetic resonance imaging in order to check the ejection fraction (EF) of the LV or myocardial disease or defect causing VT. CAD should be ruled in or out with stress testing or angiography. Occasionally specific testing for particular situations, such as endomyocardial biopsy or genetic testing should be obtained.

Usually the work-up for a patient with VT is complex. The patient should be talked to in detail about the risks and benefits, the alternative options, etc. An informed patient should ask his or her doctor this question: Could you tell me the purpose and the diagnostic accuracy of this test?

Electrocardiography A 12-lead ECG may assist in the differentiation of VT from SVT, since the presence of BBB or ventricular pre-excitation during sinus rhythm increases the likelihood that an episode of WCT might have been caused by SVT, especially if the QRS morphologies during sinus rhythm and during tachycardia are similar. On the other hand, the diagnosis of VT is supported if the ECG during sinus rhythm indicates the presence of underlying structural heart disease such as Q waves indicative of ischemic heart disease or infiltrative cardiomyopathy. Furthermore, the ECG during sinus rhythm should be inspected to see if it indicates the presence of factors that might contribute to VT, such as electrolyte disturbances, left ventricular hypertrophy, and ischemia or acute myocardial infarction (MI). Finally, the ECG during sinus rhythm should be inspected for signs of genetic syndromes associated with VT and VF, such as the long QT syndrome (LQTS), the short QT syndrome (SQTS), the Brugada syndrome, or arrhythmogenic right ventricular dysplasia/cardiomyopathy (ARVD/C).

The ECG that is obtained during WCT serves several functions. It documents the episode, and provides a template against which future episodes can be compared, such as episodes that might be induced during EPS, when the question might arise as to whether the induced arrhythmia is clinically significant. Also, the ECG obtained during WCT contains diagnostic clues as to whether the patient has VT or SVT (see below).

CLINICAL PEARLS
Identification of the site origin of VT The
ECG obtained during VT may point to the site of origin
of the VT [1]. In general, a left bundle branch block
(LBBB)-type QRS morphology during VT indicates a right ventricular origin of the tachycardia, and a right bundle branch block (RBBB)-type QRS morphology during VT indicates a left ventricular origin [2]. Septal VTs and VTs in patients with extensive scarring or infiltration of the septum can have indeterminate QRS morphology (i.e., neither RBBB-type nor LBBB-type). The axis of the VT depends on the principle that activation spreads away from the site of origin [4]. Therefore, VTs that originate in the outflow tracts have an inferior axis; VTs that originate in the inferior wall have a superior axis; VTs that originate in the anterior wall or apex have negative QRS complexes across the precordium; and VTs that originate in the posterior wall have positive QRS complexes across the precordium [6]. Finally, the ECG obtained during VT may indicate whether the site of origin is endocardial or epicardial, which is important information when ablative therapy is being considered.

Since mechanistically different types of VT favor certain anatomic locations within the heart, the site of origin can indicate important mechanistic and prognostic information. For example, a monomorphic VT with relatively narrow QRS complexes arising from the inferior septal LV (RBBB morphology with leftward axis deviation) in an otherwise healthy patient is likely a fairly benign idiopathic VT that is caused by re-entry involving fascicles of the LV specialized conduction system including a verapamil-sensitive portion of the circuit.

In another example, the RV outflow tract (LBBB morphology with inferior axis) is the site of origin for two important types of VT: the most common form of idiopathic VT, which is produced by cyclic AMP-dependent triggered automaticity and is almost always benign; and a rare and potentially lethal type of VT caused by re-entry around and through zones of fibrofatty replacement of the myocardium caused by arrhythmogenic right ventricular dysplasia/cardiomyopathy (ARVD/C). In patients who have monomorphic VT in the setting of a prior MI, it is common for the VT to have its site of origin in the ventricular region that was scarred by the infarction.

Rapid wide complex signals can be caused by VT but also by conditions that mimic VT, such as aberrantly conducting SVT, electrocardiographic artifact, and rapid ventricular pacing (as in atrial triggered ventricular pacing in a patient with a dual chamber pacemaker who develops atrial flutter or fibrillation, or pacemaker-mediated tachycardia). Artifacts can be identified readily by the presence of native QRS complexes at the cycle length of the base-line rhythm within the artifact [2]. Rapid ventricular pacing can readily be identified as the cause of a WCT in a patient with a pacemaker or defibrillator, by interrogating and reprogramming the device.

CLINICAL PEARLS
Differential diagnoses of wide QRS complex tachycardia Multiple algorithms have been advanced for distinguishing VT from SVT in patients with WCT, using the 12-lead ECG that has been recorded during tachycardia [3]. Findings that support or exclude a diagnosis of VT are shown in Table 9.2.

Table 9.2 EKG features suggestive of ventricular tachycardia

1. Atrioventricular dissociation.
2. Concordance of positivity or negativity of QRS complexes in all the precordial leads.
3. Absence of an R/S complex in any of the precordial leads.
4. Onset of R to nadir of S greater than 100 ms in any precordial lead.
5. Onset of QRS to first change in polarity (either nadir Q or peak R) in lead II of greater than or equal to 50 ms.
6. Initial R wave in aVR.
7. Absence of a typical BBB pattern.
8. LBBB: rS or QS wave in leads V1 and V2, delay to S wave nadir < 70 ms, and R wave and no Q wave in lead V6.
9. RBBB: rSR′ wave in lead V1 and an RS wave in lead V6, with R wave height greater than S wave depth.

The electrocardiographic findings that support a diagnosis of SVT include the presence of a typical BBB pattern, irregularity of the rhythm (which suggests aberrant conduction during AF or atrial flutter with variable atrioventricular response). VT should always be the default diagnosis, especially in patients with structural heart disease or prior MI, unless there is very compelling evidence of SVT.

Cardiac imaging Echocardiography is the preferred method for evaluation of structural heart disease, receiving a class I recommendation (level of evidence B) on the American College of Cardiology/American Heart Association/ European Society of Cardiology (ACC/AHA/ESC) 2006 guidelines [4]. Echocardiography is favored because of its widespread availability, accuracy in diagnosing a variety of structural cardiac defects (myocardial, valvular, congenital), safety to the patients, and relatively low expense. In addition, LV systolic function and regional wall motion can be evaluated, and in a majority of patients, EF can be determined [5]. Magnetic resonance imaging (MRI), cardiac computed tomography (CT), or radionuclide angiography can be useful in patients with ventricular arrhythmias when echocardiography does not provide accurate assessment of LV and right ventricular (RV) function and/or evaluation of structural changes (Class IIa) [4].

Exercise testing In patients with VT, exercise testing is used for detection of silent ischemia in patients suspected of having underlying CAD [6]. The current ACC/AHA guidelines recommend exercise testing in adult patients with ventricular arrhythmias who have an intermediate or greater probability of having CAD by age, gender, and symptoms to provoke ischemic changes or ventricular arrhythmias (Class I, level of evidence B). Exercise testing with an imaging modality (echocardiography or single-photon emission computed tomography [SPECT]) is recommended for detection of silent ischemia in patients with VT who have an intermediate probability of having CAD by age, symptoms, and gender and in whom ECG assessment is less reliable because of digoxin use, left ventricular hypertrophy, >1-mm ST-segment depression at rest, Wolff-Parkinson-White (WPW) syndrome, or LBBB. (Class I, Level of Evidence: B) [4].

Exercise testing is also useful in patients with known or suspected exercise-induced ventricular arrhythmias, in order to provoke the arrhythmia, achieve a diagnosis, and determine the patient's response to tachycardia (Class I, level of evidence B). Moreover, exercise testing can be useful in evaluating the response to medical or ablation therapy in patients with known exercise-induced ventricular arrhythmias (Class IIa, level of evidence B).

Electrophysiological testing Invasive electrophysiological studies (EPS) have multiple diagnostic and therapeutic applications in patients with known or suspected VT. During diagnostic EPS, multipolar electrode catheters are advanced transvenously to the RV and other intracardiac locations such as the right atrium and the His bundle position. These electrode catheters are connected to recording equipment and to a programmable stimulator that delivers sequences of stimuli in order to induce clinically relevant tachycardias. When a tachycardia is induced, the mechanism of tachycardia can be identified and the site of origin of the tachycardia can be pin-pointed by mapping.

The induction of sustained monomorphic VT carries prognostic significance in various settings, including in patients who have presented with syncope, and asymptomatic patients with a history of prior MI, LV systolic dysfunction with an EF of less than or equal to 40%, and non-sustained VT recorded by electrocardiographic monitoring. On the other hand, the induction of VF is a non-specific finding, with little prognostic significance in most patients.

EPS have been advocated as a means of risk stratification of patients with the BrS, but registries have indicated that inducibility of VT/VF does not predict arrhythmic events [7]. Recently it has been proposed that the presence of a ventricular effective refractory period less than 200 ms may be a marker of increased risk; [8] this awaits further evaluation.

DIAGNOSES

In order to assess a patient's prognosis and to select the best therapy for the patient, the physician must accurately identify which type of arrhythmia the patient possesses. Therefore, the physician must be armed with an awareness of the differential diagnosis of patients with WCT, including conditions that mimic VT, and various VT syndromes. The approach to patients with VT is different than the approach to patients with electrocardiographic artifact or with supraventricular tachycardia (SVT) conducting with wide QRS complexes.

Electrocardiographic artifact
Electrocardiographic artifact can mimic VT, causing patients to be subjected to a broad range of unnecessary diagnostic procedures, including cardiac catheterization and the implantation of cardiac devices [2].

An electrocardiographic signal must be recognized as artifact if it reveals native QRS complexes at the cycle length base-line rhythm 'marching through' the artifact. Suspicion must also be raised if the signal in question does not appear to be physiologic – for example, if the rate is too fast or the signals are squared-off.

Supraventricular tachycardia with wide QRS complexes

These can mimic VT, causing patients to be given inappropriate therapy. The QRS complexes can be wide because of bundle branch block (BBB) that is fixed (i.e., present during sinus rhythm), rate-dependent, or dependent on a sudden change in QRS cycle length (i.e., the Ashman's phenomenon) [9]. Antegrade conduction over an accessory atrioventricular pathway during SVT, atrial fibrillation, or atrial flutter can also cause a WCT that mimics VT in the presence of an antegradely conducting accessory pathway, for instance in patients with Wolff-Parkinson-White (WPW) syndrome. If WCT is difficult to different VT or SVT, should consider to manage like VT.

Re-entrant monomorphic ventricular tachycardia

This can be caused by re-entry within or around a ventricular scar, most commonly the product of a prior MI. Other causes of myocardial scar (and monomorphic VT) include surgical or traumatic ventriculotomy, sarcoidosis, arrhythmogenic right ventricular dysplasia (ARVD), and Chagas disease. Usually the re-entrant circuit includes a segment that is a narrow isthmus between two separate scars, or a narrow pathway that wends its way through an otherwise dense scar.

Bundle branch re-entry ventricular tachycardia

Bundle branch re-entry ventricular tachycardia is a monomorphic VT in which the re-entering wavefront typically uses the following activation sequence: the right bundle branch (RBB) in the antegrade direction, the interventricular septum between the distal RBB and the distal left bundle branch (LBB), the LBB in the retrograde direction, and the portion of the specialized intraventricular conduction system where the distal His bundle bifurcates into the LBB and the RBB. Since the ventricles are activated by antegrade conduction over the RBB, this tachycardia has a LBBB pattern and can be mistaken for SVT conducting with functional LBBB. Because the re-entrant circuit of this tachycardia consists almost entirely of the specialized conduction system, the rate of the tachycardia is usually high. Furthermore, it often occurs in patients with significant structural heart disease. Therefore, if untreated it carries an adverse prognosis and can cause syncope or even cardiac arrest.

Verapamil-sensitive fascicular tachycardia

This is a monomorphic VT that is caused by re-entry in a circuit that likely incorporates both a septal fibromuscular false tendon and the left ventricular fascicular system [10]. The re-entrant circuit is located most often near the left posterior fascicle but occasionally near the left anterior fascicle. Because of its origin in the fascicular system, the QRS complexes are relatively narrow and are often confused for SVT. It is seen in patients without significant structural heart disease and usually carries a benign prognosis except that it can result in palpitations, hypotension, and the need for emergency treatment.

Outflow tract ventricular tachycardia

Outflow tract ventricular tachycardia is a monomorphic VT that can arise from either the right or the LV tract. It often coexists with frequent unifocal premature ventricular complexes (PVCs) with the same QRS morphology as seen during VT. Episodes of VT are often triggered by exercise, caffeine, emotional stress, and, in women, premenstrual or perimenopausal hormonal flux. The mechanism is triggered activity due to cyclic adenosine monophosphate (cAMP)-mediated delayed after-depolarizations (DADs). Increased cAMP can occur with either beta-adrenergic receptor stimulation or caffeine-mediated inhibition of phosphodiesterase, resulting in increased intracellular calcium and DADs, triggering PVCs or VT. These are almost always benign except when extremely frequent PVCs and VT (e.g. more than 20% of total QRS complexes) cause tachycardia-mediated cardiomyopathy. Also, rarely, short-coupled PVCs from the outflow tract trigger *torsades de pointes* (a rapid polymorphic VT), and in these rare cases there is a high mortality risk if the PVCs are not completely eliminated [11].

A scoring system that uses electrocardiographic criteria can be used in order to distinguish the usually benign syndrome of idiopathic RV outflow tract VT from the much more dangerous syndrome of arrhythmogenic right ventricular dysplasia/cardiomyopathy (ARVD/C) [12]. In this scoring system, three points are provided for anterior T wave inversions in V_1 to V_3 during sinus rhythm; two points are provided for QRS duration greater than 120 ms in lead I during VT; two points are provided for QRS notching in multiple leads during VT; and 1 point is awarded for precordial transition in V_5 or later during VT. ARVD/C is indicated when the score is 5 or more.

Papillary muscle and mitral annulus ventricular tachycardia

These are usually benign, except cases with significant structural abnormalities. VTs originating from papillary muscles should be taken into account when an ablation procedure is offered for patients, since additional imaging modalities would be required (for instance, intracardiac echo visualization).

Polymorphic ventricular tachycardia

Polymorphic ventricular tachycardia arises from a variety of causes, including congenital and acquired long QT (LQT) syndromes, the Brugada syndrome, catecholaminergic polymorphic VT (CPVT), and acute ischemia.

Long QT syndrome   Patients with LQTS are susceptible to a form of polymorphic VT called *torsades de pointes* and have prolonged QT intervals during sinus rhythm. Congenital LQT syndromes are caused by mutations in genes that encode cardiac ion channel subunits or proteins, thus modulating ionic currents. These mutations result in delayed cardiac repolarization (hence the long QT), which is highly arrhythmogenic, probably by causing cardiac cells to be susceptible to early after-depolarizations and promoting re-entry, resulting in a polymorphic VT known as *torsades de pointes*. Corrected QT intervals (QTc) of greater than 440 ms in males and 460 ms in females are considered to be prolonged. The risk for polymorphic VT (*torsades de pointes*) increases with longer QT intervals, especially when the QTc exceeds 500 ms. Mutations in 13 different genes have been identified as causing LQT syndromes; by far the most common of the LQT syndromes, representing over 90% of cases, are LQT1, LQT2, and LQT3.

The risk of developing VT (in this case, *torsades de pointes*) or sudden cardiac death (SCD) increases as the QT gets longer, especially when QTc exceeds 500 to 550 ms. Besides QT prolongation, T wave abnormalities are common in LQTS, including notched T waves and beat-to-beat alternation of T wave amplitude or polarity. The appearance of the T wave can suggest which type of LQTS might be present. Smooth, broad-based T waves are seen in patients with LQT1 or LQT5, who have mutations in the *KCNQ1* and *KCNE1* genes, respectively, that encode the proteins of subunits of the slow delayed rectifier potassium current. Low-amplitude and notched T waves are seen in patients with LQT2 and LQT6 who have mutations in the *KCNH2* and *KCNE2* genes, respectively, that encode proteins of subunits of the fast delayed rectifier potassium current. Long isoelectric ST segments with late onset of T waves are seen in patients with

LQT3, who have mutations of the *SCN5A* gene that encodes the protein of the cardiac sodium channel.

In LQT1, the KCNQ1 gene is mutated. This gene codes for a subunit of the potassium channel that conducts the I_{Ks} delayed rectifier current, which contributes to cardiac repolarization. The normal I_{Ks} current is increased by sympathetic activation and is essential for QT shortening at faster heart rates during exercise. When I_{Ks} is defective, the QT interval fails to shorten appropriately during tachycardia, and exercise-induced induced *torsades de pointes* may ensue. Numerous different mutations of this gene are known, which have varying severity depending on the part of the protein that is affected, whether or not the defective subunits can co-assemble with wild peptides, and whether the mutation prevents the defective subunit from being trafficked to the membrane. Beta adrenergic receptor blocking drugs reduce the tendency to *torsades de pointes* in patients with LQT1. Patients who are homozygous for mutations in KCNQ1 are likely to have congenital deafness in addition to cardiac arrhythmias; this is the Jervell and Lange–Nielsen syndrome.

In LQT2 there is a mutation in the KCNH2 gene, which encodes the alpha subunit of the potassium channel that conducts the I_{Kr} delayed repolarizing current (also known as HERG). Normally this gene contributes to repolarization. Loss of function of this channel leads to reduction of the I_{Kr} current and prolongation of the action potential, predisposing the patient to *torsades de pointes*.

In LQT3 there is a mutation in the SCN5A gene, which encodes the protein of the channel that conducts the I_{Na} depolarizing sodium current which produces the rapid upstroke of the action potential. These mutations in patients with LQT3 cause the channel not to fully close after the beginning of the action potential, so that an inward sodium current persists during the plateau of the action potential, prolonging depolarization and delaying repolarization. Sodium channel blocking drugs such as mexiletine can normalize the QT interval in patients with LQT3, but it is not known how effectively these drugs prevent *torsades de pointes* in these patients. Patients with LQT3 may have sudden long pauses in their sinus rhythm.

The different LQT syndromes differ in their clinical presentations. In LQT1, episodes of syncope and cardiac arrest typically occur during exercise; in long QT2, episodes occur during noxious auditory stimuli (e.g., telephone ringing or alarm clock going off and startling the patient) and other forms of emotional stress; and in LQT3, episodes tend to occur when the patient is sleeping. Also, the ECGs during sinus rhythm tend to be different according to the syndrome. Patients with LQT2 and LQT3 are at low risk during exercise, since they have a preserved I_{Ks} current

Table 9.3 Scoring system for assessing presence of LQTS based on clinical and electrocardiographic characteristics

Electrocardiographic findings	Points
QTc greater than or equal to 480 ms	3
between 460 and 479 ms	2
between 450 and 459 ms (male only)	1
QTc in the fourth minute of recovery after an exercise stress test greater than or equal to 480 ms	1
Torsades de pointes	2
T wave alternans	1
Notched T waves in three ECG leads	1
Low heart rate for age	0.5
Clinical history	
Syncope With stress	2
Without stress	1
Congenital deafness	0.5
Family history	
Family members with definite LQTS	1
Unexplained sudden cardiac death below age 30 among immediate family members	0.5

Score: Patients with less than or equal to 1 point have a low probability of LQTS; patient with more than one point and up to 3 points are at intermediate risk of LQTS; and patients with more than or equal to 3.5 points have a high probability of LQTS.

so their QT intervals shorten appropriately during exercise. For unknown reasons, females with LQT2 are at increased risk for events in the postpartum period, the menopausal transition, and the postmenopausal period (5 years before and after the onset of menopause).

Table 9.3 lists the diagnostic criteria for LQT, with a scoring system. Patients with less than or equal to 1 point have a low probability of LQTS; patients with more than one point and up to 3 points are at intermediate risk of LQTS; and patients with more than or equal to 3.5 points have a high probability of LQTS. Patients with intermediate probability for LQTS should have serial ECGs and repeated Holter recordings because the QTc value can vary from day to day and day to night.

Short QT syndrome   Patients with SQTS are susceptible to VF and have short QT intervals (less than or equal to 330 ms) during sinus rhythm with tall, symmetric peaked T waves. Three different genetic variants have been described. Causes of acquired short QT such as hyperkalemia, digitalis toxicity, acidosis, hypercalcemia, androgen use, and increased vagal tone must be excluded. The cutoff lower limit of normal QTc has not been defined and there is considerable overlap of QTc intervals between the normal population and patients with SQTS. Patients with SQTS have tall peaked T waves in the precordial leads.

Brugada syndrome   Brugada syndrome (BrS) encompasses patients with transient or persistent electrocardiographic changes in the right precordial ECG leads. Some of these patients are asymptomatic, but others are subject to lethal polymorphic VT and VF. Three different ECG patterns have been recognized.

Type I, which is the only pattern that is diagnostic for BrS, consists of coved (downward concave) ST segment elevation greater than 2 mm followed by a descending negative T wave in at least one right precordial lead (V_1 to V_3).

Type II and type III are saddleback-shaped patterns, with high J-point elevation followed by ST elevation greater than 2 mm for type II and less than 2 mm for type III. Other ECG criteria that support a diagnosis of BrS include: presence of first-degree AV block and left-axis deviation of the QRS; presence of AF; fragmented QRS; late potentials in the signal-averaged ECG; and ST-T wave alternans and spontaneous PVC's with LBBB-type morphology.

MANAGEMENT

Strategic mapping

Management can be stratified into acute management that aims to terminate an ongoing episode of VT or VF or to suppress incessant VT; and maintenance management that aims to prevent recurrent VT and protect the patient from SCD. The best approach to the acute management of VT depends on the hemodynamic status of the patient. In hemodynamically unstable patients (such as when VT causes hypotension, shock, angina, congestive HF, or cerebral hypoperfusion), VT should be treated promptly with cardioversion/defibrillation. In patients who are hemodynamically stable during VT, defibrillation should be deferred until pharmacologic interventions have been tried. After the resolution of VT, a search for reversible conditions contributing to the initiation and persistence of VT should be made and the conditions corrected such as cardiac ischemia, HF, electrolyte abnormalities, or drug toxicities.

Patients who have VT due to a transient or reversible cause may not have a poor long-term prognosis, if the offending cause can be thoroughly eradicated. These patients may not require prophylactic therapy

Table 9.4 Questions to discuss with clinicians before treatment

1. What are the levels of certainty of evidence regarding risks and benefits?
2. How do these risks and benefits compare with potential alternatives?
3. What are the treatment options available?
4. What are the rates of success or failure of these treatment options?
5. What are the side-effects or complications with these treatment options?
6. What would be the comparative cost or cost-effectiveness of the treatment?
7. What happens if this treatment approach does not work for me?
8. How will you help me balance my treatment with the demand of active life?

after the index episode. Other patients may have a VT (such as idiopathic LV VT or RV outflow tract VT) that is curable by catheter ablation. Chronic prophylactic therapy is initiated after ruling out reversible transient causes and specific syndromes which may be amenable to curative treatment.

Unfortunately, however, most patients with VT do not have a transient, reversible, or curable condition. These patients require maintenance therapy to prevent recurrent VT and/or arrhythmic SCD. Treatment options include anti-arrhythmic drug therapy or ICD therapy. Radiofrequency catheter ablation (RFCA) may be used for in order to make episodes of VT less likely to occur, even when the RFCA is not expected to fully eliminate the risk of recurrent VT. Frequently, a combination of the above options is required for management of patients with an ongoing risk of VT.

For patients with VT, the treatment plan should be discussed in detail concerning indications, risks and benefits, and alternate options. A well-informed patient should ask about treatment options and question the success and potential complications of the proposed treatment. The detailed questions are listed in Table 9.4.

Acute management

Acute management of sustained VT depends on the hemodynamic status. In the acute treatment of VT, direct current (DC) shock is usually successful. If distinct QRS and T waves are identified in the monitoring ECG, the shock can be synchronized to the QRS complex. The desire to terminate VT with a shock that has the lowest possible energy must be balanced by the desire to avoid the need for multiple shocks when the first shock(s) are ineffective. As a result, guidelines recommend that the initial synchronized shock in these circumstances should be 100 joules with a biphasic waveform, and 200 joules with a monophasic waveform, with titration of the energy upward as needed [13].

The DC shock should not be synchronized. If the QRS complex and T wave cannot be distinguished accurately, or if the QRS complexes are wide and bizarre, or if the VT is polymorphic, such patients should be treated with immediate defibrillation (unsynchronized shock) using 360 joules [monophasic] or 200 joules [biphasic]). The only definitive treatment for VF is defibrillation. When defibrillation is performed promptly, the success rate for terminating VF can be as high as 95% [14–17]. However, the success rate falls substantially as the duration of VF increases, probably due to myocardial ischemia, acidosis, and other metabolic changes. These cellular changes are associated with deterioration of VF [18]. Certain specific precautions are needed during cardioversion in specific populations and these are summarized in Table 9.5.

If the patient is hemodynamically stable, acute termination of VT may be achieved by intravenous administration of amiodarone, lidocaine, or procainamide, followed by an infusion of the successful drug [19]. In patients in whom procainamide is ineffective or in whom procainamide may be problematic (severe HF, renal failure), intravenous amiodarone is often effective. Amiodarone is the preferred drug.

Treatment of coexisting precipitating factors

If VT recurs or persists following initial attempts at cardioversion, suppression of the arrhythmia by pharmacologic means should be attempted and further evaluation should focus upon the presence of arrhythmia triggers (e.g. ischemia, electrolyte abnormalities, and drug toxicity). Cardioversion or defibrillation should be repeated as necessary in patients who are hemodynamically unstable. Multiple recurrences of VT should raise concern about cardiac ischemia, hypokalemia, digitalis toxicity, and polymorphic VT with or without QT prolongation, all of which have specific appropriate therapy including withdrawal of the offending agent and infusion of magnesium sulfate.

Extreme hyperkalemia (with serum potassium concentration >8 mEq/L) can cause an incessant VT with a sinusoidal morphology. It should be treated with IV calcium (10–30 mL 10% calcium gluconate given over 1–5 minutes), hypertonic glucose plus insulin, and sodium bicarbonate (44–132 mEq, or 1–3 ampules).

Class IC anti-arrhythmic drugs (flecainide, encainide, and propafenone) cause a similar VT, which occasionally responds to lidocaine but can be highly refractory. Theoretically, this arrhythmia might respond best to hypertonic sodium, which would counteract the sodium channel blocking effects of the Class IC drug [51, 52].

Table 9.5 Electrical cardioversion in specific populations

Pregnant women

- Can be performed during pregnancy without affecting the rhythm of the fetus [14].
- Fetal heart rate should be monitored during the procedure using standard fetal monitoring techniques.

Patients with ICD or pacemaker

- Defibrillation in these patients can damage the pulse generator, the lead system, or the myocardial tissue, resulting in device dysfunction.
- The electrode paddle (or patch) should be at least 12 cm from the pulse generator and an anteroposterior paddle position is recommended.
- Elective cardioversion should be initiated with the lowest indicated energy (which will vary depending on the arrhythmia) in order to avoid damage to the device circuitry and the electrode-myocardial interface.
- After cardioversion, the pacemaker should be interrogated and evaluated to ensure normal pacemaker function.
- It is possible to defibrillate with less energy directly via an implanted ICD.

Patients with digoxin toxicity

- There is a relative contraindication to cardioversion in the setting of digitalis toxicity since digitalis sensitizes the heart to the electrical stimulus and, hence, cardioversion could trigger additional arrhythmias, most importantly ventricular fibrillation.
- If cardioversion must be performed for a life-threatening ventricular arrhythmia, prophylactic lidocaine (1 mg/kg up to a maximum dose of 100 mg IV push) should be given and the lowest indicated energy levels used.

Anti-arrhythmic drugs

Beta-blockers   Beta-blockers (BB) are increasingly being utilized in patients with ventricular arrhythmias for their anti-arrhythmic and anti-fibrillatory effects per se. This class of drugs has been shown to be useful as solitary agents in patients with specific VT/VF syndromes, such as RVOT VT or exercise-induced VT, and in those with reversible myocardial ischemia [20, 21]. BBs have been a mainstay in patients with HF, CAD, and ventricular arrhythmias. In the Multicenter Automatic Defibrillator Implantation (MADIT)-II trial, patients receiving higher doses of BBs had a significant reduction in the risk for VT or VF requiring ICD therapy, while also improving survival [22]. BBs exert a synergistic effect in combination with amiodarone, but no clear mechanism has been identified for this beneficial interaction. Finally, BBs have also been used in patients with ICDs for suppression of excessive ICD discharges.

Calcium channel antagonists   Calcium channel antagonists have been shown to be of use in therapy of idiopathic RVOT VT and idiopathic left VT [23].

Class II and III anti-arrhythmic drugs   Broadly speaking, class II and III anti-arrhythmic drugs have become the mainstay of drug therapy for prevention of VT recurrences. The first drugs to be used for prevention of recurrences of VT were the class I anti-arrhythmic agents. However, quinidine and procainamide not only failed to reduce the probability of recurrent VT, but by their pro-arrhythmic effects, increased the risk of VT/VF and sudden death recurrence. Class IC anti-arrhythmics also can be detrimental in patients with structural heart disease.

The Cardiac Arrhythmia Suppression (CAST) trial evaluated the effect of encainide and flecainide in patients with asymptomatic or mildly symptomatic ventricular arrhythmia after myocardial infarction (MI). During an average of 10 months of follow-up, patients treated with drug had a higher rate of death from arrhythmia and higher total mortality than the patients assigned to placebo [24]. In the Electrophysiologic Study versus Electrocardiographic Monitoring (ESVEM) trial, seven anti-arrhythmic drugs (imipramine, mexiletine, pirmenol, procainamide, propafenone, quinidine and sotalol) were randomly tried until one was effective in suppressing the inducible arrhythmia (in the electrophysiology group) or in suppressing premature ventricular complexes (in the Holter monitoring group). In the electrophysiology group 242 patients (45%) received a prediction of efficacy while 185 patients (77%) did so in the Holter-monitoring group. However, despite these predictions of efficacy the arrhythmia recurrence rate was very high. Importantly sotalol, which was not as effective as class I anti-arrhythmic drugs (such as mexiletine) in suppressing non-sustained VT on Holter monitor, was more effective in reducing mortality than other class I anti-arrhythmic agents [26]. This showed the dissociation between arrhythmia suppression and total mortality. The Multicenter Unsustained Tachycardia (MUSTT) trial compared standard medical therapy to electrophysiologically guided treatment with anti-arrhythmic drug (AAD) or ICD for the prevention of sudden death in patients with monomorphic VT induced at electrophysiology study in patients with ICM and non-sustained VT clinically. There was no statistically significant difference when compared to patients receiving standard medical therapy in terms of sudden death and ventricular arrhythmia occurrence [27].

Amiodarone Amiodarone has now emerged as the most effective anti-arrhythmic drug for the short- and long-term treatment of VT. Numerous small trials in the 1980s indicated the efficacy of amiodarone in patients with ventricular arrhythmia and the drug significantly reduced the incidence of deaths due to arrhythmia in subsequent large randomized trials [28–30]. The clinical benefits of amiodarone persist despite persistent inducibility of VT at EPS on steady-state oral therapy [31].

Currently, for acute management amiodarone, 150 mg IV over 10 minutes followed by an infusion of 1 mg/minute for 6 hours, then 0.5 mg/minute, is recommended in most settings, for VT. Alternatives include procainamide (15 to 18 mg/kg administered as slow infusion over 25–30 minutes, followed by 1–4 mg/minute by continuous infusion); or lidocaine (1 to 1.5 mg/kg over 2 to 3 minutes), particularly if cardiac ischemia is suspected.

Treatment of specific genetic syndromes

Long QT syndrome BBs should be administered to all patients with LQTS whether symptomatic (syncope, cardiac arrest, or palpitations that correspond to VT on monitor) or asymptomatic [32]. There is no evidence to support cardioselective BB versus non-cardioselective BB, except in patients with asthma in whom the former would be preferred. Long-acting BBs such as nadolol or sustained-release propranolol are preferred to short-acting drugs such as atenolol, metoprolol tartrate, or carvedilol. Left cardiac sympathetic denervation (LCSD) is a therapeutic option when BBs are contraindicated.

Patients with LQT1 should avoid strenuous exercise especially swimming. On the other hand, patients may participate in with genetically proven LQTS but with borderline prolongation of the QT interval, no history of cardiac symptoms, and no family history of SCD may exercise and participate in competitive sports as long as they are closely supervised, with personnel trained in basic life support and an automatic external defibrillator nearby.

Patients with LQT2 should avoid abrupt loud noises such as alarm clocks or loud phone ringing. All patients with LQTS should avoid drugs that prolong the QT interval (www.qtdrugs.org). Electrolyte abnormalities should also be avoided, such as those that can occur during diarrhea, vomiting, metabolic conditions, and imbalanced diets or weight loss.

ICD therapy is indicated in patients with LQTS who have been resuscitated from a cardiac arrest, and in patients who have had syncope while taking beta-blockers. ICD therapy may also be considered in patients for whom beta-blockade is contraindicated. If ICD therapy cannot be used (for example, if the patient declines it), or in order to prevent shocks from an ICD, then LCSD is a reasonable option.

Brugada syndrome   The only proven effective therapy for patients with the BrS is the ICD. Unfortunately, the ICD has several disadvantages, especially in active young individuals, who are susceptible to receiving inappropriate shocks from their ICDs, and who will need multiple surgeries for generator and lead replacement during their lifetimes. Therefore, ICDs are indicated only in patients with BrS who have had syncope or have been resuscitated from cardiac arrest from VT or VF. Patients with BrS should avoid drugs that may induce or aggravate ST segment elevation in right precordial leads (Brugadadrugs.org). They should also avoid excessive alcohol intake and immediately treat fever with antipyretic drugs. Quinidine can be useful in patients with a history of 'VT storm', defined as more than three episodes of VT/VF in 24 hours. Quinidine may be used for the treatment of SVT in patients with BrS, which is important because other anti-arrhythmic drugs such as flecainide and propafenone are contraindicated in BrS. Isoproterenol infusion can be helpful in the acute management of patients with BrS and arrhythmic storm.

Prevention of sudden cardiac death   The goal of long-term therapy is to prevent SCD and recurrence of symptomatic VT. This may be categorized into two types: primary prevention (prophylactic) in which the subjects have not experienced a life-threatening ventricular arrhythmia or a symptomatic equivalent and secondary prevention where subjects who have had an abortive cardiac arrest, a life-threatening VT, or unexplained syncope with work-up suggesting a high probability that a ventricular tachyarrhythmia was the cause of the syncope.

Several prospective multicenter clinical trials have documented improved survival with ICD therapy in high-risk patients with LV dysfunction due to prior MI and non-ischemic cardiomyopathy (Table 9.6) [33–40]. ICD therapy compared with conventional or traditional anti-arrhythmic drug therapy has been associated with mortality reductions from 23% to 55% depending on the risk group participating in the trial, with the improvement in survival due almost exclusively to a reduction in SCD.

Evidence from multiple randomized controlled trials (RCT) supports the use of ICDs for secondary prevention of sudden cardiac arrest regardless of the type of underlying structural heart disease (Table 9.7). In patients resuscitated from cardiac arrest, the ICD is associated with clinically and statistically significant reductions in sudden death and total mortality

Table 9.6 Major ICD trials for primary prevention of SCD

Trial	Total number of subjects	Selection criteria	Design	Mortality, Hazard Ratio ICD
MADIT, 1996	196	Prior myocardial infarction (MI), non-sustained VT (NSVT) on monitoring, left ventricular (LV) dysfunction (LVEF <35%), and inducible sustained monomorphic VT	ICD vs. medical management	Mortality 0.46 (P = 0.009)
MUSTT, 1999	704	Prior MI (less than one month to more than three years previously), asymptomatic NSVT, an LVEF ≤40%, and inducible sustained VT	EP guided treatment with AADs vs. ICD vs. no AAD	Mortality 0.40 (P < 0.001)
MADIT II, 2002	1232	With a myocardial infarction more than 30 days prior to enrollment (and more than three months if bypass surgery was performed) and an LVEF ≤30%	3:2 ICD vs. medical management	Mortality 0.65 (P = 0.016) Survival benefit was due to prevention of SCD
CABG patch, 1997	900	Epicardial ICD implanted at the time of CABG undergoing surgery for severe CHD who had significant LV dysfunction (LVEF <36%) and a positive signal-averaged electrocardiogram (ECG)	ICD with CABG vs. no ICD with CABG	Mortality 1.07 (P = NS)
CAT, 2002	104	Recent onset (≤9 months) dilated cardiomyopathy and an LVEF ≤30%	ICD vs. no ICD	Cumulative survival was not significantly different between the two groups (93% and 80% in the control group vs. 92% and 86% in the ICD group after 2 and 4 years, respectively).

SCDHeFT, 2005	2521	NYHA class II or III heart failure (HF) due to either an ischemic or non-ischemic cardiomyopathy and LVEF ≤35% and	ICD vs. amiodarone vs. placebo	Mortality 0.77 (P = 0.007)
DINAMIT	674	MI in the preceding 6 to 40 days (mean 18 days), LVEF ≤35% and reduced heart rate variability or elevated resting heart rate (≥80 beats/min). Patients with sustained VT >48 hours post-MI, NYHA class IV HF, or CABG or three-vessel PCI post-MI were excluded.	ICD vs. no ICD	Mortality 1.08 (P = 0.66)
DEFINITE	458	Non-ischemic dilated cardiomyopathy, an LVEF ≤35%, and ventricular premature beats or NSVT	ICD vs. medical management	Mortality HR 0.65 (P = 0.08)
AMIOVERT	103	moderate to severe non-ischemic dilated cardiomyopathy as manifested by class I to III heart failure, an LVEF ≤35%, and asymptomatic NSVT	ICD, often with amiodarone, to amiodarone alone	Mortality (P = 0.8) Arrhythmia free survival (P = 0.1)
COMPANION	1520	NYHA class III–IV HF and an LVEF ≤35% who had had a hospitalization for HF within the year prior to enrollment	CRT-D vs. CRT-P	Mortality HR 0.64 (P = 0.004)
IRIS, 2009	898	MI within the preceding 5 to 31 days, and one or both of the following two criteria: • LVEF ≤40% and a resting heart rate ≥90 beats/min • Non-sustained VT at a rate of ≥150 beats/min	ICD vs. no ICD	Mortality 1.04 (P = 0.78)

Table 9.7 Major ICD trials for secondary prevention of SCD

Trial	Total no. of patients	Selection criteria	Randomization	Outcome
AVID 1997	1016	(a) Resuscitated VF; (b) sustained VT with syncope; or (c) sustained VT with BP <80 mmHg or (near-syncope, CHF, or angina with hemodynamic compromise and LVEF ≤40%	ICD vs. class III anti-arrhythmics (mainly amiodarone)	Mortality HR 0.62 ($P < 0.02$)
CASH 2000	349	Survivors of cardiac arrest due to documented VT or VF	ICD vs. amiodarone, propafenone, metoprolol	Mortality HR 0.766 ($P = 0.081$) SCD HR 0.423 $P = 0.005$).
CIDS 2000	659	Resuscitated VT/VF or syncope deemed to be secondary to VT/VF	ICD vs. amiodarone	Mortality RRR 19.7% ($P = 0.142$) SCD RRR 32.8% ($P = 0.094$)

compared with anti-arrhythmic drug therapy in prospective RCTs [41–48]. The effectiveness of ICDs on outcomes in the recent large, prospective secondary prevention trials – AVID (Anti-arrhythmics Versus Implantable Defibrillators) [42], CASH (Cardiac Arrest Study Hamburg) [44], and CIDS (Canadian Implantable Defibrillator Study) [45] were consistent with prior investigations [43]. Specifically, the ICD was associated with a 50% relative risk reduction for arrhythmic death and a 25% relative risk reduction for all-cause mortality [47]. Thus, secondary prevention trials have been robust and have shown a consistent effect of improved survival with ICD therapy compared with anti-arrhythmic drug therapy across studies [47].

Sustained monomorphic VT with prior MI is unlikely to be affected by revascularization [41]. Myocardial revascularization may be sufficient therapy in patients surviving VF in association with myocardial ischemia when ventricular function is normal and there is no history of an MI [41].

Unless electrolyte abnormalities are proven to be the sole cause of cardiac arrest, survivors of cardiac arrest in whom electrolyte abnormalities are discovered in general should be treated in a manner similar to that of cardiac arrest survivors without electrolyte abnormalities [41]. Patients who experience sustained monomorphic VT in the presence of anti-arrhythmic drugs or electrolyte abnormalities should also be evaluated and treated in a manner similar to patients with VT or VF without electrolyte abnormalities or anti-arrhythmic drugs [41].

Primary prevention   Primary prevention of SCD refers to the use of ICDs in individuals who are at risk for but have not yet had an episode of sustained VT, VF, or resuscitated cardiac arrest. Clinical trials have evaluated the risks and benefits of the ICD in prevention of sudden death and have improved survival in multiple patient populations, including those with prior MI and HF due to either CAD or non-ischemic dilated cardiomyopathy (DCM). Prospective registry data are less robust but still useful for risk stratification and recommendations for ICD implantation in selected other patient populations, such as those with HCM, ARVD/C, and the long-QT syndrome. In less common conditions (e.g., Brugada syndrome, catecholaminergic polymorphic VT, cardiac sarcoidosis, and LV non-compaction), clinical reports and retrospectively analyzed series provide evidence in support of current recommendations for ICD use [49].

Catheter ablation   Anti-arrhythmic therapy, although commonly used to complement ICD therapy in patients with recurrent VT, is incompletely successful in preventing VT episodes and may cause important cardiac and non-cardiac side effects [50]. Moreover, ICD shocks have deleterious effects on morbidity. As a result, catheter ablation of VT is becoming a more frequently utilized option. Ablation is most often performed as adjunctive therapy in patients with ICDs and frequently taking AAD.

Catheter ablation has been very effective in certain specific types of ventricular arrhythmias such as idiopathic VT and bundle branch re-entrant VT [51, 52]. The success of radiofrequency ablation in therapy of idiopathic VT is very high with infrequent complications and excellent long term results. Complications during ablations for VT include development of complete left or right BBB, aortic regurgitation, left main coronary artery occlusion, and, rarely, death [53, 54]. Although it is typically reserved for patients who have failed or are intolerant to therapy with

---

Table 9.8 Indications for catheter ablation

Current ACC/AHA guidelines give Class I recommendation for ablation in:

1. Patients who are otherwise at low risk for SCD and have sustained predominantly monomorphic VT that is drug resistant, who are drug intolerant, or who do not wish long-term drug therapy (Level of Evidence: C).
2. Patients with bundle-branch re-entrant VT (Level of Evidence: C).
3. As adjunctive therapy in patients with an ICD who are receiving multiple shocks as a result of sustained VT that is not manageable by reprogramming or changing drug therapy or who do not wish long-term drug therapy [67, 68] (Level of Evidence: C).
4. Patients with Wolff-Parkinson-White syndrome resuscitated from sudden cardiac arrest due to atrial fibrillation and rapid conduction over the accessory pathway causing VF [69] (Level of Evidence: B) [4].
5. For above group of patients with non-sustained VT, ablation procedure is given Class IIa recommendation with Level of Evidence C.

---

anti-arrhythmic agents, ablation is an attractive initial treatment strategy in selected patients with idiopathic VT.

However, ablation of VT in patients with CAD disease remains extremely challenging [55]. VT ablation is more technically difficult and subject to a higher risk for complications than many other ablation procedures. Limitations also arise due to presence of re-entrant circuits with broad paths that may be located subendocardially, intramurally or even in subepicardial regions of the myocardium [56, 57]. Also more than one re-entrant circuit may exist with multiple morphologies of VT [58]. As a result, curative ablation of post-infarct VT is achieved in only a small group of patients [58–62]. Most patients have additional VTs which are induced in the electrophysiology laboratory besides their 'clinical' VT. Available data suggest that these 'non-clinical' VTs are likely to manifest during follow-up suggesting that all inducible VTs should be ablated. Rothman et al [58]. showed that all inducible VTs could be ablated in only 30% of patients. Recurrences of VT during follow-up are rare among these patients. Almost all patients would thus still need ICD therapy after radiofrequency catheter ablation. Hence, currently the most frequent indication for radiofrequency catheter ablation is in patients with ICDs who are experiencing frequent VT episodes which require repeated electrical shocks. Nevertheless, ablation for VT in patients after MI is important, not for its relative frequency, but for the profound influence this procedure has on quality of life [63, 64]. Most patients who undergo VT ablation have ICDs and have frequent episodes leading to ICD shocks. Patients who present with uniform tolerated VT typically receive ICDs after successful ablation because even after the most complete form of substrate modification, subendocardial resection, there is a significant residual risk for sudden death (2.1% per year) [65]. This is consistent with the observation from the Electrophysiologic Study Versus Electromagnetic Monitoring (ESVEM) trial that presentation with uniform tolerated VT does not predict presentation with recurrent tolerated VT as opposed to cardiac arrest [66]. Anti-arrhythmic therapy, although commonly used to complement ICD therapy in patients with recurrent VT, is incompletely successful in preventing VT episodes and may cause important cardiac and non-cardiac side effects [50]. The indications for catheter ablation are listed in Table 9.8.

ACTION POINTS

Treatment for VT in patients with both ischemic and non-ischemic cardiomyopathy has progressed greatly over the past few decades, from medical, to ICD, to ablative therapy. While ICDs have been a tremendous advance in the prevention of sudden death and anti-arrhythmic medications can help minimize ICD therapies, the continued evolution of catheter ablation may allow for greater success in greater numbers of patients.

REFERENCES

1. Tracy CM, Epstein AE, Darbar D, et al. 2012 ACCF/AHA/HRS focused update of the 2008 guidelines for device-based therapy of cardiac rhythm abnormalities: a report of the American College of Cardiology Foundation/American Heart Association Task Force on Practice Guidelines and the Heart Rhythm Society. *Circulation.* 2012 Oct 2;126(14):1784–1800.
2. Knight BP, Pelosi F, Michaud GF, Strickberger SA, Morady F. (1999). Clinical consequences of electrocardiographic artifact mimicking ventricular tachycardia. *New Engl J Med.* 1999;341(17):1270–1274. doi:10.1056/NEJM199910213411704.
3. Brugada P, Brugada J, Mont L, et al. A new approach to the differential diagnosis of a regular tachycardia with a wide QRS complex. *Circulation.* 1991;83:1649–1659.
4. ACC/AHA/ESC 2006 guidelines for management of patients with ventricular arrhythmias and the prevention of sudden cardiac death: a report of the American College of Cardiology/American Heart Association Task Force and

the European Society of Cardiology Committee for Practice Guidelines (Writing Committee to Develop Guidelines for Management of Patients With Ventricular Arrhythmias and the Prevention of Sudden Cardiac Death) *J Am Coll Cardiol.* 2006;48(5):e247–346.

5. Schiller NB, Shah PM, Crawford M, et al. Recommendations for quantitation of the left ventricle by two-dimensional echocardiography. American Society of Echocardiography Committee on Standards, Subcommittee on Quantitation of Two-Dimensional Echocardiograms. *J Am Soc Echocardiogr.* 1989;2:358–367.

6. Gibbons RJ, Balady GJ, Bricker JT, et al. ACC/AHA 2002 guideline update for exercise testing: summary article: a report of the American College of Cardiology/American Heart Association Task Force on Practice Guidelines (Committee to Update the 1997 Exercise Testing Guidelines). *J Am Coll Cardiol.* 2002;40:1531–1540.

7. Probst V, Veltmann C, Eckardt L, Meregalli PG, Gaita F, Tan HL, Wilde AAM. Long-term prognosis of patients diagnosed with Brugada syndrome: Results From the FINGER Brugada Syndrome Registry. *Circulation.* 2010;121(5):635–643. doi: 10.1161/circulationaha.109.887026.

8. Priori SG, Gasparini M, Napolitano C, Della Bella P, Ottonelli AG, Sassone B, Colombo M. Risk stratification in Brugada syndrome: Results of the PRELUDE (PRogrammed ELectrical stimUlation preDictive valuE) Registry. *J Am Coll Cardiol.* 59(1):37–45. doi: 10.1016/j.jacc.2011.08.064.

9. Gouaux JL, Ashman R. Auricular fibrillation with aberration simulating ventricular paroxysmal tachycardia. *Am Heart J.* 1947;34:366–373.

10. Nogami A1, Naito S, Tada H, Taniguchi K, et al. Demonstration of diastolic and presystolic Purkinje potentials as critical potentials in a macrore-entry circuit of verapamil-sensitive idiopathic left ventricular tachycardia. *J Am Coll Cardiol.* 2000 Sep;36(3):811–823.

11. Noda T, Shimizu W, Taguchi A, et al. Malignant entity of idiopathic ventricular fibrillation and polymorphic ventricular tachycardia initiated by premature extra systoles originating from the right ventricular outflow tract. *J Am Coll Cardiol.* 2005;46(7):1288–1294.

12. Hoffmayer KS, Bhave PD, Marcus GM, et al. (2013). An electrocardiographic scoring system for distinguishing right ventricular outflow tract arrhythmias in patients with arrhythmogenic right ventricular cardiomyopathy from idiopathic ventricular tachycardia. *Heart Rhythm.* 2013;10(4), 477–482. doi: 10.1016/j.hrthm.2012.12.009.

13. Link MS, Atkins DL, Passman RS, Halperin HR, Samson RA, White RD, Cudnik MT, Berg MD, Kudenchuk PJ, Kerber RE. Part 6: electrical therapies: automated external defibrillators, defibrillation, cardioversion, and pacing: 2010 American Heart Association Guidelines for Cardiopulmonary Resuscitation and Emergency Cardiovascular Care. *Circulation.* 2010;122(18 Suppl 3):S706–719.

14. Faddy SC, Powell J, Craig JC. Biphasic and monophasic shocks for transthoracic defibrillation: a meta-analysis of randomized controlled trials. *Resuscitation.* 2003;58(1):9–16.

15. Morrison LJ, Dorian P, Long J, Vermeulen M, Schwartz B, Sawadsky B, Frank J, Cameron B, Burgess R, Shield J, Bagley P, Mausz V, Brewer JE, Lerman BB, Steering Committee, Central Validation Committee, Safety and Efficacy Committee.

Out-of-hospital cardiac arrest rectilinear biphasic to monophasic damped sine defibrillation waveforms with advanced life support intervention trial (ORBIT). *Resuscitation*. 2005;66(2):149–157.

16. Martens PR, Russell JK, Wolcke B, Paschen H, Kuisma M, Gliner BE, Weaver WD, Bossaert L, Chamberlain D, Schneider T. Optimal Response to Cardiac Arrest study: defibrillation waveform effects. *Resuscitation*. 2001;49(3):233–243.

17. Stothert JC, Hatcher TS, Gupton CL, Love JE, Brewer JE. Rectilinear biphasic waveform defibrillation of out-of-hospital cardiac arrest. *Prehosp Emerg Care*. 2004;8(4):388–392.

18. Tovar OH, Jones JL. Electrophysiological deterioration during long-duration ventricular fibrillation. *Circulation*. 2000;102(23):2886–2891.

19. Singh SN, Fletcher RD, Fisher SG, et al. Amiodarone in patients with congestive heart failure and asymptomatic ventricular arrhythmia. *N Engl J Med*. 1995;333:77.

20. Moss AJ, Hall WJ, Cannom DS, et al. Improved survival with an implanted defibrillator in patients with coronary disease at high risk for ventricular arrhythmia. *N Engl J Med*. 1996;335:1933.

21. Buxton AE, Lee KL, Fisher JD, Josephson ME, Prystowsky EN, Hafley G. A randomized study of the prevention of sudden death in patients with coronary artery disease. Multicenter Unsustained Tachycardia Trial Investigators. *N Engl J Med*. 1999;341:1882–1890.

22. Brodine WN, Tung RT, Lee JK, et al. Effects of beta-blockers on implantable cardioverter defibrillator therapy and survival in the patients with ischemic cardiomyopathy (from the Multicenter Automatic Defibrillator Implantation Trial-II). *Am J Cardiol*. 2005;96:691–695.

23. Gill JS, Mehta D, Ward DE, et al. Efficacy of flecainide, sotalol and verapamil in the treatment of right ventricular tachycardia in patients without overt cardiac abnormality. *Br Heart J*. 1992;68:392–397.

24. The Cardiac Arrhythmia Suppression Trial (CAST) Investigators. Preliminary report: effect of encainide and flecainide on mortality in a randomized trial of arrhythmia suppression after myocardial infarction. *N Engl J Med*. 1989;321:406–412.

25. Mason JW, for the Electrophysiologic Study versus Electrocardiographic Monitoring Investigators. A comparison of electrophysiologic testing with Holter monitoring to predict anti-arrhythmic-drug efficacy for ventricular tachyarrhythmias. *N Engl J Med*. 1993;329:445–451.

26. Mason JW, for the Electrophysiologic Study versus Electrocardiographic Monitoring Investigators. A comparison of seven anti-arrhythmic drugs in patients with ventricular tachyarrhythmias. *N Engl J Med*. 1993;329:52–58.

27. Buxton AE, Lee KL, Fisher JD, Josephson ME, Prystowsky EN, Hafley G. A randomized study of the prevention of sudden death in patients with coronary artery disease. Multicenter Unsustained Tachycardia Trial Investigators. *N Engl J Med*. 1999;341:1882–1890.

28. Julian DG, Camm AJ, Frangin MJ, et al. for the European Myocardial Infarct Amiodarone Trial Investigators. Randomized trial of effect of amiodarone on mortality in patients with left-ventricular dysfunction after recent myocardial infarction: EMIAT. *Lancet*. 1997;349:647–674.

29. Cairns JA, Conrolly SJ, Roberts R, et al. for the Canadian Amiodarone Myocardial Infarction Arrhythmia Trial Investigators. Randomized trial of outcome after myocardial infarction in patients with frequent or repetitive ventricular premature depolarisations: CAMIAT. *Lancet.* 1997;349: 675–682.

30. Amiodarone Trials Meta-Analysis Investigators. Effect of prophylactic amiodarone on mortality after acute myocardial infarction and in congestive heart failure: meta-analysis of individual data from 6500 patients in randomised trials. *Lancet.* 1997 Nov 15;350 (9089):1417–1424.

31. Nasir N, Swarna US, Boachene KA, et al. Therapy of sustained ventricular arrhythmias with amiodarone: prediction of efficacy with serial electrophysiologic studies. *J. Cardiovasc Pharmacol Ther.* 1996;1:123–133.

32. Priori SG, Wilde AA, Horie M, Cho Y, Behr ER, Berul C, Tracy C. HRS/EHRA/APHRS Expert Consensus Statement on the Diagnosis and Management of Patients with Inherited Primary Arrhythmia Syndromes. *Heart Rhythm.* 10(12):1932–1963. doi: 10.1016/j.hrthm.2013.05.014.

33. Buxton AE, Lee KL, Fisher JD, Josephson ME, Prystowsky EN, Hafley G. A randomized study of the prevention of sudden death in patients with coronary artery disease. Multicenter Unsustained Tachycardia Trial Investigators. *N Engl J Med.* 1999;341:1882–1890.

34. Bardy GH, Lee KL, Mark DB, et al. Amiodarone or an implantable cardioverter-defibrillator for congestive heart failure. *N Engl J Med.* 2005;352:225–237.

35. The Anti-arrhythmics versus Implantable Defibrillators (AVID) Investigators. A comparison of anti-arrhythmic-drug therapy with implantable defibrillators in patients resuscitated from near-fatal ventricular arrhythmias. *N Engl J Med.* 1997;337:1576–1583.

36. Moss AJ, Hall WJ, Cannom DS, et al. Improved survival with an implanted defibrillator in patients with coronary disease at high risk for ventricular arrhythmia. Multicenter Automatic Defibrillator Implantation Trial Investigators. *N Engl J Med.* 1996;335:1933–1940.

37. Bigger JT Jr. Prophylactic use of implanted cardiac defibrillators in patients at high risk for ventricular arrhythmias after coronary-artery bypass graft surgery. Coronary Artery Bypass Graft (CABG) Patch Trial Investigators. *N Engl J Med.* 1997;337:1569–1575.

38. Moss AJ, Zareba W, Hall WJ, et al. Prophylactic implantation of a defibrillator in patients with myocardial infarction and reduced ejection fraction. *N Engl J Med.* 2002;346:877–883.

39. Lee DS, Green LD, Liu PP, et al. Effectiveness of implantable defibrillators for preventing arrhythmic events and death: a metaanalysis. *J Am Coll Cardiol.* 2003;41:1573–1582.

40. Ezekowitz JA, Armstrong PW, McAlister FA. Implantable cardioverter defibrillators in primary and secondary prevention: a systematic review of randomized, controlled trials. *Ann Intern Med.* 2003;138: 445–452.

41. ACC/AHA/ESC 2006 guidelines for management of patients with ventricular arrhythmias and the prevention of sudden cardiac death: a report of the American College of Cardiology/American Heart Association Task Force and the European Society of Cardiology Committee for Practice Guidelines (Writing

Committee to Develop Guidelines for Management of Patients With Ventricular Arrhythmias and the Prevention of Sudden Cardiac Death) *J Am Coll Cardiol.* 2006;48(5):e247–346.

42. The Anti-arrhythmics versus Implantable Defibrillators (AVID) Investigators. A comparison of anti-arrhythmic-drug therapy with implantable defibrillators in patients resuscitated from near-fatal ventricular arrhythmias. *N Engl J Med.* 1997;337:1576–1583.

43. Wever EF, Hauer RN, van Capelle FL, et al. Randomized study of implantable defibrillator as first-choice therapy versus conventional strategy in postinfarct sudden death survivors. *Circulation.* 1995;91:2195–2203.

44. Siebels J, Kuck KH. Implantable cardioverter defibrillator compared with anti-arrhythmic drug treatment in cardiac arrest survivors (the Cardiac Arrest Study Hamburg). *Am Heart J.* 1994;127:1139–1144.

45. Connolly SJ, Gent M, Roberts RS, et al. Canadian implantable defibrillator study (CIDS): a randomized trial of the implantable cardioverter defibrillator against amiodarone. *Circulation.* 2000;101:1297–1302.

46. Kuck KH, Cappato R, Siebels J, Ruppel R. Randomized comparison of anti-arrhythmic drug therapy with implantable defibrillators in patients resuscitated from cardiac arrest: the Cardiac Arrest Study Hamburg (CASH). *Circulation.* 2000;102:748–754.

47. Connolly SJ, Hallstrom AP, Cappato R, et al. Meta-analysis of the implantable cardioverter defibrillator secondary prevention trials. AVID, CASH and CIDS studies. Anti-arrhythmics vs. Implantable Defibrillator study. Cardiac Arrest Study Hamburg. Canadian Implantable Defibrillator Study. *Eur Heart J.* 2000;21:2071–2078.

48. Lee DS, Austin PC, Rouleau JL, Liu PP, Naimark D, Tu JV. Predicting mortality among patients hospitalized for heart failure: derivation and validation of a clinical model. *JAMA.* 2003;290:2581–2587.

49. Epstein AE, DiMarco JP, Ellenbogen KA, Freedman RA, et al.ACC/AHA/HRS 2008 Guidelines for Device-based therapy of cardiac rhythm abnormalities: A Report of the American College of Cardiology/American Heart Association Task Force on Practice Guidelines (Writing Committee to Revise the ACC/AHA/NASPE 2002 Guideline Update for Implantation of Cardiac Pacemakers and Antiarrhythmia Devices). *Circulation.* 2008;117:e350–e408.

50. Connolly SJ, Dorian P, Roberts RS, et al. Comparison of beta-blockers, amiodarone plus beta-blockers, or sotalol for prevention of shocks from implantable cardioverter defibrillators. The OPTIC Study: a randomized trial. *JAMA.* 2006;295:165–171.

51. Klein LS, Shih HT, Hackett K, et al. Radiofrequency catheter ablation of ventricular tachycardia in patients without structural heart disease. *Circulation.* 1992;85:1666–1674.

52. Coggins DL, Lee RJ, Sweeney J, et al. Radiofrequency catheter ablation as a cure for idiopathic tachycardia of both left and right ventricular origin. *J Am Coll Cardiol.* 1994;23:1333–1341.

53. Zhu D, Maloney JD, Simmons TE, et al. Radiofrequency catheter ablation for management of symptomatic ventricular ectopic activity. *J Am Coll Cardiol.* 1995;26:843–849.

54. Friedman PL, Stevenson WG, Bihl JA, et al. Left main coronary artery occlusion during radiofrequency catheter ablation of idiopathic outflow tract tachycardia. *Pacing Clin Electrophysiol.* 1997;20:1184.

55. Stevenson WG, Khan H, Sager P, et al. Identification of re-entry circuit sites during catheter mapping and radiofrequency ablation of ventricular tachycardia late after myocardial infarction. *Circulation* 1993; 88: 1647–1670.

56. Kaltenbrunner W, Cardinal R, Dubuc M, et al. Epicardial and endocardial mapping of ventricular tachycardia in patients with myocardial infarction: is the origin of the tachycardia always subendocardially localized? *Circulation.* 1991;84: 1058–1571.

57. Downar E, Kimber S, Harris L, et al. Endocardial mapping of ventricular tachycardia in the intact human heart II. Evidence for multiuse re-entry in a function sheet of surviving myocardium. *J Am Coll Cardiol.* 1992;20:869–878.

58. Rothman SA, Hsia HH, Cossu SF, et al. Radiofrequency catheter ablation of post infarction ventricular tachycardia: long-term success and the significance of inducible nonclinical arrhythmias. *Circulation.* 1997;96:3499–3508.

59. Morady F, Harvey M, Kalbfleisch SJ, et al. Radiofrequency catheter ablation of ventricular tachycardia in patients with coronary artery disease. *Circulation.* 1993;87:363–372.

60. Bogun F, Bahu M, Knight BP, et al. Comparison of effective and ineffective target sites that demonstrate concealed entrainment in patients with coronary artery disease undergoing radiofrequency ablation of ventricular tachycardia. *Circulation.* 1997;95:183–190.

61. El-Shalakany A, Hadjis T, Papageorgion P, et al. Entrainment/mapping criteria for the prediction of termination of ventricular tachycardia by single radiofrequency lesion in patients with coronary artery disease. *Circulation.* 1999;99:2283–2289.

62. Stevenson WG, Friedman PL, Kocovic D, et al. Radiofrequency catheter ablation of ventricular tachycardia after myocardial infarction. *Circulation.* 1998; 98:308–314.

63. Strickberger SA, Man KC, Daoud EG, et al. A prospective evaluation of catheter ablation of ventricular tachycardia as adjuvant therapy in patients with coronary artery disease and an implantable cardioverter-defibrillator. *Circulation.* 1997;96:1525–1531.

64. Calkins H, Bigger JTJ, Ackerman SJ, et al. Cost-effectiveness of catheter ablation in patients with ventricular tachycardia. *Circulation.* 2000;101:280–288.

65. Sarte BH, Finkle JK, Gerszten RE, et al. What is the risk of sudden cardiac death in patients presenting with hemodynamically stable sustained ventricular tachycardia after myocardial infarction?. *J Am Coll Cardiol.* 1996;28:122–129.

66. Caruso AC, Marcus FI, Hahn EA. et al. Predictors of arrhythmic death and cardiac arrest in the ESVEM trial. Electrophysiologic Study Versus Electromagnetic Monitoring. *Circulation.* 1997;96:1888–1892.

67. Silva RM, Mont L, Nava S, et al. Radiofrequency catheter ablation for arrhythmic storm in patients with an implantable cardioverter defibrillator. *Pacing Clin Electrophysiol.* 2004;27:971–975.

68. Brugada J, Brugada R, Brugada P. Determinants of sudden cardiac death in individuals with the electrocardiographic pattern of Brugada syndrome and no previous cardiac arrest. *Circulation.* 2003;108: 3092–3096.
69. Pappone C, Santinelli V, Manguso F, et al. A randomized study of prophylactic catheter ablation in asymptomatic patients with the Wolff-Parkinson-White syndrome. *N Engl J Med.* 2003;349:1803–1811.

CHAPTER 10

Syncope

Christopher M. Bianco, Rajasekhar Nekkanti, Faisal Latif,
Phan Nam Hung, Phillip Tran, Hy Tat An and Thach Nguyen

Management of Complex Cardiovascular Problems, Fourth Edition. Edited by
Thach N. Nguyen, Dayi Hu, Shao Liang Chen, Moo Hyun Kim and Cindy L. Grines.
© 2016 John Wiley & Sons, Ltd. Published 2016 by John Wiley & Sons, Ltd.

BACKGROUND

Syncope is defined as abrupt, transient loss of consciousness (T-LOC) with loss of postural tone, followed by complete, rapid recovery [1]. The term syncope is an umbrella of several different pathophysiologic states; each leads to a common pathway of cerebral hypoperfusion via depressed cardiac output and/or decreased peripheral vascular resistance. The most common cause of syncope is neurally mediated syncope, followed by orthostatic syncope, then by cardiac origin. Seizure or any syncope due to neurological problems is rare.

CHALLENGES

The **first challenge** is to make a diagnosis of syncope, while differentiating true syncope from other mimicking conditions. Once a diagnosis of syncope is established, the **second challenge** is to determine its etiology. The highest diagnostic yield comes from the history and physical exam [2], but some further testing may still be needed. As syncope of cardiovascular (CV) origin is a harbinger of significant morbidity and even sudden cardiac death (SCD), the **third challenge** lies in ruling out the cardiac causes, in an inpatient or outpatient setting. Because non-discriminating order of diagnostic tests will give misleading results with low diagnostic yield, the **fourth challenge** is to find a judicious, logical and cost-effective investigating approach. The **final challenge** is that treatment options are limited for certain etiologies of syncope and yield variable results.

STRATEGIC MAPPING

In general, the majority of syncope is caused by the neurally mediated, orthostatic hypotensive, cardiac and neurological mechanisms. Therefore, the best diagnostic yield is to rule in or rule out the above four mechanistic etiologies according to their incidence (common to rare) when asking

Table 10.1 Questions to guide the history, physical examination and ordering of tests

1. Is it a neurally mediated syncope?
2. Is it orthostatic hypotension?
3. Is there an intrinsic cardiac problem causing hypotension (acute coronary syndrome, aortic stenosis, mitral stenosis, dilated cardiomyopathy or any significant arrhythmia?)
4. Does the patient have seizure?

the history, performing the physical examination and ordering tests. The questions which guide all the investigations are listed in Table 10.1.

This is the best strategy to formulate a working diagnosis and to establish the most likely etiology. Subsequent, focused diagnostic testing would confirm the working diagnosis. After the diagnosis and etiology are confirmed, treatments then could be planned.

CLINICAL PEARLS
Rules of thumb when ordering a test If the patient is suspected for CAD, then stress test may be indicated. If the patient has structural heart disease (after aortic stenosis or significant ischemia in CAD are ruled out), then electrophysiologic study may be indicated. If the patient has no structural heart disease, tilt table may be indicated. If syncope remains unexplained, prolonged rhythm monitoring is the best choice.

HIGH-RISK MARKERS

Anyone may have vaso-vagal syncope, while elderly patients often have syncope due to bradyarrhythmias, orthostatic hypotension, aortic stenosis and medication intolerance. Young patients usually have reflex syncope. Any patient with significant heart disease having syncope is at high risk for SCD due to ventricular tachycardia (VT) or ventricular fibrillation (VF).

HIGH-RISK PREDICTORS

There are high-risk features and prognostic scoring formulae which are helpful. The high-risk predictors are listed in Table 10.2.

Table 10.2 High-risk predictors

1. Known significant cardiac disease
2. Suspected cardiac arrhythmia or ischemia
3. Family history of sudden cardiac death
4. Event associated with physical exercise
5. Event associated with serious injury.

Generally accepted 'low risk':
1. Absence of structural heart disease.
2. History of recurrent syncope over many years.

INVESTIGATIONS

Although syncope is a confusing syndrome, almost all etiologies belong to one of the four most common problems: neurally mediated, ortho-static, cardiac and neurological. Therefore, the first strategy is to look for any symptoms or signs pointing towards these four groups of causes when asking a detailed history and performing the physical examination. Once a working diagnosis is formulated, for neurally-mediated syncope patients, the second step is to find the three factors which create the appearance of syncope: a susceptible terrain, an appropriately inappro-priate reflex causing vasodilation with or without bradycardia and a trig-gering factor. This second step is discussed in the critical thinking section below.

CRITICAL THINKING
Need of a trigger on a susceptible terrain to ignite a syncopal episode In real world practice, the most common cause for syncope is neurally mediated syncope which is initiated by anything that leads to strong myocardial contractions in an 'empty' heart. Emotional stress, reduced venous return (from dehydration or prolonged standing), or vasodilation (caused by a hot environment) stimulates the sympathetic nervous system and reduces the left ventricular cavity size, which leads to strong hyperdynamic contractions in a relatively empty heart. This hyperdynamic cavity obliteration activates myocardial mechanoreceptors, initiating a paradoxical vagal reflex

with vasodilation and relative bradycardia, and ending up with hypotensive syncope [3].

In any patient, first, there is a need to have a susceptible terrain such as moderate aortic stenosis, a new acute illness (e.g. gastrointestinal bleed, dehydration from diarrhea) or a new destabilizing situation such vasodilation from alcohol intake, or prolonged supine position, etc. These acute illnesses and destabilizing situations, could by themselves cause hypotension. Standing up may unmask low blood pressure and the patient develops syncope due to hypovolemic hypotension. In this situation, there is no vasovagal reflex, just pure hypotension causing syncope from low BP.

In these same situations such as moderate aortic stenosis, a new acute illness (e.g. gastrointestinal bleed, or dehydration from diarrhea) or a new destabilizing situation such as vasodilation from alcohol intake, or prolonged supine position, the blood pressure may not be low enough to cause hypovolemic hypotension. In these cases, a stronger trigger needs to arrive to spark the vasodilating reflex with or without bradycardia and decrease the return of blood to the right heart. These vasodilating and bradycardic reflexes and subsequent hypotension are appropriate in answering the strong ventricular contraction on an empty heart (from a local perspective); however, it is inappropriate because it precipitates generalized low blood pressure (from a global (whole body) perspective). This is why this reflex is labeled to be 'appropriately inappropriate' in the context of a neurally mediated syncope. The triggering factors could be intense emotional stimuli, physical activity, pain or any physical stressors such as sneezing, coughing, straining during bowel movement, etc. This sudden trigger ignites inappropriate bradycardia and vasodilation cascade culminating into sudden loss of blood pressure and producing the classic syncopal episode.

In order to create or recreate a scenario of hypovolemic hypotension, only two factors need to be present. In the case of a vasovagal syncopal episode, all three factors need to be positive or present. Without the susceptible terrain, even with the arrival of a trigger, there is no syncope (e.g. the patient could pass out due to sneezing while standing up but not when lying down). If there is no trigger, with a very strong susceptible terrain, there is no syncope (as seen in patient with severe aortic stenosis). The unfortunate trigger needs to induce enough severe vasodilation without bradycardia or moderate vasodilation with bradycardia in order to produce hypotension and create the syncopal episode. If only two factors are positive or present, then syncope will not happen. The formula for confirming a neurally mediated syncope is shown in Table 10.3.

Table 10.3 Formula confirming the diagnosis of hypovolemic syncope and neurally mediated syncope

Hypovolemic syncope needs a total of 2 to be positive	
Susceptible terrain	1
Triggering factor	1
Neurally mediated syncope needs a total of 3 to be positive	
Susceptible terrain	1
New appropriately un-appropriate reflex	1
Triggering factor	1

Practical examples are shown in Table 10.4. Therefore, in the investigation of a patient with syncope, there is need to identify a chronic susceptible terrain, a moderate destabilizing situation and a triggering factor.

Age

Syncope can occur at any age although on a population level, the first syncopal events tend to occur in a bimodal distribution with the first peak

Table 10.4 Identification of the susceptible terrain, a new destabilizing situation and a triggering factor

Event	Terrain	New destabilizing situation	Triggering factor		Result
Urinating	**Old age**	**Prolonged standing**	**Straining**		
	+	+	+	=	Syncope
	− (young)	+	+	=	No syncope
	+	+	−	=	No syncope
	+	−	+	=	No syncope
Exercise	**Moderate AS**	**Exercise**	**Heart rate**		
	Yes	Prolonged	High	=	Syncope
	No	Prolonged	High	=	No syncope
	Yes	Short	Not too high	=	No syncope

around age 15 and the second peak around age 70 [4]. Neurally mediated (reflex syncope) is the most common cause in all age groups.

In the young (<40 years old), neurally mediated (reflex) syncope accounts for approximately half of cases [5]. Conversely orthostatic syncope (<3%), CV syncope (approximately 1%) [5] and carotid sinus syndrome [6] are quite rare. Although benign causes of syncope predominate in the young, particular attention to genetic/congenital causes need to be considered (e.g. long QT syndrome [LQTS], Wolf-Parkinson-White [WPW] syndrome, Brugada syndrome, hypertrophic obstructive cardiomyopathy [HOCM], and congenital coronary anomalies).

In the elderly, there is a higher frequency of CV causes, particularly bradyarrhythmias, and orthostatic hypotensive syncope, each accounting for one-third of the cases in patients aged >75 years [3, 8]. Medication intolerance and polypharmacy should be strongly considered in elderly patients.

CLINICAL PEARLS

Syncope in the elderly Complete amnesia is present in up to 40% of elderly patients with syncope [9] and therefore witness accounts are essential. Although bradyarrhythmias and medication-induced orthostasis are common causes, unique causes such as postprandial orthostatic hypotension and degenerative vasomotor disease should be considered [10]. Regardless of the cause of syncope, elderly patients are at greater risk for syncope related injury and poor quality of life [4]. Always consider, and rule out, medications as a primary cause of syncope in an elderly patient even when cardiovascular disease is present before undertaking an aggressive, and perhaps risky, evaluation.

Presence of cardiac disease

Cardiac causes of syncope portend a poor prognosis with 1 year mortality rates between 18–33% [12], therefore a thorough work-up for both tachy- and bradyarrhythmia as well as non-arrhythmic causes should be pursued in those with known cardiac disease (Table 10.5). The structural heart disease which could cause syncope include: aortic stenosis, mitral stenosis, left atrial myxoma, hypertrophic cardiomyopathy (HOCM), pulmonary artery hypertension, dilated cardiomyopathy. Ventricular arrhythmias should be suspected in patients with cardiomyopathy. Tachycardia–bradycardia syndrome should be considered in patients with atrial fibrillation (AF). Although quite uncommon, pacemaker failure should be

Table 10.5 Causes of arrhythmia-related syncope

1. Sinus bradycardia <40 bpm while awake.
2. Repetitive sinoatrial blocks or sinus pauses >3 seconds.
3. Mobitz II 2nd degree atrioventricular block.
4. Third degree atrioventricular block.
5. Alternating left and right bundle branch block.
6. Rapid paroxysmal supraventricular tachycardia.
7. Ventricular tachycardia.
8. Non-sustained polymorphic ventricular tachycardia associated with long or short QT interval.
9. Pacemaker malfunction.

considered in patients with implantable electronic cardiac devices. Even so, non-cardiac causes still account for a number of patients with known cardiac disease.

CLINICAL PEARLS
Non-cardiac syncope in patients with structural heart disease Even if the probability of syncope in patients with a structural cardiac problem is of arrhythmic origin, these patients can develop neurally mediated syncope when the circumstances allow. A patient with moderate aortic stenosis who is not qualified for aortic valve replacement may pass out after having dehydration from diarrhea. A patient with dilated cardiomyopathy and low ejection fraction could develop orthostatic hypotensive syncope after a large meal. This patient may not have non-sustained ventricular tachycardia triggering syncope. Therefore, there is a need to investigate the possibility of neurally-mediated or orthostatic hypotensive syncope even in patients with documented structural heart disease.

Pertinent medical history

In order to rule out a non-cardiac cause of syncope, a complete personal and familial history for epilepsy should be sought. Young patients with recurrent syncope may be previously misdiagnosed with epilepsy, so supporting clinical evidence should be scrutinized. It is not uncommon for patients to suffer myoclonic jerks during syncope, so called 'convulsive syncope'. Neurological diseases (Parkinson disease, multiple system atrophy, diabetic neuropathy) can result in primary autonomic nervous system impairment leading to orthostatic syncope. Secondary autonomic failure from systemic illness such as amyloidosis, diabetes, hyperthyroidism, or oncologic neuropathies should be considered [13]. Signs of potential autonomic failure include disturbed micturition, erectile dysfunction, and labile heart rate/blood pressure. Uncommon syncope related conditions include cataplexy, Meniere's disease, and disequilibrium syndromes. Although migraine attacks rarely lead to T-LOC, patients with migraine headaches have a higher lifetime prevalence of syncope [14].

CLINICAL PEARLS
Differential diagnoses of seizure from syncope
In seizure, unconsciousness often lasts longer than 5 minutes. After a seizure, the patient may experience post-ictal confusion or paralysis. Seizure may include prolonged tonic–clonic movements; although these movements may be seen with any form of syncope lasting more than 30 seconds, the movements during syncope are more limited and brief, lasting less than 15 seconds. Tongue biting strongly suggests seizure. Urinary incontinence does not help distinguish the two, as it frequently occurs with syncope as well as seizure.

Family history

Unexplained sudden death at a young age in a family member is the key question. Potential malignant familial syndromes include HOCM, long QT syndrome, Wolf-Parkinson-White syndrome, Brugada syndrome, arrhythmogenic right ventricular cardiomyopathy (ARVC), and familial cardiomyopathy. Genetic syndromes of vasovagal syncope have recently been described; it is likely that other heritable syncope syndromes exist [15].

Medications

Several medications have been implicated in syncope; particular culprits include vasodilators, volume depleting drugs (i.e. laxatives, diuretics), psychotropic drugs, QT prolonging drugs (i.e. antihistamines, antifungals, antibiotics), and paradoxically anti-arrhythmics. Herbals/over the counter drugs (i.e. Ma Huang, anoretics) or other unregulated substances should be identified.

Table 10.6 Causes of syncope during exercise

1. Critical coronary artery disease.
2. Severe aortic stenosis.
3. Hypertrophic obstructive cardiomyopathy.
4. Congenital coronary artery anomaly.
5. High-grade atrioventricular block.
6. Long QT syndrome.
7. Subclavian steal syndrome associated with arm exercise.

Event characteristics

Activities surrounding the event   Syncope during a lying posture argues against orthostatic or neurally mediated (reflex) causes. Fainting spells upon standing suggest orthostatic syncope. Syncope during exercise primarily suggests cardiac causes (Table 10.6). Syncope following exercise may be associated with arrhythmia as well as poor vascular tone.

CLINICAL PEARLS

Syncope after exercise When exercise ceases, venous blood stops getting pumped back to the heart by peripheral muscular contraction. Yet the heart is still exposed to the catecholamine surge induced by exercising, and it hypercontracts on an empty cavity. This triggers a vagal reflex [16].

Diving, swimming, exercise, stress-related emotions, or sleep may trigger torsades de pointes in patients with particular types of LQTS. Syncope following abrupt neck movements, particularly looking upward, may point to carotid sinus syndrome.

Rarely throat or facial pain may be associated with syncope due to glossopharyngeal or trigeminal neuralgia. Concomitant chest pain may be suggestive of coronary vasospasm or ischemic heart disease perhaps leading to ischemia mediated arrhythmia. Repeated visual stimuli, sleep deprivation, or particular mental activities (i.e. arithmetic, reading, or listening to music) may trigger seizure or cataplexy.

Precipitating events   Precipitating events (e.g. pain, fear, sign of blood, instrumentation, prolonged standing) can be associated with typical prodromal symptoms (nausea, vomiting, sweating, cold, tiredness) and suggest vagal stimuli leading to a neurally mediated mechanism.

Provocating situations A provocating situation occurs during or immediately after a typical situational cause of reflex syncope (e.g. cough, sneeze, gastrointestinal stimulation, defecation, swallowing, visceral pain, micturition, post-exercise, post-prandial, laughter, weightlifting, wind instrument playing).

Event description Bystander description of the event may be helpful. Syncope is typically brief (reflex syncope lasts <20 s), and rarely lasts up to several minutes. Prolonged states of lost or altered consciousness are more typical of metabolic causes or seizure disorder. Sudden, flaccid collapse is more typical of syncope while rigid; keeling over posture suggests seizure. Prolonged (>30 s), synchronous movements, perhaps concomitant with LOC suggest seizure. Automatisms, tongue biting, blue face, or horizontal eye deviation all suggest seizure. Injury or potential injury suggests true involuntary LOC, while a faint that avoids injury is suggestive of a psychogenic episode.

CLINICAL PEARLS
Caveats for cardiac syncope Syncope often occurs suddenly without any warning signs, in which case it is called *malignant syncope*. Unlike that which occurs in neurally mediated syncope, the post-recovery period is not usually marked by lingering malaise [16]. Besides the usual structural heart diseases or arrhythmias mentioned before, bradyarrhythmias can occur with or without underlying structural heart disease. They are most often related to degeneration of the conduction system or to medications rather than to cardiomyopathy. When a patient with a history of heart failure presents with syncope, the top considerations are ventricular tachycardia and bradyarrhythmia. Nevertheless, about half of cases of syncope in patients with cardiac disease have a non-cardiac cause, including the hypotensive or bradycardiac side-effects of drugs [17, 18].

Prodromal symptoms Prodromal symptoms may all occur minutes to just prior to reflex syncope, although about one-third of reflex syncope occurs without a prodrome. Premonitory symptoms of orthostatic syncope include lightheadedness, blurring of vision, and muscular aches in a coat-hanger distribution (neck/shoulders/occiput). Palpitations may precede tachyarrhythmia, while fatigue with nausea may precede bradycardic syncope. Prodromal auras or premonitions, senses of strange smell or unprovoked fear, or abnormal limb movements leading up to LOC suggest seizure.

Post-syncope symptoms (symptoms on awakening)   Reflex syncope is often associated with nausea, sweating, or pallor following the event. Seizures may be associated with post-ictal confusion.

Event history
Previous episodes   A complete account of all previous LOC events should be reviewed. Multiple syncopal episodes starting early in life generally indicate benign etiologies. The one-year recurrence rates in low-risk patients of benign etiologies is 15% vs. 36% (in those with two or less previous episodes versus three of more previous episodes, respectively) [19].

Syncope-related morbidity   One of the major goals in syncope care is recognition and avoidance of significant injury or poor quality of life related to recurrent syncope. Nearly one-third of patients presenting to the emergency department with syncope suffer some form of minor injury [20]. Fractures or motor vehicle accidents occur in about 6% of patients [21]. The majority of patients with recurrent syncope self-reports significant anxiety, depression, or changes in their daily activities of life. Driving restrictions and job changes are not uncommon in patients with recurrent syncope and may hamper patient independence.

Physical examination
Although the physical exam is less likely to provide guidance in the evaluation of syncope, key findings include cardiovascular signs, neurologic signs, or the presence of orthostatic hypotension.

Orthostatic hypotension   Orthostatic intolerance is assessed by active standing or head up tilt table testing. Manual blood pressure (BP) checks with a sphygmomanometer in the supine position then during active standing for three minutes or longer should be performed during part of the initial evaluation to screen for orthostatic intolerance. Orthostasis is present when there is a fall in systolic BP of >20 mmHg or diastolic BP >10 mmHg or a decrease in systolic BP to <90 mmHg within 3 minutes of standing. More subtle sign of orthostasis may be noted when compensatory increase in heart rate occurs.

CLINICAL PEARLS
Differential diagnoses of orthostatic hypotension
Orthostatic hypotension should be associated
with reproduction of syncope (or presyncope) to be
considered diagnostic for orthostatic syncope. Classic orthostatic
hypotension occurs within 3 minutes of orthostatic stress. An initial
normal adaptation reflex followed by a relatively rapid fall in BP and
heart rate (HR) between 3–5 minutes characterizes classic reflex
syncope. Delayed (progressive) orthostatic hypotension is observed
between 3–30 minutes after orthostatic stress is introduced and
characterized by a slow fall in BP without reflex tachycardia.

When orthostatic hypotension is abrupt and associated with reflex
tachycardia, volume depletion should be suspected. When it is gradual
and unaccompanied by tachycardia, autonomic dysfunction is the likely
diagnosis.

Continue checking BP longer than 3 minutes after standing. An
increase in heart rate >30 bpm (or rate exceeding 120 bpm) with orthostatic symptoms, notably often without any significant BP change, within
10 minutes of standing is suggestive of postural orthostatic tachycardia
syndrome (POTS). POTS patients often concomitantly suffer from recurrent reflex syncope [22].

CLINICAL PEARLS
Postural orthostatic tachycardia syndrome This
autonomic dysfunction does not affect the heart, which
manifests a striking compensatory increase in rate of
more than 30 beats per minute within the first 10 minutes of
orthostasis, or an absolute heart rate greater than 120 beats per
minute. Unlike in orthostatic hypotension, blood pressure and
cardiac output are maintained through this increase in heart rate,
although the patient still develops symptoms of severe fatigue or
near-syncope, possibly because of flow maldistribution and reduced
cerebral flow [22].

Cardiovascular examination Common findings are murmurs of
aortic stenosis and HOCM. Less common signs include the tumor plop

of atrial myxoma, snap and click of mitral valve prolapse, diastolic rumble of mitral stenosis, and the systolic murmur of tricuspid regurgitation potentially related to primary valvular disease (e.g. carcinoid syndrome) or pulmonary hypertension. Gallops, narrow pulse pressure, heaves, or displaced points of maximal impulse may indicate underlying cardiomyopathy. Volume status is crucial and can be ascertained via jugular vein assessment as well as skin turgor and oral mucosa.

Neurologic examination Signs of neuropathy, dysautonomia, and/or primary degenerative disease might indicate autonomic failure, which is the most common neurogenic cause of syncope. Cerebrovascular disease is an uncommon cause of syncope. Vertebrobasilar insufficiency due to subclavian steal or critical multivessel (bilateral carotid and vertebral arteries) cerebrovascular disease is a potential cause, thus arterial auscultation and potential provocative arm manipulation can elicit an explanation.

Carotid sinus massage Carotid sinus hypersensitivity (CSH) is defined by a ventricular pause >3 s and/or >50 mmHg fall in systolic blood pressure (SBP) induced by carotid sinus massage (CSM). A diagnosis of carotid sinus syndrome (CSS) requires reproduction of syncope or significant symptoms associated with CSH. Although CSM should probably be avoided in patients with known or suspected carotid disease or cerebrovascular accident (CVA), neurologic complications related to CSM are exceedingly rare (<0.29%) [23]. CSS more commonly affects older individuals, primarily males, and is quite rare in patients <40 years old [23].

CLINICAL PEARLS
How to perform carotid massage The head of the patient is turned to the left and the carotid artery is palpated at the angle of the right jaw. This is where the carotid sinus is located. Press this area with your index and middle finger (some physicians prefer to use their thumb) and feel for carotid pulsation. Stop the pressure immediately if a response is obtained. An electrocardiogram should record the rhythm strip. Remember not to use prolonged carotid sinus stimulation, since serious consequences can occur, such as prolonged cardiac asystole, and even death. Instead, press over the carotid sinus for 3 to 5 seconds, then let up for 5 to 10 seconds. Repeat this several times.

When carotid sinus pressure is not effective, it usually means that the exact spot of the carotid arterial pulsation at the angle of the jaw has not been located.

A normal response to carotid sinus massage is a transient decrease in the sinus rate, slowing of atrioventricular (AV) conduction, or both. Carotid sinus hypersensitivity is defined as a sinus pause longer than 3 seconds in duration and a fall in systolic blood pressure of 50 mmHg or more. The response to carotid sinus massage can be classified as cardioinhibitory (asystole), vasodepressive (fall in systolic blood pressure), or mixed. Carotid sinus hypersensitivity is detected in approximately one-third of elderly patients who present with syncope or after falls. It is important to recognize, however, that carotid sinus hypersensitivity is also commonly observed in asymptomatic elderly patients [23].

 CLINICAL PEARLS
Precautions when performing carotid massage Do not use carotid sinus pressure in a patient who has known cerebro-vascular disease. Do not use simultaneous carotid sinus pressure over both right and left sides of the neck. Even though pressure over the eyeballs has been used and advocated as vagus nerve stimulation in the past, don't use it. Serious injury to the eye can and has resulted. Carotid sinus hypersensitivity has been noted in some patients with advanced aortic stenosis.

WORKING DIAGNOSES

The working diagnoses could be a neurally mediated syncope, orthostatic hypotension, structural cardiac or arrythmia induced syncope. Other non-cardiac problems could be severe hypovolemia or gastrointestinal bleeding, large pulmonary embolus with hemodynamic compromise, tamponade, aortic dissection, or hypoglycemia. Other exotic vascular causes are listed below.

Bilateral critical carotid disease or severe vertebrobasilar disease very rarely cause syncope, and, when they do, they are associated with focal neurologic deficits [2]. Vertebrobasilar disease may cause 'drop attacks', i.e., a loss of muscular tone with falling but without loss of consciousness [24].

Severe proximal subclavian disease leads to reversal of the flow in the ipsilateral vertebral artery as blood is shunted toward the upper extremity. It manifests as dizziness and syncope during the ipsilateral upper extremity activity, usually with focal neurologic signs (subclavian steal syndrome) [25].

Psychogenic pseudosyncope is characterized by frequent attacks that typically last longer than true syncope and occur multiple times per day or week, sometimes with a loss of motor tone. It occurs in patients with anxiety or somatization disorders.

Following the initial evaluation, a presumptive diagnosis can be reached in approximately one-half of cases. In the case of an uncertain diagnosis, the next step involves risk stratification. Several prognostic scores predict risk of recurrence and/or serious adverse outcomes and assist in disposition following initial medical contact. The generally accepted criteria for hospital admission for further diagnostic work-up are listed in Table 10.2. Patients with recurrent or complex events, particularly those associated with injury, should be considered for referral to a specialized syncope center [26].

SMART TESTING

After reasonable exclusion of a cardiac cause for syncope, further testing may be unnecessary for a single or rare syncopal episode in a low-risk patient. There is no test for vasovagal syncope because vasovagal syncope is a clinical diagnosis. Recurrent syncopal events or those associated with injury or significant impairment may warrant further evaluation.

Strategic mapping

Broadly speaking, two general approaches to further diagnostic testing exist, provocative testing versus observational testing [26]. Perceived risk and frequency of episodes dictates which strategy is best utilized, as each has shortcomings. Provocative tests attempt to reproduce syncope in an artificial setting with the assumption that a positive response is due to the same mechanism as the original event. Common provocative tests include tilt-table testing, exercise testing, and electrophysiology study. The downside to this approach lies in the assumption of a common mechanism between the original and reproduced event. Observational testing through documentation of another spontaneous event avoids this

Table 10.7 Strategy for sequential test ordering in patients with syncope

STEP 1	**Scenario A** If neurally-mediated syncope is strongly suspected, supported by good history, or if there is no strong cause suspected, then check structural heart disease to be sure no severe cardiac problems are missed.
	1. Electrocardiogram **2.** Echocardiography
	If both are negative, work-up can stop here. **Scenario B** If neurally-mediated syncope is vaguely suspected, supported by weak history, then after severe structural heart disease is ruled out, clinician could order:
	3 Tilt table test
STEP 2	**Scenario C** If the patient is suspected for coronary artery disease induced severe arrhythmia then clinician could order:
	4 Stress test
STEP 3	**Scenario D** If the four above tests are negative and syncope remains unexplained, prolonged rhythm monitoring is the best choice:
	5 Implantable loop recorder
	Scenario E If the patient has no structural heart disease and ventricular arrhythmia is strongly suspected then clinician may ask for:
	6 Electrophysiologic study

potential bias; however it exposes the patient to risk associated with another event. The strategy of sequential test ordering for patient with syncope is listed in Table 10.7.

Observational tests

An ECG monitoring is the prototypical observational test and is indicated when there is significant suspicion for arrhythmic syncope based on the clinical scenario and/or suggestive EKG findings (Table 10.8). The absence of arrhythmia during syncope by ECG monitoring excludes arrhythmic

Table 10.8 EKG findings suggestive (but NOT diagnostic) of arrhythmic syncope [1]

1. Bifascicular block (defined as either RBBB combined with either LAFB or LPFB or LBBB).
2. QRS >120 ms.
3. Mobitz 1 II degree atrio-ventricular block.
4. Asymptomatic inappropriate sinus bradycardia (<50 bpm).
5. Pre-excited QRS.
6. Long or short QT intervals.
7. Early repolarization.
8. RBBB pattern with STE in leads V1-3 (Brugada pattern).
9. Negative T waves in right precordial leads, Epsilon waves, and ventricular late potentials suggestive of ARVC.
10. Q waves suggesting MI.

Note: RBBB, right bundle branch block; LAFB: left anterior fascicular block; LPFB: left posterior fascicular block; LBBB; left bundle branch block; STE: ST segment elevation; ARVC: Arrhythmogenic right ventricular cardiomyopathy; MI: myocardial infarction.

syncope. The rare findings suggestive (but NOT diagnostic) of severe arrhythmic seen incidentally in EKG patients are listed in Table 10.8. Rarely, the EKG finding of sinoatrial block or sinus pauses >3 s in the absence of negative chronotropic drugs or non-sustained ventricular tachycardia can be seen.

Echocardiogram Echocardiography is suggested as a screening test if the history, physical exam, and EKG fail to provide a diagnosis or if underlying heart disease is suspected [27]. The structural heart diseases to be ruled out by echocardiography are: aortic stenosis, HOCM, mitral stenosis, pulmonary hypertension, etc.

Holter and 'event' monitoring Diagnostic yield of the Holter monitor for syncope is generally quite low. However, Holter monitoring may be useful in frequently occurring symptoms or suspected 'psychogenic pseudo syncope' to disprove an arrhythmic etiology of these events. 30-day event monitors should be considered in patients who have an inter-symptom interval <4 weeks. The diagnostic utility may be limited by improper patient use. The diagnostic yield associated with external recorders may be as high as 25% at one month [26].

Table 10.9 Indications for head up tilt testing

1. Unexplained single syncopal episode in high risk settings (physical injury potential or occupational implications).
2. Recurrent episodes in the absence of organic heart disease or in the presence of heart disease after cardiac causes have been excluded.
3. Discriminate between reflex and orthostatic syncope.
4. Discriminate syncope with jerking movements from epilepsy.
5. Evaluate patients with recurrent unexplained falls.
6. Suspected recurrent psychogenic syncope.

Implantable loop recorder Implantable loop recorders (ILRs) allow for longer monitoring periods. ILR implantation is a minor procedure, particularly now given new injectable ILRs. ILR is indicated in high-risk patients in whom a comprehensive basic evaluation fails to demonstrate a cause. Diagnostic yield associated with ILRs range from 35% to nearly 90% at 6 months in selected patient populations. ILR is superior to tilt testing in identifying reflex syncope patient who will benefit from cardiac pacing [28]. Classification of ECG recordings obtained with ILR is listed in Table 10.8.

Provocative tests
Tilt table testing Head up tilt testing (HUTT) allows the clinician to investigate the response of the autonomic nervous system to orthostatic stress. Protocols may also incorporate pharmacologic provocation with

Table 10.10 Classification of hypotensive results based on head up tilt table test

Response	Hemodynamics
Type 1: Mixed	BP and HR fall without severe bradycardia or asystole
Type 2 Cardio-inhibition type A	Severe bradycardia or asystole with BP fall before HR fall
Type 2 Cardio-inhibition type B	Severe bradycardia or asystole with BP fall at the same time or after HR fall
Type 2: vasodepression	BP fall without HR fall

Adapted from *Eur J Cardiac Pacing Electrophysiol* 1992;3:180–183. Source: Sutton 1992 [61]. Reproduced with permission of Oxford University Press.

isoproterenol or nitroglycerine. Contraindications to isoproterenol provocation include ischemic heart disease, LV outflow tract obstruction, sick sinus syndrome, and uncontrolled HTN.

Traditionally HUTT has been employed to evaluate for reflex syncope; however non-classical forms of delayed orthostatic intolerance may be uncovered with tilt testing Generally accepted indications for HUTT are listed in Table 10.9. Various types of responses to HUTT are listed in Table 10.10.

CLINICAL PEARLS
When I should I do a tilt table test? Consider a tilt table test:
1 When episodes suggest, but do not indicate, a neurocardiogenic cause
2 If there is recurrent syncope with no apparent cause at any age
3 When other evaluation is unrevealing
4 When therapies directed at other potential causes are ineffective
5 There is no reason to do a tilt table test when the etiology is clear from the history

---

Exercise stress test   Exercise stress testing (EST) is indicated in patients who experience syncope during or shortly after exertion, otherwise EST is of extremely low diagnostic yield and cost ineffective. In addition to ischemia evaluation, EST may demonstrate chronotropic incompetence, exercise induced heart block, or catecholaminergic polymorphic VT. Finally, for patients treated with class IC antiarrhythmic drugs, widening of the QRS during exercise can signal a propensity for proarrhythmia.

CLINICAL PEARLS
Advanced AV block during exercise Exercise induced second or third degree AV block is an ominous sign associated with progression to permanent AV block. Coronary artery disease may be a contributory factor to exercise induced block and warrants diagnostic angiography.

Electrophysiology study   The electrophysiology study (EPS) is used to confirm a clinical suspicion of cardiac arrhythmias or cardiac conduction disease. Although appropriate in select cases, the EPS is generally a poor

Table 10.11 Indications for electrophysiologic studies

Known CAD when initial evaluation suggests an arrhythmic cause (unless there is already an established indication for ICD).

1. Syncope preceded by palpitations.
2. Evaluate the exact nature of a presumed arrhythmia [1].
3. Select patients with HCM, ARVC, or Brugada syndrome.
4. Select patients with high-risk occupations.
5. Select patients with a family history of sudden cardiac death.
6. Select cases of suspected sinus node dysfunction.

Note: CAD: coronary artery disease; ICD: Implantable cardioverter defibrillator; HCM: hypertrophic cardiomyopathy; ARVC: Arrhythmogenic right ventricular cardiomyopathy.

predictor of outcomes in patients with 'channelopathies' (LQTS, Brugada syndrome, etc). Indications for EPS are listed in Table 10.11, when non-invasive tests failed to make a diagnosis.

MANAGEMENT

Strategic mapping

Various components of management of patients with syncope include education for injury prevention, lifestyle and behavioral changes and pharmacologic and device-based interventions in certain specific etiologies. The principal goal of treatment is to prevent mortality and morbidity associated with subsequent syncopal events. Then, employ strategies to improve quality of life and prevent injury, such as physical maneuvers to counter an eminent vasovagal episode, or generalized, such as placing driving restrictions in appropriate cases.

Orthostatic hypotension Lifestyle measures including physical counter-pressure maneuvers (PCM), and avoidance of sudden postural changes should be stressed. Iatrogenic predisposing medications include diuretics, vasodilators, and medications including sympathomimetic amines. First-line management involves volume expansion via adequate hydration (2–3 L fluids) and salt intake (10 g NaCl) in the absence of HTN or HF [29]. Head-up sleeping at night may also help expand intravascular volume. Compression stockings and abdominal binders may help prevent venous pooling [30].

Mineralocorticoids and alpha agonist vasoconstrictors represent effective adjunct pharmacologic therapies for many patients with orthostatic syncope. Midodrine (5–20 mg thrice daily) has been shown to decrease orthostatic symptoms [31–33]. Fludrocortisone (0.1–0.3 mg once daily) has also been shown to decrease recurrence of orthostatic symptoms [34–36].

Neurally mediated reflex syncope

Non-pharmacological measures   Lifestyle modification and patient education are paramount. Key points include identification and avoidance of syncope triggers, as well as recognition of prodromal symptoms and the subsequent use of PCM [37–39]. Tilt testing may be used to teach the patient to recognize prodromal symptoms. Tilt training may be considered for vasovagal syncope associated with an orthostatic stress trigger, as depicted in Figure 10.1 [40–43]. Finally, volume expansion may be beneficial in reflex as well as orthostatic syncope (Figure 10.2).

EVIDENCE BASED MEDICINE
Physical Counterpressure Maneuvers Trial (PC-Trial) A multicenter, prospective, randomized trial included 223 patients with recurrent reflex syncope and recognizable prodromal symptoms randomized to conventional therapy versus conventional therapy plus PCM. The median yearly syncope burden during follow-up was significantly lower in the group trained in PCM than in the control group ($P = 0.004$). During a mean follow-up period of 14 months, overall 50.9% of the patients with conventional treatment and 31.6% of the patients trained in PCM experienced a syncopal recurrence ($P = 0.005$). Actuarial recurrence-free survival was better in the treatment group (log-rank $P = 0.018$), resulting in a relative risk reduction of 39% (95% confidence interval, 11% to 53%) [39].

Pharmacologic therapy   Pharmacologic therapy is indicated if syncopal episodes impair quality of life, or are associated with physical injury or motor vehicle accident. Therapy may also be warranted in patients with high-risk occupations. Although multiple pharmacological agents have been employed over the years, few have consistently demonstrated

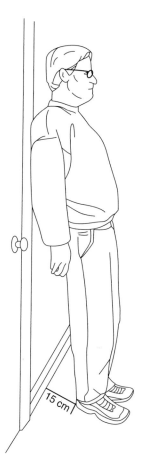

Figure 10.1 Tilt training (Standing training). Source: Benditt 2009 [50].
Reproduced with permission of Elsevier.

efficacy in reflex syncope. Midodrine, an alpha agonist vasoconstrictor, is
perhaps the only drug to demonstrate efficacy for reflex syncope in multiple small randomized trials [45–47]. Another oral alpha agonist, etilefrine,
has failed to show benefit over placebo [48].

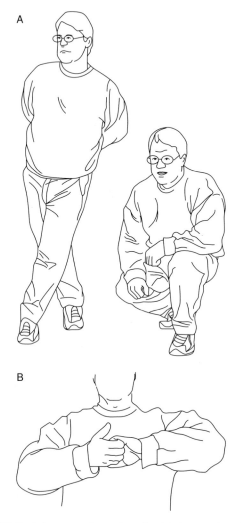

Figure 10.2 Physical maneuvers to counter an imminent vasovagal or orthostatic faint. Source: Benditt 2009 [50]. Reproduced with permission of Elsevier.

EVIDENCE BASED MEDICINE
Usefulness of Midodrine in Patients
with Severely Symptomatic Neurocardiogenic
Syncope – A randomized control study A total of
61 patients with at least monthly occurrences of syncope and a
positive tilt-table test were randomized to treatment either with
midodrine or with fluid, salt tablets, and counseling. Midodrine was
given at a starting dose of 5 mg three times a day and increased up
to a dose of 15 mg three times a day when required. At the
6-month follow-up, 25 (81%) of 31 midodrine-treated patients and
4 (13%) of the 30 fluid-therapy patients had remained
asymptomatic ($P < 0.001$). Only one patient had to discontinue
taking midodrine due to side-effects. When using midodrine one
should be careful especially in the elderly and dosing should avoid
risks associated with supine hypertension [49].

Beta-blockade is thought to blunt stimulation of mechanoreceptors involved in the Bezold–Jarisch reflex, as well as reduce adrenaline-induced hypotension. However, several trials of beta-blockers have failed to show benefit in reflex syncope, and thus carry a class III recommendation in the ESC guidelines.

EVIDENCE-BASED MEDICINE
No Benefits by Beta-blockers in
Prevention of Syncope Trial (POST) The multicenter
Prevention of Syncope Trial (POST) was a randomized,
placebo-controlled, double-blind, trial designed to assess the effects
of metoprolol in vasovagal syncope over a 1-year treatment period.
The main outcome measure was the first recurrence of syncope. A
total of 208 patients (mean age 42 ± 18 years) with a median of
nine syncopal spells over a median of 11 years were randomized,
108 to receive metoprolol and 100 to the placebo group. There
were 75 patients with ≥1 recurrence of syncope. The likelihood of
recurrent syncope was not significantly different between groups.
Neither the age of the patient nor the need for isoproterenol to
produce a positive tilt test predicted subsequent significant benefit
from metoprolol. The conclusions of the study are that metoprolol
was not effective in preventing vasovagal syncope in the patients
with orthostatic hypotension [50].

Fludrocortisone, a mineralocorticoid, has long been used for the treatment of reflex syncope although no clinical data support its efficacy. Selective serotonin reuptake inhibitors (SSRI) are thought to blunt an abnormal hypersensitivity serotonin response, which may contribute to neurally-mediated syncope. Paroxetine demonstrated efficacy over placebo in one randomized trial [48]. Fluoxetine however failed to demonstrate any benefit over placebo in a subsequent trial.

EVIDENCE BASED MEDICINE
Effects of Paroxetine Hydrochloride on Refractory Vasovagal Syncope – A randomized, double-blind, placebo-controlled study Sixty-eight patients with recurrent syncope and positive head-up tilt test in whom standard therapies with beta-blockers, vagolytic, negative inotropic or mineral corticoid agents were ineffective or poorly tolerated were enrolled. The patients were randomly assigned to either paroxetine at 20 mg once a day or a placebo. A head-up tilt test was then repeated after one month of treatment, and the clinical effect was noted over a mean follow-up of 25.4 ± 7.9 months. The response rates (negative tilt test) after one month of treatment were 61.8% versus 38.2% ($P < 0.001$) in the paroxetine and placebo groups, respectively. During follow-up, spontaneous syncope was reported in six patients (17.6%) in the paroxetine group as compared to 18 patients (52.9%) in the placebo group ($P < 0.0001$). Only one patient (2.9%) asked to be discontinued from the drug for severe side effects [48].

Invasive management
Cardiac pacing Reflex syncope may result from transient asystolic/bradyarrhythmic periods related to cardioinhibitory as well as vascular collapse related to vasodilatory mechanisms. Although a cardioinhibitory response may be effectively treated with cardiac pacing, vasodilatory mechanisms will be unaffected. Tilt testing does not reliably detect all who will have asystole during a spontaneous syncopal event, thus may not accurately identify patients who will benefit from cardiac pacing. However, ILR may better identify patients with spontaneous transient asystole who will benefit from cardiac pacing [28]. Finally, carotid sinus syndrome related syncope can be effectively treated with cardiac pacing [49–52].

EVIDENCE BASED MEDICINE
ISSUE 3 Double-blind, randomized
placebo-controlled study This was conducted in
29 centers. Patients were >40 years, had experienced
three syncopal episodes in the previous 2 years. Initially,
511 patients, received an implantable loop recorder; 89 of these had
documentation of syncope with 3 second asystole or 6 second
asystole without syncope within 1210 months and met criteria for
pacemaker implantation; 77 of 89 patients were randomly assigned
to dual-chamber pacing with rate drop response or to sensing only.
The data were analyzed on intention-to-treat principle. There was
syncope recurrence during follow-up in 27 patients, 19 of whom
had been assigned to pacemaker OFF and 8 to pacemaker ON. The
2-year estimated syncope recurrence rate was 57% (95% CI, 40–74)
with pacemaker OFF and 25% (95% CI, 13–45) with pacemaker ON
(log rank: $P = 0.039$ at the threshold of statistical significance of
0.04). The risk of recurrence was reduced by 57% (95% CI, 4–81). It
was concluded that the observed 32% absolute and 57% relative
reduction in syncope recurrence support pacemaker treatment for
selected patients with neurally mediated syncope.

ACTION POINTS

1 History and physical examination are the cornerstone of diagnosis.
2 Reflex syncope is the most common cause of syncope.
3 Only 60% of patients presenting with syncope need to be admitted to hospital for inpatient work up, predominantly due to risk of cardiac causes.
4 Non-pharmacologic lifestyle changes generally have a more important role when compared to medical therapy, in patients with reflex syncope.
5 Use diagnostic testing judiciously.
6 Beware of supine hypertension in patients treated with midodrine, or fludrocortisone.

REFERENCES

1. Task Force for the Diagnosis and Management of Syncope, European Society of Cardiology (ESC), European Heart Rhythm Association (EHRA), et al. Guidelines

for the diagnosis and management of syncope (version 2009). *Eur Heart J* 2009; 30:2631–2671.

2. Linzer M, Yang EH, Estes NA III, et al. Diagnosing syncope, part 1: value of history, physical examination, and electrocardiography: Clinical Efficacy Assessment Project for the American College of Physicians. *Ann Intern Med.* 1997;126:989–996.

3. Grubb BP Neurocardiogenic syncope and related disorders of orthostatic intolerance. *Circulation.* 2005; 111:2997–3006.

4. Kenny RA, Bhangu J, King-Kallimanis BL. Epidemiology of syncope/collapse in younger and older Western patient populations. *Prog Cardiovasc Dis.* 2013 Jan–Feb;55(4):357–363.

5. Olde Nordkamp LAR, van Dijk N, Ganzeboom KS, Reitsma JB, Luitse JSK, Dekker LRC, Shen WK, Wieling W. Syncope prevalence in the ED compared to that in the general practice and population: a strong selection process. *Am J Emerg Med.* 2009;27:271–279.

6. Puggioni E, Guiducci V, Brignole M, et al. Results and complications of the carotid sinus massage performed according to the 'methods of symptoms'. *Am J Cardiol* 2002;89:599–560.

7. Ungar A, Mussi C, Del Rosso A, Noro G, Abete P, Ghirelli L, Cellai T, Landi A, Salvioli G, Rengo F, Marchionni N, Masotti G. Diagnosis and characteristics of syncope in older patients referred to geriatric departments. *J Am Geriatr Soc.* 2006;54:1531–1536.

8. Del Rosso A, Alboni P, Brignole M, Menozzi C, Raviele A. Relation of clinical presentation of syncope to the age of patients. *Am J Cardiol.* 2005;96:1431–1435.

9. Kenny RA. Syncope in the elderly: diagnosis, evaluation, and treatment. *J Cardiovasc Electrophysiol.* 2003; 14: S74–S77.

10. Sim V, Pascual J, Woo J. Evaluating elderly patients with syncope. *Arch Gerontol Geriatr.* 2002 Sep–Oct;35(2):121–135.

11. Costantino G, Perego F, Dipaola F, Borella M, Galli A, Cantoni G, Dell'Orto S, Dassi S, Filardo N, Duca PG, Montano N, Furlan R; STePS Investigators. Short- and long-term prognosis of syncope, risk factors, and role of hospital admission: results from the STePS (Short-Term Prognosis of Syncope) study. *J Am Coll Cardiol.* 2008;51:276–283.

12. Kapoor W. Evaluation and outcome of patients with syncope. *Medicine.* 1990;69:160–175.

13. Goldstein DS, Robertson D, Esler M, et al. Dysautonomias: Clinical Disorders of the Autonomic Nervous System. *Ann Intern Med.* 2002;137(9):753–763.

14. Thijs RD, Kruit MC, van Buchem MA, Ferrari MD, Launer LJ, van Dijk JG. Syncope in migraine: the population-based CAMERA study. *Neurology.* 2006;66:1034–1037.

15. Klein KM1, Bromhead CJ, Smith KR, O'Callaghan CJ, Corcoran SJ, Heron SE, Iona X, Hodgson BL, McMahon JM, Lawrence KM, Scheffer IE, Dibbens LM, Bahlo M, Berkovic SF. Autosomal dominant vasovagal syncope: clinical features and linkage to chromosome 15q26. *Neurology.* 2013 Apr 16;80(16):1485–1493.

16. Seger JJ. Syncope evaluation and management. *Tex Heart Inst J*. 2005;32(2): 204–206.
17. Brignole M, Hamdan MH. New concepts in the assessment of syncope. *J Am Coll Cardiol*. 2012; 59:1583–1591.
18. Brignole M, Menozzi C, Moya A, et al. International Study on Syncope of Uncertain Etiology 3 (ISSUE-3) Investigators. Pacemaker therapy in patients with neurally mediated syncope and documented asystole: Third International Study on Syncope of Uncertain Etiology (ISSUE-3): a randomized trial. *Circulation*. 2012; 125:2566–2571.
19. Brignole M, Vardas P, Hoffman E, Huikuri H, Moya A, Ricci R, Sulke N, Wieling W. Indications for the use of diagnostic implantable and external ECG loop recorders. *Europace*. 2009;11;671–687.
20. Brignole M, Alboni P, Benditt DG, Bergfeldt L, Blanc JJ, Bloch Thomsen PE, van Dijk JG, Fitzpatrick A, Hohnloser S, Janousek J, Kapoor W, Kenny RA, Kulakowski P, Masotti G, Moya A, Raviele A, Sutton R, Theodorakis G, Ungar A, Wieling W; Task Force on Syncope, European Society of Cardiology. Guidelines on management (diagnosis and treatment) of syncope – update 2004. *Europace*. 2004;6:467–537.
21. Bartoletti A, Fabiani P, Bagnoli L, Cappelletti C, Cappellini M, Nappini G, Gianni R, Lavacchi A, Santoro G. Physical injuries caused by a transient loss of consciousness: main clinical characteristics of patients and diagnostic contribution of carotid sinus massage. *Eur Heart J*. 2008;29:618–624.
22. Task Force for the Diagnosis and Management of Syncope; European Society of Cardiology (ESC); European Heart Rhythm Association (EHRA); Heart Failure Association (HFA); Heart Rhythm Society (HRS), Guidelines for the diagnosis and management of syncope (version 2009). *Eur Heart J*. 2009; 30:2631–2671.
23. Puggioni E, Guiducci V, Brignole M, Menozzi C, Oddone D, Donateo P, Croci F, Solano A, Lolli G, Tomasi C, Bottoni N. Results and complications of the carotid sinus massage performed according to the 'methods of symptoms'. *Am J Cardiol*. 2002;89:599–560.
24. Savitz SI, Caplan LR. Vetebrobasilar disease. *N Engl J Med*. 2005;352:2618–2626.
25. Potter BJ, Pinto D. Subclavian steal syndrome. *Circulation*. 2014;129:2320–2323.
26. Brignole M, Hamdan MH. New Concepts in the Assessment of Syncope. *J Am Coll Cardiol*. 2012;59:1583–1591.
27. Maisel W. Specialized syncope evaluation. *Circulation*. 2004;110:3621–3623.
28. Michele Brignole, MD; Carlo Menozzi, MD; Angel Moya, MD; on behalf of the International Study on Syncope of Uncertain Etiology 3 (ISSUE-3) Investigators Pacemaker Therapy in Patients With Neurally Mediated Syncope and Documented Asystole Third International Study on Syncope of Uncertain Etiology (ISSUE-3) A Randomized Trial. *Circulation*. 2012;125:2566–2571.
29. Claydon VE, Hainsworth R. Salt supplementation improves orthostatic cerebral and peripheral vascular control in patients with syncope. *Hypertension* 2004;43: 809–813.

30. Smit AA, Wieling W, Fujimura J, Denq JC, Opfer-Gehrking TL, Akarriou M, Karemaker JM, Low PA. Use of lower abdominal compression to combat orthostatic hypotension in patients with autonomic dysfunction. *Clin Auton Res.* 2004; 14:167–175.

31. Jankovic J, Gilden JL, Hiner BC, Kaufmann H, Brown DC, Coghlan CH, Rubin M, Fouad-Tarazi FM. Neurogenic orthostatic hypotension: a double-blind, placebo-controlled study with midodrine. *Am J Med.* 1993;95:38–48.

32. Low PA, Gilden JL, Freeman R, Sheng KN, McElligott MA. Efficacy of midodrine vs placebo in neurogenic orthostatic hypotension. A randomized, double-blind multicenter study. Midodrine Study Group. *JAMA.* 1997;277:1046–1051.

33. Wright RA, Kaufman HC, Perera R, Opfer-Gehrking TL, McEllogott MA, Sheng KN, Low PA. A double-blind, dose–response study of midodrine in neurogenic orthostatic hypotension. *Neurology.* 1998;51:120–124.

34. van Lieshout JJ, ten Harkel AD, Wieling W. Fludrocortisone and sleeping in the head-up position limit the postural decrease in CO in autonomic failure. *Clin Auton Res.* 2000;10:35–42.

35. Finke J, Sagemueller I. Fludrocortisone in the treatment of orthostatic hypotension: ophthalmodynamography during standing. *Dtsch Med Wochenschr.* 1975; 100:1790–1792.

36. ten Harkel AD, van Lieshout JJ, Wieling W. Treatment of orthostatic hypotension with sleeping in the head-up tilt position, alone and in combination with fludrocortisones. *J Intern Med.* 1992;232:139–145.

37. Linzer M, Pritchett EL, Pontinen M, McCarthy E, Divine GW. Incremental diagnostic yield of loop electrocardiographic recorders in unexplained syncope. *Am J Cardiol.* 1990;66:214–219.

38. Livanis EG1, Kostopoulou A, Theodorakis GN, Aggelopoulou N, Adamopoulos S, Degiannis D, Kremastinos DT. Neurocardiogenic mechanisms of unexplained syncope in idiopathic dilated cardiomyopathy. *Am J Cardiol.* 2007 Feb 15;99(4):558–562. Epub 2007 Jan 2.

39. Zaidi A, Clough P, Cooper P, Scheepers B, Fitzpatrick AP. Misdiagnosis of epilepsy: many seizure-like attacks have a cardiovascular cause. *J Am Coll Cardiol.* 2000;36:181–184.

40. Heitterachi E, Lord SR, Meyerkort P, McCloskey I, Fitzpatrick R. BP changes on upright tilting predict falls in older people. *Age Ageing.* 2002;31:181–186.

41. Petersen ME, Williams TR, Sutton R. Psychogenic syncope diagnosed by prolonged head-up tilt testing. *QJM.* 1995;88:209–213.

42. Sarasin FP1, Junod AF, Carballo D, Slama S, Unger PF, Louis-Simonet M. Role of echocardiography in the evaluation of syncope: a prospective study. *Heart.* 2002 Oct;88(4):363–367.

43. Brignole M, Croci F, Menozzi C, Solano A, Donateo P, Oddone D, Puggioni E, Lolli G. Isometric arm counter-pressure maneuvers to abort impending vasovagal syncope. *J Am Coll Cardiol.* 2002;40:2053–2059.

44. Krediet CT, van Dijk N, Linzer M, van Lieshout JJ, Wieling W. Management of vasovagal syncope: controlling or aborting faints by leg crossing and muscle tensing. *Circulation.* 2002;106:1684–1689.

45. van Dijk N, Quartieri F, Blanc JJ, Garcia-Civera R, Brignole M, Moya A, Wieling W; PC-Trial Investigators. Effectiveness of physical counterpressure maneuvers in preventing vasovagal syncope: the Physical Counterpressure Manoeuvres Trial (PC-Trial). *J Am Coll Cardiol.* 2006;48:1652–1657.

46. Foglia-Manzillo G, Giada F, Gaggioli G, Bartoletti A, Lolli G, Dinelli M, Del Rosso A, Santarone M, Raviele A, Brignole M. Efficacy of tilt training in the treatment of neurally mediated syncope. A randomized study. *Europace.* 2004;6:199–204.

47. Kinay O, Yazici M, Nazli C, Acar G, Gedikli O, Altinbas A, Kahraman H, Dogan A, Ozaydin M, Tuzun N, Ergene O. Tilt training for recurrent neurocardiogenic syncope: effectiveness, patient compliance, and scheduling the frequency of training sessions. *Jpn Heart J.* 2004;45:833–843.

48. On YK, Park J, Huh J, Kim JS. Is home orthostatic self-training effective in preventing neurocardiogenic syncope? A prospective and randomized study. *Pacing Clin Electrophysiol.* 2007;30:638–643.

49. Duygu H, Zoghi M, Turk U, Akyuz S, Ozerkan F, Akilli A, Erturk U, Onder R, Akin M. The role of tilt training in preventing recurrent syncope in patients with vasovagal syncope: a prospective and randomized study. *Pacing Clin Electrophysiol.* 2008;31:592–596.

50. Benditt DG, Nguyen JT. Syncope: Therapeutic Approaches. *J Am Coll Cardiol.* 2009;53:1741–1751.

51. Samniah N, Sakaguchi S, Lurie KG, Iskos D, Benditt DG. Efficacy and safety of midodrine hydrochloride in patients with refractory vasovagal syncope. *Am J Cardiol.* 2001;88:80–83.

52. Perez-Lugones A, Schweikert R, Pavia S, Sra J, Akhtar M, Jaeger F, Tomassoni GF.Saliba W, Leonelli FM, Bash D, Beheiry S, Shewchik J, Tchou PJ, Natale A. Usefulness of midodrine in patients with severely symptomatic neurocardiogenic syncope: a randomized control study. *J Cardiovasc Electrophysiol.* 2001;12: 935–938.

53. Ward CR, Gray JC, Gilroy JJ, Kenny RA. Midodrine: a role in the management of neurocardiogenic syncope. *Heart.* 1998;79:45–49.

54. Raviele A, Brignole M, Sutton R, Alboni P, Giani P, Menozzi C, Moya A. Effect of etilefrine in preventing syncopal recurrence in patients with vasovagal syncope: a double-blind, randomized, placebo-controlled trial. The Vasovagal Syncope International Study. *Circulation.* 1999;99:1452–1457.

55. Di Girolamo E, Di Iorio C, Sabatini P, Leonzio L, Barbone C, Barsotti A. Effects of paroxetine hydrochloride, a selective serotonin reuptake inhibitor, on refractory vasovagal syncope: a randomized, double-blind, placebo-controlled study. *J Am Coll Cardiol.* 1999;33:1227–1230.

56. Kerr SR, Pearce MS, Brayne C, Davis RJ, Kenny RA. Carotid sinus hypersensitivity in asymptomatic older persons: implications for diagnosis of syncope and falls. *Arch Intern Med.* 2006;166:515–520.

57. Brignole M, Menozzi C, Lolli G, Bottoni N, Gaggioli G. Long-term outcome of paced and non-paced patients with severe carotid sinus syndrome. *Am J Cardiol.* 1992;69:1039–1043.

58. Claesson JE, Kristensson BE, Edvardsson N, Wahrborg P. Less syncope and milder symptoms in patients treated with pacing for induced cardioinhibitory carotid sinus syndrome: a randomized study. *Europace.* 2007;9:932–936.

59. Morley CA, Perrins EJ, Grant PL, Chan SL, Mc Brien DJ, Sutton R. Carotid sinus syncope treated by pacing. Analysis of persistent symptoms and role of atrioventricular sequential pacing. *Br Heart J.* 1982;47:411–418.

60. Russo AM, Stainback RF, Bailey SR, et al. ACCF/HRS/AHA/ASE/HFSA/SCAI/SCCT/SCMR 2013 Appropriate Use Criteria for Implantable Cardioverter-Defibrillators and Cardiac Resynchronization Therapy. *J Am Coll Cardiol.* 2013;61(12):1318–1368.

61. Sutton R, Petersen M, Brignole M. Proposed classification for tilt induced vasovagal syncope. *Eur J Cardiac. Pacing Electrophysiol.* 1992;3:180–183 (table 9).

CHAPTER 11

Aortic Stenosis

Rajiv Goswami, Phillip Tran, Nguyen Lan Hieu, Aravinda Nanjundappa and Neal Kleiman

Management of Complex Cardiovascular Problems, Fourth Edition. Edited by Thach N. Nguyen, Dayi Hu, Shao Liang Chen, Moo Hyun Kim and Cindy L. Grines.
© 2016 John Wiley & Sons, Ltd. Published 2016 by John Wiley & Sons, Ltd.

BACKGROUND

Aortic stenosis (AS) is narrowing of the aortic valve with consequent limitation in the heart's ability to augment cardiac output and match physiologic demand. AS is the most common valvular heart disease in developed countries with a prevalence that increases with age, affecting 2% to 9% in the over 65 population. The most common cause is '*senile calcific aortic stenosis*', which results from years of mechanical stress on the aortic valve causing degeneration of the collagen structure and pathologic 'repair' with calcium deposition, impairing leaflet mobility.

CHALLENGES

There are several challenges faced by the clinician managing patients with AS. The **most important first challenge** is the assessment of the severity of AS, since this will determine prognosis and management. The slow insidious progression of AS allows time for physiologic compensation and gradual reduction in physical activity. The patient will often not report symptoms giving the clinician the impression of being asymptomatic.

The **second challenge** is the physical findings (in this case, it is the intensity of the AS murmur) do not always correlate with the severity of AS for a variety of reasons, for example, if left ventricular (LV) ejection fraction (EF) declines, the intensity of the murmur will lessen due to low flow. The problem becomes more problematic when the patient has low-flow low-gradient AS. In this situation, the severity of stenosis can be underestimated by the commonly used Doppler velocity and gradient measurements since they are flow-dependent. Other criteria such as the Doppler-velocity index or dobutamine-stress echocardiography must be used to accurately assess severity.

The **third challenge** is the management of patients with severe AS and severe coronary artery disease (CAD) at high surgical risk. While they maybe candidates for trans-catheter aortic valve replacement (TAVR), there is currently no evidence base to guide the management strategy for concomitant severe CAD. Whether revascularization is performed before TAVR, after TAVR or deferred entirely will depend on local practice and physician judgement.

The **fourth challenge** is in the management of the very elderly patient (80 years of age and older) with severe AS. They have higher risk for vascular access complications, for stroke and a prolonged course of recovery due to frailty. The recently reported 5-year results from the Placement of Aortic Transcatheter Valve (PARTNER) I trial showed a 93.6% mortality with standard therapy that included balloon aortic valvuloplasty versus a 71.8% mortality with TAVR [1]. Despite the reduction, the high overall post-procedural mortality over five years due to other co-morbidities makes proper patient selection an important issue from the resource utilization perspective.

HIGH-RISK MARKERS

Patients with severe AS and clinical evidence of congestive heart failure (HF) and low cardiac output manifested by syncope are risk markers for short-term mortality. These patients should be managed aggressively by surgical or trans-catheter valve replacement. Important co-morbidities such as chronic obstructive lung disease (COPD), advanced chronic kidney disease (CKD), peripheral vascular disease (PVD) and severe liver disease will increase surgical risk. Frailty, dementia, prior amputation, history of stroke with significant residual deficits, connective tissue disease, prior radiation treatment, musculoskeletal deformities are all factors that will complicate surgical management and postoperative recovery.

HIGH-RISK PREDICTORS

The Society for Thoracic Surgery (STS) score is the surgical risk score based on demographic, clinical, anatomic and procedural factors used to determine the risk of significant operative morbidity and mortality during surgery. The predictors of 2-year mortality for the patient undergoing surgery for aortic valve replacement (SAVR) are: prior CABG, STS score, liver disease, moderate or severe mitral regurgitation. Decreased body-mass index (BMI), prior stroke and chronic obstructive lung disease (COPD) requiring supplemental oxygen are significant predictors of death at 2 years for patients undergoing TAVR. One important predictor for SAVR and TAVR is frailty. Frailty can be classified by a 5-meter walk greater than 6 seconds, handgrip strength less than 18 kg, and a Katz Index of Independence in Activities of Daily Living (ADL) score less than 4 out of 6.

INVESTIGATIONS

Symptoms to look for

Generally patients develop the typical symptoms of AS when the aortic valve area decreases below 1 cm^2, but there is considerable individual variation in the valve area at the time of index symptoms [2].

Angina is the first symptom in approximately one-third of patients. Angina due to severe AS is usually exertional and improves with rest. The cause is a mismatch between oxygen supply and demand. There is increased oxygen demand due to increased LV mass; however, the supply is limited due to vascular compression by the hypertrophic LV and a decrease in the coronary perfusion gradient due to elevation in LV diastolic filling pressure.

Syncope or near syncope occurs during exertion when arterial pressure falls due to systemic vasodilatation in the setting of a fixed cardiac output. There is some evidence to support an abnormal baroreceptor mechanism and vasodepressor response to extreme elevations in LV systolic pressure during exercise [3].

Dyspnea is the most ominous symptom since it represents pressure overload of the LV and failure of compensatory mechanisms. The rising filling pressure of the LV translates back into the pulmonary vasculature giving rise to the sensation of dyspnea and orthopnea. The neurohormonal activation in HF will produce volume overload with the attendant congestive symptoms of edema. Fatigue is commonly attributable to AS, but the insidious onset and non-specific nature limit the diagnostic utility of this symptom.

No symptoms Some patients remain 'asymptomatic' despite hemodynamically significant AS because of a gradual and subtle decrement in their activity level to match their decline in cardiovascular (CV) capacity. Detailed interrogation often reveals a subtle decrease in exertional tolerance. The presence of significant AS may not become apparent until the occurrence of a concurrent illness such as infection or trauma, which then causes hemodynamic decompensation, especially with loss of the atrial transport ('kick') if atrial fibrillation (AF) occurs.

Signs to look for

The jugular venous pulse usually shows a prominent *a* wave indicating reduced right ventricular compliance from ventricular septal hypertrophy [4]. In advanced stages, development of pulmonary hypertension (HTN), right ventricular failure and tricuspid regurgitation, *v* waves may become prominent [5]. The arterial pulse is weak and delayed ('*parvus et tardus*'), with an anacrotic notch in the upstroke. This can best be appreciated with simultaneous palpation of the cardiac apical and carotid impulse or by simultaneous comparison of the patient's carotid pulse with examining physician's own (assuming he or she also does not have the disease).

With LV failure, the point of maximal cardiac impulse is sustained and displaced inferiorly and laterally [5]. If present, a systolic thrill can be palpated in the second intercostal space on either side of the sternum or in the suprasternal notch with the patient leaning forward in full expiration [5].

Auscultation of the heart sounds reveals a normal or soft S_1 and prominent S_4, due to the '*atrial kick*' and partial closure of the mitral valve in presystole [6]. There are various plausible explanations for the diminished intensity of S_2, including the prolongation of ventricular systole making A_2 and P_2 coincide, the systolic murmur obscuring P_2, or the immobility of the aortic valve making A_2 inaudible [5].

CLINICAL PEARLS
Caveat of aortic stenosis murmur Classically, the systolic murmur of AS is harsh, late peaking with a crescendo–decrescendo quality best heard over the second right intercostal space, radiating to the carotid arteries. The intensity of the murmur will decrease in tandem with declining cardiac output from LV failure. It can be differentiated from the murmur of hypertrophic obstructive cardiomyopathy by its diminished intensity with a Valsalva maneuver. The AS murmur will decrease with isometric exercise unlike the systolic murmur of mitral

regurgitation (MR) and also display beat to beat variability when the diastolic filling period varies with AF or premature contractions unlike MR which will be constant.

SMART TESTING

The electrocardiogram in severe AS shows the non-specific findings of LV hypertrophy and left atrial enlargement. The cornerstone of diagnostic testing remains echocardiography. Two-dimensional echocardiography provides an important morphologic characterization of the stenotic aortic valve. The aortic valve leaflets will appear thickened and calcified; systolic doming and reduced leaflet separation during systole are also well appreciated.

Calculation of the aortic valve area   The quantitative assessment of AS severity is reliant upon Doppler interrogation. The modified Bernoulli equation makes the assumptions that the flow acceleration and viscous friction components of the Bernoulli equation are not clinically relevant and the velocity distal to the stenosis is much greater than the velocity proximal [7]. Using continuous wave Doppler, the *simplified Bernoulli equation* for calculation of the pressure gradient becomes:

$$\Delta P = 4V^2$$

The calculation of aortic valve area (AVA) relies upon the *continuity equation* and measurement of the LV outflow tract (LVOT) diameter. The formula is:

$$AVA = (LVOT_{area} \times LVOT_{TVI})/AV_{TVI}$$

TVI is time-velocity integral, a measurement of blood flow. The advantage of this calculation is that it is flow-independent since the calculation accounts for volume flow. This is particularly important with low cardiac output states such as low gradient AS with reduced ejection fraction or preserved ejection fraction in a small hypertrophied LV.

Classification of severity   The definition of severe AS is derived from natural history studies indicating a worse prognosis in patients with peak aortic valve velocity greater than 4 m/s, mean gradient greater than 40 mmHg and aortic valve area (AVA) less than 1 cm^2. The definitions of severe, moderate and mild AS are defined in Table 11.1 below [8]:

Table 11.1 Classification of aortic stenosis

Severity	Peak velocity (m/s)	Mean gradient (mmHg)	Valve area (cm²)
Normal	<2.5	–	3–4
Mild	2.5–2.9	<25	1.5–2
Moderate	3–4	25–40	1–1.5
Severe	>4	>40	<1

The advantages of using aortic velocity as a marker of AS severity are that it is relatively simple, does not require calculations and is less affected by inter-observer variability, as opposed to AVA. Compared with valve area, peak aortic velocity is a stronger predictor of outcome in asymptomatic patients with severe AS [2]. A disadvantage of using peak aortic velocity is that it reflects volume flow rate across the valve, which may be artificially elevated if concomitant aortic regurgitation is present or if cardiac output is increased as in patients with anemia, or low if LV failure has developed. Sometimes LV dysfunction results in low ventricular systolic pressures which fail to separate adequately the aortic valve leaflets, causing the echocardiographic appearance of AS, the so-called 'pseudo-AS'. In this circumstance, dobutamine stress echocardiography (DSE) will increase ventricular performance so the aortic valve gradient will increase if AS is present but not in the case of pseudo-stenosis.

DSE is the next appropriate test in the low-flow/low-gradient symptomatic AS group.

The most recent iteration of the ACC/AHA valvular heart disease guidelines have advocated defining AS in stages [9] since the appropriate classification of the patient will guide management. There are four categories: at risk of AS (bicuspid or aortic valve sclerosis); progressive AS (mild or moderate hemodynamic findings); asymptomatic severe AS; and symptomatic severe AS. The Table 11.2 below summarizes the details of three important subgroups within the symptomatic severe category that warrant closer attention:

CLINICAL PEARLS
How to interpret the results of dobutamine stress echocardiography Starting at a dose of 5 mcg/kg/min, dobutamine is progressively increased by an increment of 5 mcg to a maximum dose of 20 mcg/kg/min. The change in

trans-aortic stroke volume, mean pressure gradient, AVA and LV contractility will distinguish severe AS with LV systolic dysfunction from primary myocardial dysfunction and moderate AS with reduced leaflet excursion ('pseudo-AS'). If severe AS is present, the maximum velocity will increase above 4 m/s with increasing LV contractility; however the AVA will remain fixed at less than 1 cm². If primary myocardial dysfunction without severe AS is present, the AVA will increase with only a modest increase in maximum trans-aortic velocity and gradient. Patients that fail to develop a 20% increase in stroke volume represent a third group called 'lack of contractile reserve'. This group has a very poor prognosis with either medical or surgical therapy.

Left heart catheterization   In cases where the image quality is substandard or Doppler assessment is limited by a non-parallel intercept angle, echocardiography may underestimate the severity of AS. If this results in a discrepancy between the non-invasive data and clinical evaluation, left heart catheterization is indicated. Simultaneous measurement of LV and aortic pressure will yield a peak-to-peak and a mean gradient. Since the aortic pressure peak is time delayed, the peak-to-peak gradient measured invasively underestimates the true peak instantaneous gradient

Table 11.2 Classification of severe symptomatic aortic stenosis

Symptomatic severe AS:	Hemodynamics	LV characteristics	Dobutamine
High gradient	AVA <1 cm² V_{max} >4 m/s ΔP_{mean} >40 mmHg	Normal LVEF Diastolic dysfunction	n/a
Low-flow/ Low-gradient	AVA <1 cm² with V_{max} <4 m/s or ΔP_{mean} <40 mmHg	LVEF <50% LVH Diastolic dysfunction	V_{max} >4 m/s
Paradoxical low flow	AVA <1 cm² with V_{max} <4 m/s or ΔP_{mean} <40 mmHg Indexed AVA <0.6 cm²/m² SV <35 mL/m²	LVEF > 50% Small/hypertrophic Reduced SV Restrictive diastolic filling	n/a

measured by Doppler echocardiography. However, the mean gradients obtained by invasive and non-invasive techniques are directly comparable. The AVA is calculated using the *Gorlin equation* below:

$$\textit{Aortic valve area} = CO/(SEP \times HR \times 44.3 \times \Delta P)$$

CO is the cardiac output measured during right heart catheterization by Fick or thermo-dilution method, *SEP* is the systolic ejection period and ΔP is the mean trans-aortic pressure gradient. In low flow states, the catheterization-derived gradient may underestimate that obtained with echocardiography. In some circumstances, dobutamine stress may be performed in the cardiac catheterization laboratory.

MANAGEMENT

Medical treatment

There is no effective medical therapy for AS. Despite the significant overlap in the CV risk factors for AS and atherosclerosis, trials to date have not shown benefit in AS from commonly used medical therapies for atherosclerosis. Three randomized controlled trials (RCT) of HMG-CoA Reductase inhibitors (statins) failed to show benefit in AS [10–12]. While the early pathogenesis of AS involves lipid deposition and inflammation, once osteogenesis has been activated the disease process is driven by the molecular signaling involved in bone metabolism rather than atherosclerosis. This may explain why lipid modification did not affect the progression of AS but the degree of calcification predicted progression [13].

Balloon aortic valvuloplasty

Balloon aortic valvuloplasty was first introduced as an alternative to aortic valve replacement [14]. Currently, the indications are bridging therapy to foster clinical improvement until definitive therapy such as surgical or trans-catheter aortic valve replacement; symptom palliation in patients deemed inoperable due to extreme risk; treatment of cardiogenic shock due to severe AS [15]. The procedure improves AS by creating microfractures in the calcific nodules, separating the fused commissures and stretching the aortic annulus [16]. However it offers only a partial relief of the stenosis, generally resulting in a 0.4 cm^2 gain in aortic valve area and a 50% decrease in trans-valvular gradient. The results only last a few months due to elastic recoil of the aortic annulus and restenosis; furthermore, it does not alter long-term mortality [17].

In a relatively recent retrospective observational study of balloon aortic valvuloplasty in high risk or inoperable patients, the mortality was approximately 50% at a median follow-up of 6 months and a final valve area >1 cm^2 was associated with improved long-term mortality [18]. This study reported less improvement in AVA in patients who underwent repeat valvuloplasty compared with initial valvuloplasty (increase of 0.2 cm^2 vs. 0.45 cm^2), similar to previous studies [19]. Considering the generally transient benefit of balloon aortic valvuloplasty and the risk for complication such as severe aortic regurgitation, it can be considered an option as a bridge to SAVR or TAVR but not routinely recommended [9].

Multidisciplinary aortic valve replacement approach

The integrated approach to management of AS involves the heart valve team consisting of a structural valve interventionalist, CV surgeon, CV imaging specialist and an anesthesiologist. This multidisciplinary approach offers a comprehensive assessment of valve disease, identification of the various treatment options available, and consideration of the associated risks and benefits to optimize outcomes.

Risk assessment involves calculation of the operative mortality using the Society of Thoracic Surgeons (STS) risk estimator and the evaluation of frailty. Some measures of frailty are as follows: time to 5 meter walk ≥6 s; grip strength ≤18 kg; cognitive dysfunction defined as a score <4 on the mini-cognitive assessment for dementia. Other indicators are the ability to perform activities of daily living (Katz ADLs score <4), consideration of the number of organ systems with dysfunction and procedure specific impediments. Table 11.3 below, taken from the recent AHA/ACC guideline for valvular heart disease [9], summarizes the risk assessment.

Indications for surgical aortic valve replacement

The indication for intervention in severe AS is based on the presence of symptoms; since once even mild symptoms are present, prognosis is

Table 11.3 Classification according to risks for aortic valve replacement

	Low	Intermediate	High	Prohibitive
STS pred. mortality	< 4%	4–8%	>8%	>50%
Frailty indices	None	1 (mild) or	≥2 or	
Compromised organ systems	None	1 or	≤2	≥3
Procedure specific impediments	None	possible	Possible	Severe

poor unless the outflow obstruction is corrected. SAVR is recommended in patients with: decreased systolic opening of a calcified or congenitally stenotic aortic valve; and aortic valve velocity ≥4 m/s or mean gradient ≥40 mmHg; and symptoms of heart failure, syncope, angina or pre-syncope on exercise testing [9]. Calculations of AVA are not necessary when the velocity and gradient are high, but most patients will have a valve area ≤1.0 cm^2 or a valve area indexed to body surface area of ≤0.6 cm^2/m^2. The valve area calculation becomes paramount with either low ejection fraction or stroke volume. SAVR is reasonable in symptomatic patients with low-flow/low-gradient AS (stroke volume ≤35 mL/m^2) with LV function ≥50% but aortic velocity <4 m/s or mean gradient <40 mmHg if the indexed valve area is ≤0.6 cm^2/m^2 [20, 21]. SAVR is also reasonable in low-flow/low-gradient AS with LVEF <50% if dobutamine stress echocardiography shows an increase in velocity ≥4 m/s or mean gradient ≥40 mmHg with a valve area ≤1 cm^2 [22], It is important that the measurements are obtained when the patient is normotensive with a systolic blood pressure less than 140 mmHg. Although there is no randomized trial data, post hoc analysis of this subset of patients has suggested improved outcome with surgical or trans-catheter aortic valve replacement over medical management alone [23].

In asymptomatic patients with a calcified aortic valve with decreased systolic opening and severe stenosis (velocity >4 m/s or gradient >40 mmHg), aortic valve replacement is indicated if LV function is less than 50% [22]. SAVR is reasonable in very severe asymptomatic AS (velocity is ≥5 m/s and gradient ≥60 mmHg) and the patient is at low risk for SAVR (STS predicted mortality <4%). This recommendation is based on observational studies that demonstrated a higher rate of symptom onset and major adverse CV events in patients with very severe compared with severe AS [24] as well as a propensity-score matched study showing reduced mortality with early SAVR [25]. SAVR is also considered to be reasonable in asymptomatic calcific AS with valve velocity of 4 to 4.9 m/s and mean gradient 40 to 59 mmHg if an exercise test demonstrates a fall in systolic blood pressure (or failure to rise at least 20 mmHg), or decreased exercise tolerance compared to age/sex matched controls [1, 26]. Table 11.4 below summarizes the recommendations for SAVR in AS.

CLINICAL PEARLS
Indications for surgery of moderate aortic stenosis
In patients undergoing cardiac surgery for another reason, SAVR is indicated at the time of surgery for

Table 11.4 Recommendations of surgeries for aortic stenosis

Type of AS	Criteria	LVEF	Symptoms or circumstance	Dobutamine	Recommendation
Severe	V_{max} >4 MG >40	>50	Symptomatic	n/a	Indicated
Severe	Same	<50	Asymptomatic	n/a	Indicated
Severe	Same	>50	Other CV surgery	n/a	Indicated
Low-flow Low-gradient	V_{max} <4 MG <40 AVA_{index} <0.6 SV <35	>50	Symptomatic	n/a	Reasonable
Low-flow Low-gradient	Same	<50	Symptomatic	V_{max} >4 MG >40 AVA <1	Reasonable
Very severe	V_{max} >5 MG >60	>50	Asymptomatic	n/a	Reasonable
Very severe	V_{max} 4–4.9 MG 40–59	>50	Asymptomatic	↓ SBP w/exercise or <20 mm rise ↓ exercise capacity	Reasonable
Moderate	V_{max} 3–3.9 MG 20–39	>50	Other CV surgery		Reasonable
Severe	Same w/ V_{max}↑> 0.3 m/s/yr.	>50	Asymptomatic		Consider

severe AS and is considered to be reasonable for moderate AS (velocity 3 to 3.9 m/s or mean gradient 20 to 39 mmHg) [9]. These recommendations are based on the likelihood of symptom onset within the next 5 years balanced against the risk for repeat surgery [27,28]. SAVR may be considered for asymptomatic severe AS if there are risks for rapid disease progression such as older age, severe valvular calcification and increase in aortic valve velocity of ≥0.3 m/s/year [29]; however there is uncertainty due to the lack of supportive evidence.

Trans-catheter aortic valve replacement

The first human case description of percutaneous trans-catheter aortic valve replacement (TAVR) for calcific AS was published in 2002 [30]. This experience ultimately set the stage for TAVR as a less invasive therapeutic alternative for non-operable or high-risk patients who were studied in the Placement of Aortic Trans-catheter Valves (PARTNER) trial. This multicenter RCT compared TAVR with standard therapy in high-risk patients with severe AS, including a pre-specified cohort of patients considered inoperable. Patients with symptomatic severe AS were divided into cohorts A and B. *Cohort A* is a high surgical risk group as guided by a STS risk of mortality at 30 days ≥10%. *Cohort B* is a group not considered to be suitable for surgery due to co-morbidities that would be associated with a predicted probability of death or disability ≥50%. The Edwards *SAPIEN* heart-valve system (Edwards Lifesciences, Irvine, CA) used in the PARTNER study is a balloon-expandable tri-leaflet bovine pericardial valve mounted on stainless steel support frame that can be delivered retrograde via a 22 or 24 F trans-femoral access or through a direct apical puncture under general anesthesia and trans-esophageal echocardiography guidance. Inoperable patients (*cohort B*) were randomly assigned to TAVR or standard therapy which included balloon aortic valvuloplasty in 83.8% of the patients by 30 days post-randomization.

The results showed significant reductions in the primary endpoint of all-cause mortality at 1 year and the co-primary endpoint of all-cause mortality or repeat hospitalization at 1 year [31]. The magnitude of this reduction in all-cause mortality becomes apparent with understanding that only five patients need to be treated with TAVR to prevent one death over the course of a year and only three patients need to be treated to prevent one death or repeat hospitalization over the same time period. The penalty for TAVR is an increased rate of strokes, major vascular complications and bleeding events. The benefits of TAVR were preserved at two-year follow-up. Notably, comparing the patients alive at the end of 1 year in both groups, there was a continued divergence in mortality rate at 2 years, 18.2% with TAVR and 35.1% with standard therapy [32]. A summary of the 1-year and 2-year results of PARTNER B is provided in Table 11.5 below.

Table 11.5 Results of the PARTNER B trial

End point	TAVR (%)	Standard (%)	HR (95% CI)	*P*
1 yr. all-cause death	**30.7**	**50.7**	0.55 (0.40–0.74)	<0.001
1 yr. all-cause death or hospitalization	42.5	71.6	0.46 (0.35–0.59)	<0.001
30 d. major vascular complications	16.2	1.1		<0.001
30 d. major bleeding	16.8	3.9		<0.001
30 d. major stroke	5.0	1.1		0.06
1 yr. major stroke	7.8	3.9		0.018
30 d. major/minor stroke	6.7	1.7		0.03
1 yr. major/minor stroke	10.6	4.5		0.04
2 yr. all-cause death	**43.3**	**68.0**	0.56 (0.43–0.73)	<0.001
2nd year all-cause death	18.2	35.1	0.58 (0.36–0.92)	0.02
2 yr. all-cause death or hospitalization	56.7	87.9		<0.001

Considering the dismal prognosis of severe symptomatic AS, the robust results of *PARTNER B* are consistent with clinical expectations. The US Food and Drug administration approved the SAPIEN heart valve system based on these results and TAVR is now recommended by the ACC/AHA guideline committee for patients with severe symptomatic AS with prohibitive risk for SAVR as defined by: risk of death or major morbidity with surgery >50% at 1 year; disease affecting ≥3 organ systems not likely to improve after surgery; or anatomic factors such as a heavily calcified (porcelain) aorta, prior irradiation or arterial bypass conduit adherent to the chest wall.

The results of the PARTNER A trial and multi-center registries from France [36] and Canada [37] have elevated the recommendation status of TAVR to *reasonable* in the high surgical risk patient, defined as an STS predicted mortality risk of 8% to 15%, anatomic factors that increase surgical risk, or significant frailty [9]. Analysis of the 2-year mortality results of cohort B by STS score revealed a significant association between the outcomes of TAVR and STS score with no benefit in patients with STS ≥15% [32]. Multivariable analysis identified decreased body-mass index, prior stroke and COPD requiring supplemental oxygen as significant predictors of death at 2 years.

SAPIEN XT   The second generation balloon-expandable percutaneous heart valve, *SAPIEN XT* (Edwards Lifesciences, Irvine, CA), is a lower profile device. The 23 mm valve can be delivered with the 18 F Novoflex system and the 26 mm valve requires 19 F. The newer SAPIEN XT valve has several key design modifications compared with the previous-generation device, including a cobalt chromium frame and modified leaflet design which may improve durability. The SAPIEN and SAPIEN XT devices were directly compared in inoperable patients in the *PARTNER II* trial (ACC 2013). Although the 30-day all-cause mortality, stroke and re-hospitalization rates were equivalent (15.3% vs. 17%, respectively, $P = 0.60$), the design improvements in the 2nd generation valve resulted in fewer major vascular complications (15.5% vs.9.6%, respectively, $P = 0.04$) including perforations, dissections and hematomas. There was also a strong trend towards reduced disabling bleeding (12.6% vs. 7.8%, respectively, $P = 0.06$). The SAPIEN XT will increase the number of patients suitable for TAVR by broadening applicability of trans-femoral access.

CoreValve aortic valve   The first-in-man experience to evaluate the feasibility and safety of implantation of the self-expanding CoreValve aortic valve prosthesis in high-risk patients with aortic valve disease (stenosis and/or regurgitation) using a retrograde percutaneous approach was a prospective, non-randomized, single-center registry study performed in Siegburg, Germany [38]. The first-generation device used bovine pericardial tissue and was constrained within a 24 F delivery sheath. The second-generation device incorporated a porcine pericardial tissue valve within a 21 F sheath. Both devices were used in this study. The procedure was performed under general anesthesia with trans-esophageal echocardiographic (TEE) guidance and with extracorporeal percutaneous femoro-femoral bypass. The CoreValve was successfully implanted without periprocedural events in 17 of 25 patients (68%), resulting in immediate hemodynamic improvement with reduction in NYHA class by 1 to 2 grades in all patients and sustained valve performance at 30-day follow-up. The theoretical benefits of a self-expanding valve are minimization of paravalvular regurgitation and treatment of AR or mixed valve disease.

The exact positioning of the trans-catheter heart valve is one the technically challenging aspects of TAVR. The degree of AR and also perhaps the chances of developing heart block from pressure on the ventricular septum, may depend on the positioning of the heart valve. The Sapien and Sapien XT heart valve is not repositionable, making precise deployment critical. The CoreValve system is partially repositionable, but the valve cannot be re-sheathed with the deployment wheel. If the valve is less than two-thirds deployed it may be withdrawn through the 18 F access sheath and re-loaded into the delivery catheter ex-vivo.

The major drawbacks of the current heart valve systems include: paravalvular AR; incidence of heart block (20% in the CoreValve group) requiring permanent pacing; and lack of repositionability.

New valves

The **Portico** percutaneous heart valve system (St. Jude Medical, Minneapolis, MN) will attempt to address some of these issues. It consists of a nitinol self-expanding frame, bovine pericardial leaflets, a porcine sealing cuff and is fully repositionable. The latter two features may reduce the incidence of paravalvular AR. Repositionability will allow for more precise placement which may decrease complications such as coronary obstruction, interference with the anterior mitral valve leaflet function and atrioventricular conduction disturbance. A first-in-human study of TAVR with Portico valve implantation in 10 high-risk patients has been published [41]. Implantation was successful in all patients and four required recapture and repositioning, which was accomplished without withdrawal of the system. None of the patients required pacemaker implantation. The *PORTICO* trial is evaluating the safety and effectiveness of the Portico trans-catheter aortic valve system in reducing the risk of death and disabling stroke in patients with high or extreme surgical risk for open-heart valve replacement surgery.

The **Lotus aortic valve system** (Boston Scientific, Natick, MA) is a second generation percutaneous aortic valve also designed to minimize paravalvular AR with an adaptive seal, allow full atraumatic repositionability due to a low-profile delivery system and complete retrievability prior to release. **REPRISE I** is a single-arm feasibility study of 11 patients from three centers in Australia with severe symptomatic AS and high risk for surgical aortic valve replacement. Six-month outcomes of this study, presented at the ACC 2013 meeting [42], described clinical procedural success in 9 of 11 patients (one patient had an ischemic stroke and another had a residual gradient >20 mmHg); however four patients required permanent pacemakers. One-year results confirmed no new CV events and no moderate to severe paravalvular AR.

The **REPRISE II** study, a single-arm, prospective, multi-center randomized trial in high surgical risk symptomatic severe AS patients, was presented at TCT 2013. The efficacy performance goal of a ≤18 mm mean aortic valve gradient was met with a mean gradient of 11.5. Three-month data, presented at ACC 2014, showed no cases of severe paravalvular AR; >85% had no AR and a constant low mean aortic pressure gradient of 11.5 mmHg at 90 days. **REPRISE III** will be a large efficacy and safety multi-center trial including sites from the US, which is intended to support the commercial approval of this trans-catheter aortic valve.

Pitfalls in TAVR

Successful delivery of a trans-catheter aortic valve without procedural complication can still be associated with technical complications.

Paravalvular aortic regurgitation   Paravalvular AR of a moderate to severe degree persisted in 6.8% and 6.1% of cases after TAVR in the PARTNER A trial and U.S. CoreValve High Risk, respectively, exceeding the rate after SAVR in both trials. Several registry studies [43–46] and two-year follow-up data from the PARTNER study [35] suggest increased morbidity and mortality in patients with more than mild paravalvular AR after TAVR. Analysis of the FRANCE-2 TAVR registry indicated a 2.5-fold increased mortality risk with greater than mild paravalvular AR [47]. However, it remains unclear whether this observation reflects the hemodynamic effects of AR or is an indicator of more advanced vascular disease resulting, among other things, in a less compliant aortic annulus and decreased ventricular compliance in this subgroup. Acute AR is not tolerated by a non-compliant, hypertrophic LV causing a quick rise in the diastolic filling pressure and consequent hemodynamic compromise.

A comprehensive multi-modality assessment of paravalvular AR after TAVR with angiography, echocardiography and invasive hemodynamics is useful to quantify the severity and identify patients that might benefit from corrective measures. Angiography can be used to characterize quickly the severity semi-quantitatively as mild, moderate or severe depending on the extent of regurgitant filling and opacification of the LV, along with the persistence of contrast. Echocardiographic assessment of AR with the usual parameters such as vena contracta and pressure half-time are best applied to transvalvular rather than paravalvular regurgitation. However, holodiastolic flow reversal in the descending thoracic aorta remains a reasonably sensitive and specific finding in significant paravalvular regurgitation. The Valve Academic Research Consortium-2 (VARC-2) has defined paravalvular AR by the circumferential extent of the jet in the short axis view [48]. The invasively obtained AR index (ARI) has an inverse relationship with the severity of paravalvular AR with a cutoff of 25 shown to optimally predict the 1-year mortality risk after TAVR and had a high negative predictive value for greater than mild paravalvular AR when used in conjunction with echocardiography or angiography [49], although this tool still needs validation in a larger and controlled study population.

$$ARI = [(Diastolic\ Aortic\ Pressure - LVEDP)/Systolic\ Aortic\ Pressure] \times 100$$

The following table summarizes the definitions of paravalvular AR severity (Table 11.6).

Table 11.6 Definitions of paravalvular aortic regurgitation severity

Severity	Echo – VARC-2	Angio	ARI
Mild	<10%	Reflux of contrast into LVOT/mid LV and clears with each beat	>25
Moderate	10–29%	Reflux fills LV with incomplete clearance with each beat	<25
Severe	≤30%	Opacification of entire LV – same intensity as aorta, persistence after a single beat	<25

If the degree of paravalvular regurgitation is more than mild, several corrective measures can be employed depending on the implantation depth, expansion of the valve and the proposed mechanism of the regurgitation. If the trans-catheter heart valve is at the right implant depth, balloon post-dilatation sized according to the aortic annulus dimension is an option to obtain better expansion of the stent frame which may provide a better seal. If the CoreValve is positioned too deeply into the LV outflow tract, use of a vascular snare to grasp an anchoring hook and pulling the valve back is an option but carries risk of valve embolization or possibly aortic dissection by the superior margin of the valve frame. If the CoreValve is positioned too shallow, implantation of another valve inside the existing valve at the proper depth is often a solution. Newer generation devices will be repositionable and incorporate sealing skirts to help conform to the irregular surfaces of the native aortic valve. In either case, care must be taken to assess the aortic diameter at the sino-tubular junction, as well as the coronary anatomy (i.e. presence of bypass grafts), as implantation of a second valve will hold the leaflets of the initially implanted valve in an open position resulting in a tube graft that risks occluding the coronary ostia.

Stroke   The rate of stroke or transient ischemic attack was higher with TAVR as compared to SAVR in the PARTNER study with both cohorts A and B but was actually lower with TAVR in the CoreValve high-risk study. This rate appears to be decreasing with time. Trans-cranial Doppler studies during TAVR have observed the highest rates of micro-embolization during crossing of the diseased aortic valve [50] and expansion of the prosthesis [51]. Three embolic protection devices have been used during TAVR: 2 deflector devices (Embrella device, Edwards Lifesciences Inc., Irvine, California; and SMT Embolic Deflection Device, SMT Research and Development Ltd., Herzliya, Israel) and a filter device (Claret dual filter system, Claret Medical Inc., Santa Rosa, California). While first-in-man studies have demonstrated feasibility, randomized studies will be needed to demonstrate efficacy in reduction of cerebrovascular events to justify the incremental cost and added procedural complexity and risk. Improvements in the delivery systems of successive generation devices including lower crossing profiles may also lower neurologic event rates by minimizing disruption of the diseased aortic valve during positioning and obviating the need for pre or post implantation balloon valvuloplasty.

Patient selection   The commercial availability of TAVR has brought forth the issue of identification of suitable candidates for TAVR. These patients will commonly be high risk with a significant burden of co-morbidities making them non-operative, but these same factors will make the risk benefit assessment extremely important from a patient outcome and cost perspective. The findings from the 2-year mortality analysis clarified some of the patient characteristics that should be taken into consideration when estimating the expected benefits of the procedure such as prior stroke, COPD requiring supplemental oxygen, and frailty. TAVR is not recommended in patients with a life expectancy <1 year or chance of 2-year survival with benefit of <25% [9].

Low flow–low gradient aortic stenosis   One particularly challenging group of patients with severe AS is the low flow–low gradient (LF-LG). Diagnosis and management are particularly vexing in this group. Low flow is defined as a cardiac index of <3.0 L/min/m^2 and a stroke volume index <35 mL/m^2. There are two subsets within this category: LF-LG with reduced LVEF ($\leq$40%); and LF-LG with preserved LVEF, known as 'paradoxical' LF-LG AS. Both subsets are characterized by aortic valve area $\leq$1.0 cm^2 or $\leq$0.6 cm^2/m^2 and low mean aortic valve gradients <40 mmHg. If there is discordance between valve area and mean gradients (AVA <1.0 cm^2 but mean gradient <40 mmHg) but normal flow, one must suspect measurement errors resulting in underestimation of valve area or gradient (improper Doppler interrogation angle), small body size or inconsistency in guidelines criteria.

In LF-LG with reduced LVEF, it is important to differentiate true severe AS where the myocardial dysfunction may be secondary to aortic valve disease from 'pseudo-severe' AS, in which primary myocardial dysfunction is causing a low flow state and incomplete opening of the aortic valve. An obvious example of the latter is a patient with severe ischemic cardiomyopathy but a non-calcified normal appearing aortic valve with reduced leaflet excursion resulting in an effective orifice area <1.0 cm^2. However, patients with CAD will sometimes also have aortic valve calcification and sclerosis since there is significant overlap in the risk factors for these diseases, hence making the diagnosis more challenging. The ACC/AHA/ESC valvular heart disease guidelines consider dobutamine stress echocardiography a reasonable next step [9]. In the presence of LV flow reserve, defined by an increase in stroke volume by ≥20% with dobutamine [52], pseudo-severe AS will respond with an increase in AVA with modest increases in aortic valve gradient but true AS will reveal a persistently low aortic valve area with an increase in gradient. A significant survival advantage can be ascertained with SAVR in the LF-LG severe AS patients with flow reserve [53]. Thus AVR is a reasonable option within both ACC/AHA and ESC/EACTS guidelines. However, LF-LG with reduced LVEF without flow reserve represents a high-risk surgical group in which TAVR may provide a better option since the data suggest that this group still may still benefit with valve replacement [52].

CLINICAL PEARLS
Calculations of the aortic valve area when the results by dobutamine echocardiography are ambiguous In cases where the stroke volume augmentation with dobutamine is ambiguous, a projected effective orifice area can be calculated at a theoretical normal flow rate of 250 mL/s using a regression line generated from a plot of serial measurements of valve area as a function of flow at each stage of the DSE [54]; a value less than 1.0–1.2 cm^2 is considered true severe AS. Another useful test is quantification of aortic valve calcification by computed tomography; a score >1650 Agatston units has been proposed as a threshold to identify true severe AS [55].

Paradoxical LF-LG severe AS is analogous to heart failure with preserved ejection fraction since both entities are associated with older age, female sex, systemic hypertension and characterized by a restrictive physiology, where LV stroke volume is reduced despite preserved systolic function [56]. This variant of severe AS is associated with more severe LV concentric remodeling and myocardial fibrosis; several studies have reported worse prognosis than in moderate AS or normal flow severe AS [57, 58]. Paradoxical LF-LG severe AS has a better prognosis with SAVR than with medical therapy in unadjusted and propensity score matched analyses [59], therefore surgery is a reasonable recommendation. The PARTNER studies included a substantial proportion of patients with low flow, specifically, 55% met criteria for low flow on the basis of a Doppler stroke volume index $\leq$35 mL/m^2. Analysis of the paradoxical LF-LG patients in PARTNER (14% of the patients) confirmed 2-year mortality benefit of TAVR over standard therapy in cohort B and similar outcomes with TAVR and SAVR in cohort A [60].

The analysis of the low flow patients from the PARTNER study showed a 50% increase in 2-year mortality compared with normal flow patients [60]. In this analysis, low flow was independently associated with outcome and a more powerful predictor than EF or mean gradient. Considering just the low flow subgroup of the PARTNER trial, the TAVR group had a lower 2-year mortality than the standard therapy group in cohort B and the TAVR and SAVR groups had similar 2-year mortality in cohort A, confirming the benefit of therapy with TAVR or SAVR in this high-risk cohort.

Coronary artery disease The frequent coexistence of AS and CAD is a result of the overlap in risk factors and strong correlation with age for both diseases. Multiple studies have shown that coronary artery bypass increases operative and short-term mortality after SAVR [61, 62]. However, omission of revascularization at the time of SAVR impairs short and long term outcomes [63]. The ACC/AHA guidelines state that coronary artery bypass or percutaneous coronary intervention (PCI) is reasonable in patients having valve repair or replacement with significant CAD ($\geq$70% diameter stenosis in a major coronary artery or $\geq$50% left main stenosis) [9]. In the FRANCE 2 multi-center registry of 3195 TAVR patients, 48% had coronary artery disease [47]. Most studies have not included data on the extent of unrevascularized severe CAD and PARTNER excluded patients with unrevascularized CAD. A study of 171 TAVR patients reported a higher 30-day (13.1% vs. 1.2%) and 1-year mortality (35.7% vs. 18.4%) in patients with CAD [64]. Another study that evaluated the outcomes after TAVR stratified by extent of CAD characterized by the Duke Myocardial Jeopardy Score found a higher 30-day mortality post-TAVR in patients with CAD compared to those without (11.5% vs.

6.3%) but the difference was not statistically significant [65], although 11% of patients had PCI prior to TAVR. A more recent study comparing outcomes after TAVR in patients with and without CAD found no difference in 30-day or 1-year mortality [66], but 17% of patients with CAD had PCI prior to TAVR. The indications for revascularization were angina and/or proximal coronary artery stenosis jeopardizing a large area of myocardium. A study comparing 30-day outcomes of PCI in patients with severe AS with propensity-matched control subjects without AS showed no difference in 30 day mortality (4.3% vs. 4.7%) [67]. However, the study did identify two subgroups with a higher mortality, patients with EF ≤30% or STS score ≥10% (15.4% and 10.4%, respectively). The available data suggest PCI can be performed carefully in patients without penalty in outcome. Intuitively, revascularization could improve outcomes after TAVR by ameliorating ischemia during rapid ventricular pacing, balloon valvuloplasty and valve deployment, although the duration of pacing is almost always limited to less than nine or ten seconds. However an observational study comparing the outcomes in patients treated with PCI before TAVR and TAVR alone found a two-fold increase in 30-day mortality in the PCI treated TAVR patients, although the difference was not statistically significant [68]. The authors concluded there is no increased risk of 30-day mortality with TAVR alone in patients with CAD compared with patients treated with PCI before TAVR. A small but important observational study comparing complete with incomplete revascularization at baseline in a registry of TAVR patients found no difference in medium term outcomes [69]. In this registry, pre-TAVR PCI was performed in 41% of patients with a reduction in SYNTAX score from a baseline median of 9 to 5 after completion of TAVR and achieving complete revascularization in 20% of patients with incomplete revascularization at baseline. The authors conclude that appropriate revascularization strategy based on heart team consensus can obviate the need for complete revascularization while maintaining medium-term success with TAVR. However, it is important to note these results are subject to the biases inherent in non-randomized observational studies without long-term follow-up. The ongoing ACTIVATION trial (Percutaneous coronary intervention prior to transcatheter aortic valve implantation) is randomizing patients with CAD (≥70% stenosis in ≥1 vessel or ≥50% stenosis in a vein graft or protected left main) to pre-TAVR PCI or deferral of PCI. The SURTAVI and PARTNER II trials of TAVR in moderate risk severe AS will include patients with CAD and therefore will provide some data on outcomes with different management strategies for CAD and severe AS. Currently there is an insufficient evidence base to offer guidance on the management of concomitant CAD during TAVR. The pragmatic approach of reserving revascularization prior to TAVR for ostial/proximal stenosis of vessels sub-tending large territories of myocardium should be practiced until more data from future randomized trials becomes available.

Unmet needs

Medical therapy   There is no medical therapy of proven benefit in AS. This is a particularly important unmet need in patients with moderate AS, since any medical therapy that can delay progression may have significant impact. The failure of statin therapy in this disease highlights an important pathophysiologic difference; progression is likely more dependent on local mediators of calcium homeostasis than atherosclerosis. Patients with osteoporosis have a greater incidence of AS and more rapid disease progression [70, 71]. The OPG/RANK/RANKL axis plays a central role in osteoporosis and the anti-RANKL monoclonal antibody denosumab is an effective and well-tolerated therapy [72]. Similar expression of this pathway has been observed in stenotic aortic valves [73] and treatment with bisphosphonates appeared to slow disease progression in a small observational study of patients being treated for osteoporosis [70]. These findings rationalize the need for a larger randomized controlled trial of these treatments specifically for AS.

Hypertension   Hypertension and AS are both characterized by increased pressure afterload resulting in LV hypertrophy. In hypertension, ACE inhibition reduces LV hypertrophy beyond reduction in blood pressure, with reduction in myocardial fibrosis [74]. Favorable data from an observational study suggesting reduction in mortality and CV events with ACE inhibitors in patients with AS [75] and published reports suggesting the tolerability of ACE inhibitors in severe AS [76] warrant further research of the novel application of this venerable therapeutic.

Anticoagulation   The optimal anticoagulation or antiplatelet regimen after implantation of a percutaneous trans-catheter aortic valve is currently unknown. Several factors highlight the importance of peri-procedural and post-procedural anti-thrombotic therapy: the incidence of clinically apparent stroke after TAVR ranges from 2.2% to 3.4% in several of the larger registries such as SOURCE XT [77], SOURCE [78], ADVANCE [79] and FRANCE-2 [47]; while about half of the cerebrovascular events occur within 24 hours post TAVR (54%), a significant percentage occur beyond 24 hours [80]; and several studies have identified peri-procedural stroke as a multivariate predictor of mortality after TAVR [35, 44, 80]. The ACCF/AATS/SCAI/STS expert consensus document on TAVR[81] recommends an activated clotting time >300 s. Heparin in most commonly used and protamine sulfate is given for reversal at procedural conclusion. After TAVR, dual antiplatelet therapy with aspirin and clopidogrel is a common and empirical practice. In the PARTNER trial, the recommendation was to use aspirin (75 mg to 100 mg per day) for life and clopidogrel (75 mg per day) for 6 months. The ACCF/AATS/SCAI/STS consensus document is consistent with these recommendations although the duration is not specified and currently there is no significant evidence available. About one-third of patients treated with TAVR will be on chronic oral anticoagulation for atrial fibrillation with warfarin, direct thrombin or factor Xa inhibitors. The consensus recommendation is use of low dose aspirin and warfarin in this circumstance. Randomized studies of single versus dual anti-platelet therapy and anti-platelet versus anti-thrombin therapies are needed to identify the optimal therapy in these high bleeding risk patients.

ACTION POINTS

1 One should take care not to miss the presence of AS in patients, especially elderly patients, in whom the systolic ejection murmur could be soft. The muffled S2 may indicate significant AS.

2 Once there is a suspicion of AS, there is a need to check for chest pain, heart failure and history of syncope. If there are symptoms, then there is indication for intervention.

3 There is a need to check for co-morbidities: chronic obstructive lung disease (COPD), advanced chronic kidney disease (CKD), peripheral vascular disease (PVD) and severe liver disease, frailty, dementia, prior amputation, history of stroke with significant residual deficits, connective tissue disease, prior radiation treatment, musculoskeletal deformities. ALL will increase surgical or interventional risks.

4 Indications for intervention are when AVA <1 cm^2; Vmax >4 m/sec; P gradient >40 mmHg.

5 If there is a suspicion of low flow AS, then the patient needs to have dobutamine echocardiography. Starting at a dose of 5 mcg/kg/min, dobutamine is progressively increased by an increment of 5 mcg to a maximum dose of 20 mcg/kg/min. At the same time, echocardiography should be carried out to check the velocity, and peak gradient in order to calculate the aortic valve area. If severe AS is present, the maximum velocity will increase above 4 m/s with increasing LV contractility; however the AVA will remain fixed at less than 1 cm^2. If primary myocardial dysfunction without severe AS is present, the AVA will increase with only a modest increase

in maximum trans-aortic velocity and gradient. Patients who fail to develop a 20% increase in stroke volume represent a group called 'lack of contractile reserve'. This group has a very poor prognosis with either medical or surgical therapy.

6 Once there is need for intervention, a multidisciplinary approach (interventional cardiology, cardiovascular surgery) offers a comprehensive assessment of valve disease, identification of the various treatment options available, and consideration of the associated risks and benefits to optimize outcomes.

REFERENCES

1. Kapadia S. Plenary Session V: Late-Breaking Clinical Trials No. 1. Presented at: *TCT* 2014; Sep. 13–17, 2014; Washington, D.C.

2. Otto, C. M., I. G. Burwash, et al. (1997). A prospective study of asymptomatic valvular aortic stenosis: clinical, echocardiographic, and exercise predictors of outcome. *Circulation*. 95: 2262–2270.

3. Grech, E. D. and D. R. Ramsdale (1991). Exertional syncope in aortic stenosis: Evidence to support inappropriate left ventricular baroreceptor response. *Am Heart J*. 121: 603.

4. Perloff, J. K. (1968). Clinical recognition of aortic stenosis. The physical signs and differential diagnosis of the various forms of obstruction to left ventricular outflow. *Prog Cardiovasc Dis*. 10(323).

5. Braunwald, E. (1997). Valvular heart disease. In: *Heart Disease: A Textbook of Cardiovascular Medicine*. Philadelphia, W.B. Saunders Company: 1007–1076.

6. Goldblatt, A., M. M. Aygen, et al. (1962). Hemodynamic–phonocardiographic correlations of the fourth heart sound in aortic stenosis. *Circulation*. 26(92).

7. Stam, R. B. and R. P. Martin (1983). Quantification of pressure gradients across stenotic valves by Doppler ulatrasound. *J Am Coll Cardiol*. (2): 707.

8. Bonow, R. O., B. A. Carabello, et al. (2006). ACC/AHA guidelines for management of valvular heart disease: a report of the American College of Cardiology/ American Heart Association Task Force on Practice Guidelines. *Circulation*. 114(5): e84–e231.

9. Nishimura, R. A., C. M. Otto, et al. (2014). 2014 ACC/AHA Guideline for the Management of Patients with Valvular Heart Disease. *JACC*. 63(22): e57–e185.

10. Rossebo, A. B., T. R. Pedersen, et al. (2008). Intensive lipid lowering therapy with simvastatin and ezetimibe in aortic stenosis. *N Engl J Med*. 359: 1343–1356.

11. Cowell, S. J., D. E. Newby, et al. (2005). A randomized trial of intensive lipid–lowering therapy in calcific aortic stenosis. *N Engl J Med*. 352: 2389–2397.

12. Chan, K. L., K. Teo, et al. (2010). Effect of lipid lowering with rosuvastatin on progression of aortic stenosis: results of the Aortic Stenosis Progression

Observation: Measuring Effects of Rosuvastatin trial (ASTRONOMER) trial. *Circulation*. 121: 306–314.

13. Messika-Zeitoun, D., L. F. Bielak, et al. (2007). Aortic valve calcification: determinants and progression in the population. *Arterioscler Thromb Vasc Biol*. 27: 642–648.

14. Cribier, A., T. Savin, et al. (1986). Percutaneous transluminal valvuloplasty of acquired aortic stenosis in elderly patients: an alternative to valve replacement? *Lancet*. 1: 63–67.

15. Moreno, P. R., I. K. Jang, et al. (1994). The role of percutaneous aortic balloon valvuloplasty in patients with cardiogenic shock and critical aortic stenosis. *J Am Coll Cardiol*. 23: 1071–1075.

16. Waller, B. F., C. McKay, et al. (1991). Catheter balloon valvuloplasty of stenotic aortic valves. Part I: Anatomic basis and mechanisms of balloon dilation. *Clin Cardiol*. 14: 836–846.

17. Lieberman, E. B., T. M. Bashore, et al. (1995). Balloon aortic valvuloplasty in adults: failure of procedure to improve long-term survival. *J Am Coll Cardiol*. 26: 1522–1528.

18. Ben-Dor, I., A. D. Pichard, et al. (2010). Complications and outcome of balloon aortic valvuloplasty in high risk or inoperable patients. *J Am Coll Cardiol Int*. 3(11): 1150–1156.

19. Kuntz, R. E., T. A. N. Kuntz R.E., Maitland L.A, et al. (1992). Immediate results and long-term follow-up after repeat balloon aortic valvuloplasty. *Cathet Cardiovasc Diagn*. 25: 4–9.

20. Tarantini, G., E. Covolo, et al. (2011). Valve replacement for severe aortic stenosis with low transvalvular gradient and left ventricular ejection fraction exceeding 0.50. *Ann Thorac Surg*. 91: 1808–1815.

21. Clavel, M. A., J. G. Dumensil, et al. (2012). Outcome of patients with aortic stenosis, small valve area and low-flow, low-gradient despite preserved left ventricular ejection fraction. *J Am Coll Cardiol*. 60: 1259–1267.

22. Pai, R. G., P. Varadarajan, et al. (2008). Survival benefit of aortic valve replacement in patients with severe aortic stenosis with low ejection fraction and low gradient with normal ejection fraction. *Ann Thorac Surg*. 86: 1781–1789.

23. Herrmann, H. C., P. Pibarot, et al. (2013). Predictors of mortality and outcomes of therapy in low–flow severe aortic stenosis: a Placement of Aortic Transcatheter Valves (PARTNER) Trial analysis. *Circulation*. (127): 2316–2326.

24. Rosenhek, R., R. Zilberszac, et al. (2010). Natural history of very severe aortic stenosis. *Circulation*. 121: 151–156.

25. Kang, D. H., S. J. Park, et al. (2010). Early surgery versus conventional treatment in asymptomatic very severe aortic stenosis. *Circulation*. 121: 1502–1509.

26. Alborino, D., J. L. Hoffman, et al. (2002). Value of exercise testing to evaluate the indication for surgery in asymptomatic patients with valvular aortic stenosis. *J Heart Valve Dis*. (11): 204–209.

27. Rosenhek, R., U. Klaar, et al. (2004). Mild and moderate aortic stenosis. Natural history and risk stratification by echocardiography. *Eur Heart J*. (25): 199–205.

28. Pereira, J. J., K. Balaban, et al. (2005). Aortic valve replacement in patients with mild or moderate aortic stenosis and coronary artery bypass surgery. *Am J Med*. (118): 735–742.

29. Lindman, B. R., R. O. Bonow, et al. (2013). Current management of calcific aortic stenosis. *Circ Res.* (113): 223–237.

30. Cribier, A., H. Eltchaninoff, et al. (2002). Percutaneous transcatheter implantation of an aortic valve prosthesis for calcific aortic stenosis first human case description. *Circulation.* (106): 3006–3008.

31. Leon, M. B., R. C. Smith, et al. (2010). Transcatheter aortic–valve implantation for aortic stenosis med in patients who cannot undergo surgery. *Med N Engl J.* (363): 1597–1607.

32. Makkar, R. R., G. P. Fontana, et al. (2012). Transcatheter aortic-valve replacement for inoperable severe aortic stenosis. *N Engl J Med.* (366): 1696–1704.

33. Smith, C. R., M. B. Leon, et al. (2011). Transcatheter versus surgical aortic-valve replacement in high risk patients. *N Engl J Med.* (364): 2187–2198.

34. Kodali, S. K., M. R. Williams, et al. (2012). Two year outcomes after transcatheter or surgical aortic-valve replacement. *N Engl J Med.* (366): 1686–1695.

35. Eltchaninoff, H., A. Prat, et al. (2011). Transcatheter aortic valve implantation: early results of the FRANCE (FRench Aortic National CoreValve and Edwards) registry. *Eur Heart J.* (32): 191–197.

36. Rodes-Cabau, J., J. G. Webb, et al. (2012). Long-term outcomes after transcatheter aortic valve implantation: insights on prognostic factors and valve durability from the Canadian multicenter experience. *J Am Coll Cardiol.* (60): 1864–1875.

37. Grube, E., J. C. LaBorde, et al. (2006). Percutaneous implantation of the CoreValve self-expanding valve prosthesis in high–risk patients with aortic valve disease: The Siegburg First-in-Man Study. *Circulation.* (114): 1616–1624.

38. Popma, J. J., D. H. Adams, et al. (2014). Transcatheter aortic valve replacement using a self-expanding bioprosthesis in patients with severe aortic stenosis at extreme risk for surgery. *J Am Coll Cardiol.* 63(19): 1972–1981.

39. Adams, D. H., J. J. Popma, et al. (2014). Transcatheter aortic-valve replacement with a self-expanding prosthesis. *N Engl J Med.* (370): 1790–1798.

40. Willson, A. B., J. Rodes-Cabau, et al. (2012). Transcatheter aortic valve replacement with the St. Jude portico valve first-in-human experience. *JACC.* 60(7): 581–586.

41. Meredith, I. T., S. Worthley, et al. (2013). The Repositionable Lotus Aortic Valve Replacement System: Six-Month Outcomes in the REPRISE I feasibility study. *JACC.* 61(10): E1868.

42. Abdel-Wahab, M., R. Zahn, et al. (2011). Aortic regurgitation after transcatheter aortic valve implantation: incidence and early outcome. Results from the German transcatheter aortic valve interventions registry. *Heart.* 97: 899–906.

43. Tamburino, C., D. Capodanno, et al. (2011). Incidence and predictors of early and late mortality after transcatheter aortic valve implantation in 663 patients with severe aortic stenosis. *Circulation.* 123: 299–308.

44. Hayashida, K., T. Lefevre, et al. (2012). Impact of post-procedural aortic regurgitation on mortality after transcatheter aortic valve implantation for severe aortic stenosis. *J Am Coll Cardiol.* (59): 566–571.

45. Gotzmann, M., M. Korten, et al. (2012). Long-term outcome of patients with moderate and severe prosthetic aortic valve regurgitation after transcatheter aortic valve implantation. *Am J Cardiol.* (110): 1500–1506.

46. Gilard, M., H. Eltchaninoff, et al. (2012). Registry of transcatheter aortic-valve implantation in high-risk patients. *N Engl J Med.* 366: 1705–1715.

47. Kappetein, A. P., S. J. Head, et al. (2012). Updated standardized endpoint definitions for transcatheter aortic valve implantation. The Valve Academic Research Consortium-2 Consensus Document. *J Am Coll Cardiol.* 60: 1438–1454.

48. Sinning, J. M., C. Hammerstingl, et al. (2012). Aortic Regurgitation index defines severity of peri-prosthetic regurgitation and predicts outcome in patients after transcatheter aortic valve implantation. *J Am Coll Cardiol.* (59): 1134–1141.

49. Kahlert, P., F. Al-Rashid, et al. (2013). Cerebral embolization during transcatheter aortic valve implantation: a transcranial Doppler study. *Circulation* (126): 1245–1255.

50. Erdoes, G., R. Bascani, et al. (2012). Transcranial Doppler detected cerebral embolic load during transcatheter aortic valve implantation. *Eur J Cardiothorac Surg.* (41): 778–783.

51. Vahanian, A., O. Alfieri, et al. (2012). Guidelines on the management of valvular heart disease (version 2012): the Joint Task Force on the Management of Valvular Heart Disease of the European Society of Cardiology (ESC) and European Association for Cardio-Thoracic Surgery (EACTS). *Eur Heart J.* 33: 2451–2496.

52. Monin, J. L., J. P. Quere, et al. (2003). Low-gradient aortic stenosis: operative risk stratification and predictors for long-term outcome: a multicenter study using dobutamine stress hemodynamics. *Circulation.* 108: 319–324.

53. Blais, C., I. G. Burwash, et al. (2006). Projected valve area at normal flow rate improves the assessment of stenosis severity in patients with low flow, low gradient aortic stenosis: the multicenter TOPAS (Truly or Pseudo Severe Aortic Stenosis) study. *Circulation.* 113: 711–721.

54. Cueff, C., J. M. Serfaty, et al. (2011). Measurement of aortic valve calcification using multislice computed tomography: correlation with haemodynamic severity of aortic stenosis and clinical implication for patients with low ejection fraction. *Heart.* 97: 721–726.

55. Dumesnil, J. G., P. Pibarot, et al. (2010). Paradoxical low flow and/or low gradient severe aortic stenosis despite preserved left ventricular ejection fraction: implications for diagnosis and treatment. *Eur Heart J.* 31: 281–290.

56. Hachicha, Z., J. G. Dumesnil, et al. (2007). Paradoxical low flow, low gradient severe aortic stenosis despite preserved left ventricular ejection fraction is associated with higher afterload and reduced survival. *Circulation.* (15): 2856–2864.

57. Clavel, M. A., J. G. Dumesnil, et al. (2012). Outcome of patients with aortic stenosis, small valve area, and low-flow, low-gradient despite preserved left ventricular ejection fraction. *J Am Coll Cardiol.* 60: 1259–1267.

58. Tarantini, G., E. Covolo, et al. (2011). Valve replacement for severe aortic stenosis with low transvalvular gradient and left ventricular ejection fraction exceeding 0.50. *Ann Thorac Surg.* 91(6): 1808–1815.

59. Herrmann, H. C., P. Pibarot, et al. (2013). Predictors of mortality and outcomes of therapy in low-flow severe aortic stenosis: A Placement of Aortic Transcatheter Valves (PARTNER) Trial Analysis. *Circulation.* 127: 2316–2326.

60. Hannan, E. L., C. Wu, et al. (2007). Risk index for predicting in-hospital mortality for cardiac valve surgery. *Ann Thorac Surg.* (83): 921–929.

61. Iung, B., M. F. Drissi, et al. (1993). Prognosis of valve replacement for aortic stenosis with or without coexisting coronary heart disease: a comparative study. *J Heart Valve Dis.* 2: 430–439.

62. Lund, O., T. T. Nielsen, et al. (1990). The influence of coronary artery disease and bypass grafting on early and late survival after valve replacement for aortic stenosis. *J Thorac Cardiovasc Surg.* 100: 327–337.

63. Dewey, T. M., D. L. Brown, et al. (2010). Effect of concomitant coronary artery disease on procedural and late outcomes of transcatheter aortic valve implantation. *Ann Thorac Surg.* 89(discussion 67): 758–767.

64. Masson, J. B., M. Lee, et al. (2010). Impact of coronary artery disease on outcomes after transcatheter aortic valve implantation. *Catheter Cardiovasc Interv.* 76: 165–173.

65. Gautier, M., M. Pepin, et al. (2011). Impact of coronary artery disease on indications for transcatheter aortic valve implantation and on procedural outcomes. *EuroIntervention.* (7): 549–555.

66. Goel, S. S., S. Agarwal, et al. (2012). Percutaneous coronary intervention in patients with severe aortic stenosis: implications for transcatheter aortic valve replacement. *Circulation.* 125: 1005–1013.

67. Wenaweser, P., T. Pilgrim, et al. (2011). Impact of coronary artery disease and percutaneous coronary intervention on outcomes in patients with severe aortic stenosis undergoing transcatheter aortic valve implantation. *EuroIntervention.* 7: 541–548.

68. Van Mieghem, N. M., R. M. van der Boon, et al. (2013). Complete revascularization is not a prerequisite for success in current transcatheter aortic valve implantation practice. *JACC Cardiovasc Intervent.* 6(8): 867–875.

69. Aksoy, Y., C. Yagmur, et al. (2005). Aortic valve calcification: association with bone mineral density and cardiovascular risk factors. *Coron Artery Dis.* 16: 379–383.

70. Persy, V. and P. D'Haese (2009). Vascular calcification and bone disease: the calcification paradox. *Trends Mol Med.* 15: 405–416.

71. Cummings, S. R., J. San Martin, et al. (2009). Denosumab for prevention of fractures in postmenopausal women with osteoporosis. *N Engl J Med.* 361: 756–765.

72. Kaden, J. J., S. Bickelhaupt, et al. (2004). Receptor activator of nuclear factor kappaB ligand and osteoprotegerin regulate aortic valve calcification. *J Mol Cell Cardiol.* 36: 57–66.

73. Brilla, C. G., R. C. Funck, et al. (2000). Lisinopril-mediated regression of myocardial fibrosis in patients with hypertensive heart disease. *Circulation.* 102: 1388–1393.

74. Nadir, M. A., L. Wei, et al. (2011). Impact of renin-angiotensin system blockade therapy on outcome in aortic stenosis. *J Am Coll Cardiol.* 58: 570–576.

75. Chockalingam, A., S. Venkatesan, et al. (2004). Safety and efficacy of angiotensin-converting enzyme inhibitors in symptomatic severe aortic stenosis: Symptomatic Cardiac Obstruction-Pilot Study of Enalapril in Aortic Stenosis (SCOPE-AS). *Am Heart J.* 147: E19.

76. Wendler, O. (2012). *The Multicenter SOURCE XT TAVR registry*, Paris, France, EuroPCR.

77. Thomas, M., G. Schymik, et al. (2011). One-year outcomes of cohort 1 in the Edwards SAPIEN Aortic Bioprosthesis European Outcome (SOURCE) registry: the European registry of transcatheter aortic valve implantation using the Edwards SAPIEN valve. *Circulation.* 124: 425–433.

78. Linke, A., U. Gerckens, et al. (2012). Treatment of high risk aortic stenosis patients with transcatheter Medtronic CoreValve implantation: results from the international multicenter ADVANCE study. *J Am Coll Cardiol.* 59: e8.

79. Nombela-Franco, L., J. G. Webb, et al. (2012). Timing, predictive factors, and prognostic value of cerebrovascular events in a large cohort of patients undergoing transcatheter aortic valve implantation. *Circulation.* 126: 3041–3053.

80. Holmes, D. R., M. J. Mack, et al. (2012). ACCF/AATS/SCAI/STS expert consensus document on transcatheter aortic valve replacement. *J Am Coll Cardiol.* 59: 1200–1254.

CHAPTER 12
Mitral Regurgitation

Deepak Joshi, Rajasekhar Nekkanti, Marvin H. Eng, Madhur Roberts, Ngoc Quang Nguyen, Xian Kai Li and Mike Rinaldi

Management of Complex Cardiovascular Problems, Fourth Edition. Edited by Thach N. Nguyen, Dayi Hu, Shao Liang Chen, Moo Hyun Kim and Cindy L. Grines.
© 2016 John Wiley & Sons, Ltd. Published 2016 by John Wiley & Sons, Ltd.

BACKGROUND

Mitral regurgitation (MR) is defined as a reversal of flow from left ventricle (LV) into the left atrium (LA) during ventricular systole due to an incompetent mitral valve (MV). MR is categorized as chronic or acute with etiology divided into primary/degenerative (due to abnormalities in the apparatus) or secondary/functional MR (due to dilation or dysfunction of the LV). MR causes long-term volume overload and depending on the etiology will lead to irreversible myocardial damage.

CHALLENGES

The first challenge in the diagnosis and management of MR is comprehensive evaluation of MR including etiology and severity. Once MR is confirmed and staged, the second challenge is that particularly with primary MR there is no medical treatment to delay the natural history of the disease process.

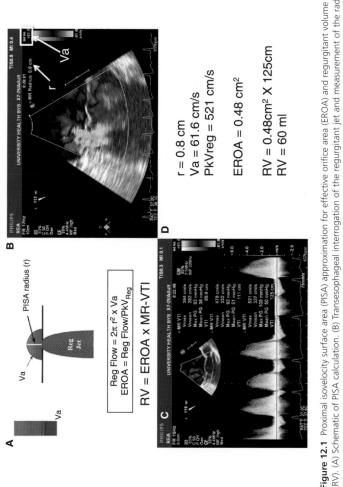

Figure 12.1 Proximal isovelocity surface area (PISA) approximation for effective orifice area (EROA) and regurgitant volume (RV). (A) Schematic of PISA calculation. (B) Transesophageal interrogation of the regurgitant jet and measurement of the radius (r) of flow convergence. (C) Measurement of MR peak velocity (PkVreg) and velocity time integral (MR-VTI). (D) Calculation for the EROA and RV based on measured values for this case. Based on the calculations, the patient has severe MR. Note that this example used the highest values, given the atrial fibrillation, there may be a need for averaging several beats. Source: Zoghbi 2003. Reproduced with permission of Oxford University Press. Chapter 12, Reference [5].

Management of Complex Cardiovascular Problems, Fourth Edition. Edited by
Thach N. Nguyen, Dayi Hu, Shao Liang Chen, Moo Hyun Kim and Cindy L. Grines.
© 2016 John Wiley & Sons, Ltd. Published 2016 by John Wiley & Sons, Ltd.

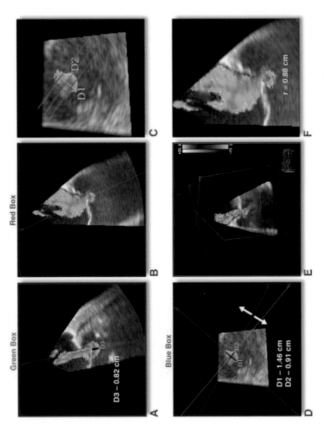

Figure 12.2 Multi-planar assessment of estimated regurgitant orifice area (EROA) using 3-dimensional (3D) Doppler. (A and B) Systolic long-axis views are optimized to visualize the MR (MR) jet. The largest systolic proximal isovelocity surface area (PISA) is used to adjust the short-axis plane (blue line) to obtain an *en face* view of the base of the PISA (C and D). (E) The color Doppler baseline is adjusted to 39.6 cm/s. (F) Multiple orthogonal view can be generated (C and D, red planes) to obtain the largest 2-dimensional PFCR. The radius, length, and width measurements are shown (A and D) and the longest PISA radius is shown (F). Source: Thavendiranathan et al. 2012. Reproduced with permission of Elsevier. Chapter 12, Reference [28].

The third challenge is the optimal time to refer patients for surgery. The reason being myocardial damage often precedes the onset of symptoms. This is why early surgical intervention improves long-term outcomes on appropriately selected patients. The parameters such as LV size, volume, ejection fraction (EF) serve as surrogates for judging appropriateness of surgical referral. Even so, LV dysfunction may still be observed despite timely referral to surgery indicating that the surrogates do not perfectly predict transition from compensated to decompensated phase of the LV [1].

STRATEGIC MAPPING

In the management of MR, the goal is to delay transition to symptomatic status as long as possible and to mitigate long-term consequences of volume overload and ventricular remodeling [2]. The strategies in the diagnosis and management of MR are summarized in Table 12.1.

At first, the evaluation of patients with chronic MR includes a comprehensive history and physical examination with attention to determining the insidious onset of decompensation and signs of congestion.

Optional tests include an electrocardiogram (EKG), a chest X-Ray (CXR) and measurement of B type natriuretic peptide (BNP) level. A baseline ECG is done for rhythm assessment, presence of chamber enlargement and severity of ST-T changes of possible ischemic origin. A CXR may be done to assess for the presence of pulmonary vascular congestion and of cardiomegaly. The level of BNP may be measured for risk stratification and is predictive of adverse outcomes.

Transthoracic echocardiography (TTE) is the primary imaging tool used for detection of MR. TTE can assess the LV function and size, including LV end diastolic pressure and EF, right ventricular (RV) function and, pulmonary artery pressures, and can delineate the mechanism and accurately

---

Table 12.1 Strategies for diagnosis and management

1 Correctly classify the stage of mitral regurgitation (acute, chronic compensated, chronic decompensated).
2 Accurately quantify the severity of mitral regurgitation.
3 Determine the mechanism of mitral regurgitation (primary versus secondary).
4 Timely referral for mitral valve repair or replacement.

quantify the severity of regurgitation [3]. If the results of TTE are inconclusive because of poor windows then trans-esophageal echocardiography (TEE) is the next step.

TEE is an essential acoustic tool for determining the exact mechanism of MR to guide surgical repair given the posterior location of the MV and better quality image resolution. However real-time three dimensional echocardiography (3DE) offers more accuracy than two dimensional echocardiography (2DE) in the measurement of LV volume and LV EF [4]. If there is equivocal information about MR, another method to detect the functional severity of MR is by exercise echocardiography.

When echocardiography is technically difficult or the results are equivocal, cardiac magnetic resonance imaging (CMR) could provide excellent MR severity quantification. Also important as part of surgical evaluation and planning, a right and left cardiac catheterization with coronary angiography should be performed. In selected patients, coronary CT angiography can provide a less invasive alternative evaluation.

HIGH-RISK MARKERS

Surgery is the standard of care for treatment of symptomatic severe degenerative MR. Some patients are at increased risk of complications or are at prohibitive risk due to concomitant co-morbidities. These included advanced age, severe lung disease, LV dysfunction, obesity, and history of heart failure (HF).

HIGH-RISK PREDICTORS

The predictors of high long-term morbidity and mortality include: pulmonary hypertension (HTN), atrial fibrillation (AF), and LV dysfunction, HF, liver disease, renal failure, morbid obesity, RV failure, active smoking and cognitive disorders.

INVESTIGATIONS

Symptoms to look for

Because most patients with MR are asymptomatic, symptoms of congestion should be elicited. The symptoms of MR could be none or point to right heart fluid overload or failure. The common symptoms of MR are listed in Table 12.2.

Table 12.2 Symptoms of mitral regurgitation

1	Symptoms	Pathophysiology mechanism
2	Shortness of breath	Pulmonary venous congestion due to high left ventricular end diastolic pressure
3	Chest pain	Pulmonary hypertension
4	Lack of energy	Liver congestion
5	Early satiety	Fluid congestion in the wall of the stomach
6	Sense of heaviness in abdomen	Abdominal wall edema
7	Nocturia	Fluid overload
8	Edema in legs	Fluid overload
10	Fatigue	Low cardiac output

Signs to look for

The signs of patients with MR could be minimal or point to HF. The typical signs of fluid overload and right HF are listed in Table 12.3.

Smart testing

In the evaluation of MR, the most important task is to quantify the degree of MR and to identify its possible etiologies. For the patient with MR, the patient could have TTE, TEE, color Doppler flow, 3DE, exercise stress testing, exercise echocardiography, cardiac magnetic resonance imaging or cardiac catheterization. The selection of a diagnostic test depends on the level of certainty of evidence regarding risks and benefits, how these risks and benefits compare with potential alternatives, and what the comparative cost or cost-effectiveness of the diagnostic test would be.

Table 12.3 Signs of mitral regurgitation

1	Rales in lungs	Transudates of fluid in the alveoli due to fluid overload from left heart
2	Loud P2	Due to pulmonary hypertension
3	Systolic murmur at apex with radiation to the back	Mitral regurgitation
4	Jugular venous distension	High right ventricular pressure
5	Hepatomegaly	Congestion in the liver due to fluid overload
6	Hard and thick abdominal wall	Abdominal wall infiltrated with fluid
7	Edema in legs	Fluid overload

Transthoracic echocardiography TTE can provide high resolution real-time imaging that is widely available and should be the first imaging modality. Two-dimensional TTE allows assessment of MV anatomy, regurgitation severity and cardiac chamber size.

The evaluation includes the anatomy of the leaflets, annulus, chordae tendinae, papillary muscles, LV dimensions and function. When the MV, annulus, and LV structure are anatomically normal, it is rare to encounter severe MR. The echocardiography techniques used for evaluating the severity of MR are summarized in Table 12.4. For accurate quantification of regurgitation severity, a combination of techniques should be used rather relying on one sole indicator for severity (Table 12.5) [3–11]. Trivial MR can be physiologic but more severe forms of MR are always pathologic [2]. The evaluation of LA size and LV function provides clues for severity and chronicity of MR while the LV size and function are important in determining the necessity and timing of surgery.

Color flow Doppler (regurgitant jet area, vena contracta, proximal isovelocity surface area), pulsed wave Doppler and continuous wave Doppler methods are used for grading the severity of MR [11]. Tables 12.4 and 12.5 are reproduced from the 2003 American Society of Echocardiograms (ASE) guidelines for native valvular regurgitations. As MR is a dynamic process, its severity is influenced by the difference in LV and LA pressure, LA compliance, volume status, duration of systole, effective regurgitant orifice (ERO) and LV contractility [12]. This is why the ERO may increase with exercise and decrease with lower preload, and thus these conditions should be considered during interpretation [13].

Trans-esophageal echocardiography While TTE often provides adequate information about MR severity and mechanism, TEE can be essential when surface windows are poor. TEE also offers more detailed characterization of MR due to its proximity to the esophagus. TEE may better delineate the mechanism of regurgitation and determine whether the anatomy is favorable for surgical repair or replacement. Additional pathology may be visualized including leaflet destruction from endocarditis or congenitally abnormal valve such as cleft MV [14, 15].

3D Echocardiography 3-Dimensional echocardiography (3DE) improves the assessment of ventricular volumes, MV apparatus and can fully characterize the abnormality on the MV. With the availability of volumetric assessment, several facets of ventricular and MV anatomy can be accurately quantified without using geometric assumptions as in case of calculating the effective regurgitant orifice area (EROA) or regurgitant fraction using the *proximal isovelocity surface area* (PISA) or volumetric

Table 12.4 Echocardiography techniques for evaluating severity of mitral regurgitation

Technique	Methodology	Advantages	Limitations
Color Doppler jet area	Jet area <4.0 cm² or <20% of LA area with the Nyquist limit of 50–60 cm/s	Excellent for excluding MR or verifying mild MR. Simple and quick screening tool.	Jet area is dependent on the mechanism of MR. Central MR yields a broad jet with a large area but eccentric MR jets may appear narrow. Jet area may significantly underestimate eccentric MR.
Vena contracta width	Smallest highest-velocity region of flow jet at or just downstream to regurgitant orifice.	Simple, quantitative, and good at identifying mild or severe MR.	Only correlates to effective regurgitant orifice area (EROA) assuming the orifice is round. May vary during systole or with hemodynamic conditions. May be difficult to align imaging plane perpendicular to vena contracta. Measurement in late systole may overestimate MR. If >1 jet present, vena contracta width cannot measure MR.

(continued)

Table 12.4 (*Continued*)

Technique	Methodology	Advantages	Limitations
Proximal isovelocity surface area (PISA)	• Flow approaching a circular orifice forms concentric, hemispheric shells of increasing velocity and decreasing surface area just proximal to the orifice. • Measure radius of flow convergence (r) and estimate the flow rate (ml/sec.) as product of the hemisphere surface area and aliasing velocity (Va) $2\pi r^2$ • Measure peak velocity of MR jet by color Doppler (PkVreg) $EROA = (2\pi r^2 \times Va)/PkVreg$ • After calculating the EROA, regurgitant volume can be calculated by multiplying the MR velocity time integral (VTI) RV= EROA X MR-VTI Note: Nyquist limit must be set at 50–60 cm/s	Technique enables quantitative instead of qualitative assessment of regurgitation.	More accurate for central jets than eccentric jets. Tends to underestimate the effective regurgitant orifice area (EROA). Measurement of the exact location of the orifice may be challenging and any error is magnified. The orifice is dynamic and may lead to errors with measurement.

Volumetric calculation	• To calculate the volume of regurgitation with MR, one can calculate the forward stroke volume and regurgitant stroke volume. • Stroke volume = cross sectional area × VTI • Stroke volume may also be calculated using difference of systolic and diastolic volumes. 3D echocardiography calculates volumes more accurately than 2D. RgV = SV mitral inflow − SV aortic outflow RgF = RgV/SV mitral inflow	Complementary quantitative technique to PISA.	Common errors: 1. Failure to measure valve annulus properly (error is squared) 2. Failure to trace modal velocity 3. Failure to position the sample volume correctly at the level of the annulus.
Pulmonary vein flow reversal	As MR severity increases, systolic velocity in the pulmonary vein decreases and eventually reverses in severe MR.	Qualitative and easy to perform.	Increased left atrial pressure of any type can cause blunting of systolic flow. Difficult to discern how accurate pulmonary vein flows are in atrial fibrillation.
Jet profile-CW	Examines Density of jet density	Simple, readily available	Qualitative; complementary data.
Peak mitral E velocity	Examines A versus E-wave dominance. Severe MR is usually E-wave dominant.	Simple, readily available, A-wave dominance excludes severe MR	Influenced by LA pressures, LV relaxation, MV area, and atrial fibrillation. Complementary data only and does not quantify MR severity.

2D = 2-Dimensional; 3D = 3-Dimensional; EROA = effective orifice area; MR = mitral regurgitation; MR-VTI = Mitral regurgitation velocity time integral; PkVreg = Peak Velocity of MR jet; RgF = Regurgitant Fraction; RgV = Regurgitant volume; SV = stroke volume; Va = aliasing velocity; VTI = velocity time integral.

Table 12.5 Specific and supportive signs and quantitative parameters in grading severity of mitral regurgitation

	Mild	Moderate	Severe
Specific signs of severity	• Small central jet <4 cm² Or < 20% of LA area[Φ] • Vena contracta width <0.3 cm • No or minimal flow convergence[Ψ]	Signs of MR > Mild present, but no criteria for severe MR	• Vena contracta width ≥0.7 cm *with large* central MR jet (area >40% of LA) *or with* a wall-impinging jet of any size, swirling in LA[Φ] • Large flow convergence[Ψ] • Systolic reversal in pulmonary veins • Prominent flail MV leaflet or ruptured papillary muscle
Supportive signs	• Systolic dominant flow in pulmonary veins • A-wave dominant mitral inflow[γ] • Soft density, parabolic CW Doppler MR signal • Normal LV size	Intermediate signs/findings	• Dense, triangular CW Doppler MR jet • E-wave dominant mitral inflow (E>1.2 m/s) [γ] Enlarged LV and LA size, (particularly when normal LV function is present)
Quantitative parameters			
Regurgitant volume (ml/beat)	<30	30–44	≥60
Regurgitant fraction (%)	<30	30–39	≥50
Effective regurgitant orifice area (EROA) cm²	<0.20	0.20–0.29	≥0.40

CW = continuous wave; LA = left atrium; LV = left ventricle; MR = mitral regurgitation.
[Φ] At a Nyquist limit of 50–60 cm/s.
[γ] Usually above 50 years of age or in conditions of impaired relaxation, in the absence of mitral stenosis or other causes of elevated LA pressure.
[Ψ] Minimal and large flow convergence defined as flow convergence radius <0.4 cm and ≤0.9 cm for central jets, respectively, with a baseline shift at a Nyquist of 40 cm/s; Cut-offs for eccentric jets are higher, and should be angle corrected.

assessment, respectively [16–18] (Figure 12.1; see insert for color representation of figure). Assessment of end-diastolic and end-systolic volume by 3DE is also more accurate and it increases the accuracy of measuring the regurgitant volume and fraction needed for determination of MR severity [19]. Using 3D Doppler interrogation, one can better quantify the EROA by directly measuring the MV orifice through post-processing biplane planimetery. An alternative technique is to calculate the PISA by examining the 3D color Doppler in a similar way (Figure 12.2; see insert for color representation of figure) [6, 20]. By utilizing 3D assessment we can better appreciate how 2DE may underestimate MR given that PISA is actually a hemi-ellipse rather than a hemisphere and therefore may be inadequately characterized with 2D assessment alone [21].

Exercise stress testing   Due to the fact that many patients with MR are asymptomatic secondary to a sedentary lifestyle or presence of subjective equivocal symptoms, an exercise stress test may unmask the presence of symptoms and the level of functional capacity. Exercise treadmill testing does not quantify regurgitation but may be useful to measure exercise capacity and determine symptomatic status. A variety of stress test protocols (Bruce, Modified-Bruce, Naughton) may be used to determine metabolic equivalents of exertion [22–24].

Exercise echocardiography   As MR is sensitive to preload and afterload, the assessment of regurgitant severity may sometimes be quantified only with provocative testing to recreate the loading conditions under stress. Exercise echocardiography on a treadmill or recumbent bike allows evaluation of exercise-related changes in LV systolic function, visualization of the regurgitant flow, the EROA, and pulmonary artery pressure. Failure of LV EF to increase or absence of contractile reserve with exercise predicts worse postoperative LV function in primary MR [25]. Changes in the EROA during exercise are not related to resting MR severity; however, increases in EROA ($\geq$13 mm^2) during exercise in functional MR have been shown to be associated with symptom status and a worsened prognosis. An increase in pulmonary artery pressure with exercise is considered a Class IIA indication for surgery in asymptomatic severe MR [22, 24, 26].

Cardiac magnetic resonance imaging   Because of its accuracy and precision in measuring LV volumes, CMR is useful for evaluation of LV remodeling in MR and can identify the presence of scar or fibrosis using delayed hyper-enhancement of gadolinium contrast agents, a finding that may be particular relevant in functional MR [15]. Limitations of CMR include cardiac arrhythmias that preclude adequate gating, pacemakers or implantable cardioverter-defibrillators, and claustrophobia. Direct measurement of the EROA by CMR may be limited by slice thickness (typically 5 mm) and cardiac translation, which may render it difficult to align the image precisely with the narrowest part of the vena contracta area (VCA) [27–29].

Cardiac catheterization   Patients with chronic MR routinely undergo pre-surgical coronary angiography to determine if concomitant coronary artery bypass grafting (CABG) should be performed. Additionally, invasive hemodynamic assessment may useful in risk stratifying patients, as pulmonary HTN is a negative predictor of functional recovery post-valve surgery [30].

In the right heart catheterization, the large V waves seen in pulmonary capillary wedge pressure (PCWP) tracing are not sensitive or specific of severe MR. Severe MR is the most common cause but large V waves can be seen in other conditions due to a combination of volume overload or poor left atrial compliance [31]. In chronic MR, increased left atrial compliance reduces the presence of V waves [14].

During the left ventriculogram (LVA) for MR investigation, the right anterior oblique (RAO) angulation 30° separates the LA from the LV perpendicularly at the mitral annulus. The regurgitant jet is qualitatively graded and scored (1+ to 4+) (Table 12.6). The grading of MR severity by LVA is only qualitative. The reliability and accuracy of this method is questionable [13].

Table 12.6 **Seller's grade for mitral regurgitation severity by angiography**

MR severity	Mitral regurgitation
1+	Contrast refluxes into the left atrium but clears on each beat.
2+	Left atrial contrast density gradually increases but never equals LV density
3+	Density of contrast in the atrium and ventricle equalize after several beats
4+	The left atrium becomes as dense as the LV on the first beat and contrast refluxes into the pulmonary veins.

LV = left ventricle.

CRITICAL THINKING
Accuracy in the assessment of severity
of mitral regurgitation 3D TTE and TEE assessment of LV volumes and EF are recommended over the use of 2D echocardiography, as 3D TTE and TEE have been clearly demonstrated to provide more accurate and reproducible measurements. If the endocardial borders are not clearly visualized, an ultrasound contrast agent should be used with 3D imaging to obtain accurate LV volumes. CMR is an excellent technique for assessment of LV volumes and should be used if the results of echocardiography are suboptimal.

In the measurement of LVEF by echocardiography, LVEF can be falsely normal in severe MR due to elevated preload while the LV end systolic dimension (LVESD) is less load-dependent. If the regurgitation fraction is to be calculated, ventriculography using biplane imaging is necessary to calculate volumes (Table 12.7).

Table 12.7 Method of calculating regurgitant fraction by ventriculography

SV = Total SV − Forward SV
Total SV = angiographic EDV − angiographic ESV
Forward SV = Total CO (Fick or Thermodilution)/heart rate
Mild <20%, Moderate 20–40%, moderate-severe 40–60%, Severe >60%

CO = cardiac output, SV = stroke volume.

PRIMARY MITRAL REGURGITATION

Management
Medical therapy   In patients with normal blood pressure and LV function (LVEF >60%), vasodilators provide no benefit and may possibly worsen the severity of primary regurgitation as the pathology is myxomatous degeneration with valvular redundancy. Lowering the afterload may decrease LV size and MV closing force, increasing the degree of prolapse. Therefore, unless the patient had HTN, treatment of MR with vasodilators carries a Class III recommendation [22, 32, 33].

Follow-up Asymptomatic patients with mild MR without LV dysfunction or pulmonary HTN can be followed on a yearly basis. Baseline exercise tolerance should be assessed and reassessed during each visit. The patient should be educated to alert the physician if symptoms develop or change. Routine follow-up TTE is not recommended for asymptomatic patients with mild MR and normal LV systolic function and size.

Patients with asymptomatic mild MR should receive a follow-up TTE every 3–4 years and moderate MR every 1–2 years as per the American College of Cardiology/American Heart Association (ACC/AHA) guidelines. For asymptomatic patients with moderate to severe MR, TTE should be done every 6 to 12 months for surveillance of LV EF and LV end systolic dimension. When there is a change of signs or symptoms, there is need to re-evaluate the MV apparatus and LV function.

Activities No restrictions to physical activity are recommended in patients with MR of any severity if the patient is asymptomatic, with normal LVEF, normal LA/LV size, and in normal sinus rhythm without pulmonary HTN. The patient should not participate in competitive sports if the patient has definite LV enlargement (LVEDD >60 mm), LV systolic dysfunction or pulmonary HTN.

Surgery Ideally, all patients should have MV surgery prior to the onset of myocardial dysfunction. Surgery is indicated when the patient has chronic severe MR and New York Heart Association (NYHA) functional class II, III or IV symptoms in the absence of severe LV dysfunction (LVEF <30% and/or LVESD >55 mm).

Although parameters of LVESD $\geq$40 mm and LVEF $\geq$60% are meant to time surgery in order to preserve LV function, a minority of patients still experience decline in LVEF after surgery. This indicates that myocardial damage may occur even before the limits of these parameters are reached [1]. The reason is that MR is a state of low afterload, so visual EF overestimates the true ventricular function; those patients with LVEF <60% will likely have some degree of permanent myocardial damage. Restoration of a competent MV will instantly increase afterload, possibly unmasking previously unappreciated LV dysfunction. The indications of surgery for mitral regurgitation are listed in Table 12.8.

High-risk patient populations MV surgery yields the best prognosis prior to the onset of irreversible myocardial dysfunction. For instance, operating on patients with severe symptoms (NYHA III–IV) as opposed

---

Table 12.8 Indications of surgery for mitral regurgitation

---

1. Asymptomatic patients with chronic severe MR and mild to moderate LV dysfunction (LVEF 30–60% and/or LVESD greater than or equal to 40 mm) also benefit from surgery [22, 34–36]

2. Patient should undergo MV repair in experienced centers for asymptomatic chronic severe MR with preserved LV systolic function (LVSF) in whom the likelihood of successful repair without residual MR is greater than 90%. MV surgery is also reasonable for asymptomatic patients with chronic severe MR, preserved LVSF and new onset AF.

3. MV surgery is reasonable for asymptomatic patients with chronic severe MR, preserved LVSF and pulmonary HTN (PA systolic pressure >50 mmHg at rest or greater than 60 mmHg with exercise). MV surgery is reasonable for patients with chronic severe MR due to primary abnormality of mitral apparatus and NYHA functional class III–IV symptoms and severe LV systolic dimension (LVSD) (LVEF <30% and/or LVESD >55 mm) in whom MV repair is highly likely.

AF = atrial fibrillation; HTN = hypertension; LV = left ventricle; LVEF = left ventricular ejection fraction; LVESD = left ventricular end systolic dimension; LVSD = left ventricular systolic dimension; LVSF = left ventricular systolic function; MR = mitral regurgitation; MV = mitral valve; NYHA = New York Heart Association; PA = pulmonary artery.

---

to patients with mild symptoms (NYHA I–II) was associated with ~30% decrease in survival at 10-year follow-up [37]. LVEF decrement portends worse mid and long-term prognosis with a >50% increase in mortality at 10 years when the LVEF <50% [38]. Severe LV dysfunction is considered a high-risk subpopulation and guideline recommendations downgrade surgical repair from class IA for LVEF 60% to class IIB for patients LVEF <30% [22, 38]. Although LV dysfunction and symptoms are the most powerful predictors of decreased postoperative survival, development of pulmonary HTN (>50 mmHg) and AF portend the worst post-repair prognosis and their presence carries a IIa recommendation for surgery if present in 'asymptomatic' patients [22, 30, 39–41].

Repair versus replacement   The presence of the native mitral apparatus assists in maintaining the prolate ellipsoid native geometry of the LV. Without the mitral apparatus, the LV cavity may become globular and less

---

Table 12.9 Advantages of MV repair over replacement

---

1. Better postoperative LV function for repair as MV apparatus is preserved.
2. No need for chronic anticoagulation for repair as opposed to replacement with mechanical prosthetic valve.
3. No risk of prosthesis failure with repair.
4. Risk of infective endocarditis is lower with repair as compared to prosthesis.
5. Operative risk is lower with repair as compared to replacement in patients with similar risk.

---

efficient [42, 43]. In practice, if the valve anatomy is suitable and the surgical skill and expertise available, MV repair is preferred over MV replacement. MV repair as compared to MV replacement has many advantages which are listed below [21, 27–29, 32]. (Table 12.9).

MV repair has its own challenges compared to MV replacement [21, 27–29, 32]. MV repair is technically more demanding. For non-rheumatic disease, the posterior mitral leaflet or degenerative ruptured chordae can usually be repaired with resection of a portion of valve and concomittant annuloplasty. Repair is more complex with anterior or bi-leaflet involvement. In general, rheumatic involvement and calcified leaflets and/or annulus diminish the possibility of repair. Higher surgical volume is correlated with higher rates of success therefore referral to centers experienced in performing MV repair is recommended.

Percutaneous therapy for mitral regurgitation The most common percutaneous therapy used for the treatment of MR consists of performing a procedure that mimics the surgical Alfieri technique of edge–edge repair to produce a double-orifice MV [44] (Figure 12.3). Known as the MitraClip® (Abbott Vascular, Santa Clara, CA), this technique uses clip devices to grasp the scallops of the anterior and posterior mitral leaflets in order to reduce MR. This anatomical defect comprises approximately 20–35% of patients with degenerative MR [45]. However, this technique could be applied to a wide spectrum of degenerative (anterior, posterior, and bileaflet prolapse) and functional regurgitant pathologies. Regardless of regurgitation etiology, the final common pathway of MitraClip implantation is the generation of a double-orifice valve. For wide regurgitant orifices, more than one clip might be needed. Given the complex structure of the subcommissural chordae a higher risk of clip entanglement can be expected. Treatment of para-commissural jets is nonetheless feasible. The benefit of the MitraClip device was evidenced by the EVEREST trial.

A

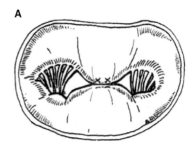

B

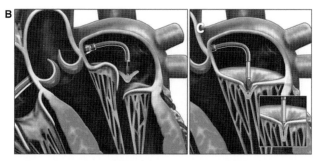

Figure 12.3 Percutaneous mitral clipping of the mitral valve using the MitraClip ®
and associated clip delivery system (CDS) (Abbott Vascular, Santa Clara, CA). (A)
Alfieri surgical technique performed to create a double orifice mitral valve and
reduce regurgitation. (B) Trans-septal access, optimization and orientating a
MitraClip with the middle scallops of the anterior and posterior leaflets, A2 and P2
respectively. (C) Successful grasping of the leaflet edges to complete an
edge-to-edge repair.

 EVIDENCE BASED MEDICINE
The EVEREST trial – MitraClip The clinical trial
EVEREST II prospectively evaluated the MitraClip
technique versus surgical MV repair or replacement in
a 2:1 fashion [46]. With respect to safety, MitraClip therapy was
equivalent to surgery with a 6% overall death rate. Mitraclip did
have a significantly lower rate of safety endpoints (MitraClip 15%
vs. surgery 48% $P < 0.001$) at 30 days primarily due to lower
transfusion requirements. However, surgery was more efficacious at

> reducing MR, as 20% of MitraClip patients ultimately required surgical intervention while 2.2% of patients randomized to surgery needed reoperation. Subsequent studies of the MitraClip in high-risk surgical cohorts found it to be efficacious in treating MR, improving hemodynamic performance, and inducing ventricular remodeling [47–49].

In face of the data accrued from EVEREST high-risk cohorts and European data, the Federal Drug Administration (FDA) approved the MitraClip Clip Delivery System. It is indicated for the percutaneous reduction of significant symptomatic MR (MR $\geq$ 3+) due to primary abnormality of the mitral apparatus (degenerative MR) in patients who have been determined to be at prohibitive risk for MV surgery by a heart team, which includes a cardiac surgeon experienced in MV surgery and a cardiologist experienced in MV disease, and in whom existing co-morbidities would not preclude the expected benefit from reduction of MR [50].

Based on the inclusion criteria of the EVEREST trial, the anatomical indications of the MitraClip device are listed in Table 12.10. The key exclusion criteria included LVEF $\leq$25%, LV end-systolic dimension >55 mm, MV orifice area <4 cm^2, or recent myocardial infarction. These EVEREST-specific clinical and anatomic criteria were used for all North American trial and registry data, but have not been consistently applied in the European experience. The contraindications for the MitraClip Device are listed in Table 12.11.

Additional supportive data can be found in several registries including the German Transcatheter Mitral Valve Interventions (TRAMI) Registry [51].

Other devices   While the MitraClip is commonly used in secondary functional MR outside the US, the data for its efficacy is more limited and led to the initiation of the Cardiovascular Outcomes Assessment of

---

Table 12.10 Anatomical indications of the MitraClip

1. Primary central regurgitant jet associated with the A2/P2 segments.
2. Coaptation length $\geq$2 mm.
3. Coaptation depth $\leq$11 mm.
4. Flail gap <10 mm.
5. Flail width <15 mm.

Table 12.11 Contraindications for the MitraClip device

1. Patients who cannot tolerate procedural anticoagulation or post-procedural antiplatelet regimen.
2. Active endocarditis of the mitral valve.
3. Rheumatic mitral valve disease.
4. Mitral stenosis.
5. Evidence of intracardiac, inferior vena cava (IVC) or femoral venous thrombus.

the MitraClip Percutaneous Therapy for Heart Failure Patients with Functional Mitral Regurgitation (COAPT) and Randomized *Study* of the Mitra-Clip Device in Heart Failure Patients With Clinically Significant Functional Mitral Regurgitation (RESHAP-HF) studies [45].

The remaining technology developed for reduction of MR includes percutaneous mitral annuloplasty through a variety of methods (direct and indirect) and investigational devices to decrease the septal-lateral dimension of the LV and remodeling the ventricle. While the CE mark has been obtained for one device (Carillon Mitral Contour System (Cardiac Dimension, Inc., Kirkland, Washington) percutaneous annuloplasty is more limited due to difficulty with inadvertent occlusion of coronary vessels because of anatomic overlap of the coronary sinus and left circumflex, and due to the less effective reduction of MR demonstrated with this technique [52]. .

Mitral regurgitation and advanced left ventricular dysfunction
Appropriate management and surgical candidacy in patients with symptomatic severe MR with advanced LV dysfunction is uncertain. The main question is whether MR is the primary problem or secondary to LV dysfunction. In primary MR, repair might improve symptoms and prevent further worsening of LVSF. If repair is highly likely, MV surgery is an ACC/AHA class IIa indication. In cases of functional MR, modification of MV geometry using an undersized annuloplasty ring can reduce mitral insufficiency. MV surgery after failure of medical therapy and biventricular pacing to relieve symptoms is a Class IIb indication. Thus far no prospective trial has been completed, comparing MV surgery with aggressive medical management and biventricular pacing in this subset of patients [37–39]. One study comparing MV repair or replacement for functional MR showed no difference between the techniques.

Atrial fibrillation   AF is an independent risk factor for development of HF and cardiac death in patients with MR. In cases with chronic AF and severe MR, the MAZE procedure along with MV repair or replacement is often performed. The MAZE procedure may help to restore sinus rhythm and may therefore decrease the risk of thromboembolism, though this has not been prospectively tested. The duration of AF prior to surgery is important. One study has demonstrated that the chance of persistence of AF after MV surgery is high if duration of AF is longer than 3 months [53–56].

Elderly population   Elderly patients with MR have a higher rate of complications with surgery. In general, the operative mortality is high if age is >75. Recovery is typically longer and concomitant co-morbidities may limit potential functional and survival benefits enjoyed by the younger patient. Thus, asymptomatic patients and those with mild symptoms may fare better with medical management [57–60]. Age alone does not perfectly predict outcomes, but must be considered along with concomitant co-morbidities.

Pregnancy   MR encountered during pregnancy is usually due to MV prolapse or rheumatic heart disease. MR is well-tolerated during pregnancy, due to a fall in systemic vascular resistance in causing afterload reduction. MR with NYHA functional class III–IV is considered high risk for both fetus and mother. Asymptomatic patients don't require any specific therapy. If symptomatic HF develops, treatment with diuretics and digoxin can be helpful. Angiotensin converting enzyme inhibitor (ACEI) or angiotensin receptor blocker (ARB) should not be used for afterload reduction due to teratogenicity; instead nitrates and hydralazine can be used. MV repair and replacement should be avoided during pregnancy because of high risk of fetal loss [61].

Endocarditis prophylaxis   The 2007 AHA guideline and 2008 focused update revised their recommendations on antibiotic prophylaxis for cardiac patients undergoing dental or other invasive procedures. For patients with MR of any cause, in the absence of prosthetic replacement of MV, antibiotic prophylaxis is not recommended.

SECONDARY MITRAL REGURGITATION

Functional or secondary MR, as opposed to degenerative or primary MR, represents disease not of the mitral leaflets, but rather of the ventricle which leads to distortion of the mitral apparatus. This results in malcoaptation of the normal mitral leaflets through papillary muscle displacement and posterior leaflet tethering or annular dilation leading to varying degrees of MR. Both cardiomyopathy and MR contribute to ventricular dilation, changing ventricular geometry from elliptical to spherical deteriorating ventricular function. Changes in the LV postulated to cause and exacerbate MR include LV enlargement, LV sphericity, baseline wall motion abnormalities of LV wall segments surrounding the papillary muscles and annular dilation [53, 62]. A vicious cycle of ventricular maladaptive changes in the LV, increasing MR and vice versa, will ultimately lead to further and progressive LV functional decline.

Thus functional MR is therefore a consequence of ventricular remodeling and associated cardiomyopathy of both ischemic and non-ischemic etiology. Occasionally focal posterolateral wall motion abnormalities can result in posterior leaflet tethering and significant MR despite globally preserved LV function. The majority of functional MR though is associated with chronic systolic HF.

Challenges

Severity of MR is associated with worsening symptoms and prognosis in a graded relationship [63]. Whether the grade of MR is simply a marker of severity of LV dysfunction or actually independently contributes to progressive LV decline and adverse outcome remains unclear, although the two are probably interdependent. Uncorrected degenerative MR clearly leads to progressive LV failure [64, 65]. Therefore it is reasonable to assume that the adverse hemodynamic consequences of functional MR similarly hasten LV decline. Unfortunately the benefits of surgical therapy for functional MR has been more difficult to show compared to the dramatic benefit evidence in symptomatic degenerative disease [66]. Conversely, while medical therapy has a limited role in degenerative disease, medical therapies targeted at the underlying systolic HF can result in dramatic benefit. Thus while degenerative MR is primarily a surgical disease, the primary therapy for functional MR is medical.

Although MR in both ischemic and dilated cardiomyopathy portend grave prognosis, the evidence that correction of MR in either disease state improves survival is mixed. The reason is because although regurgitation may improve, ischemic disease and progressing cardiomyopathy may continue and lessen the durability of a surgical repair [54–56, 67].

Medical therapy

Functional MR is a dynamic process that is dependent on volume and loading status. It is common to see MR grade improve after sedation and blood pressure reduction as well as after diuretic therapy in the setting of acute HF exacerbation. Diuretic therapy improves clinical symptoms but high doses have been associated with increased mortality [68]. Several therapies have been shown to improve HF symptoms, LV remodeling, and prognosis. These include beta-blockers, ACE inhibitors, angiotensin receptor blockers, aldosterone receptor blocker, and hydralazine nitrate combinations in selected patient populations [69–74]. Given the proven benefits of these therapies in chronic systolic HF, regardless of the presence of MR, titration to maximum tolerated dose is the first line therapy. Evidence for MR reduction is variable and therapy specific. Beta-blocker therapy with carvediolol and metoprolol has been shown to improve LV function and reduce MR grade [75, 76]. High-dose ACE inhibitors and angiotensin receptor blockers have similarly been shown to reduce MR grade [77–79]. Evidence for MR reduction following aldosterone blocker and hydralazine nitrate combinations has not been reported. Nonetheless, all of these drugs improve outcomes. There are no reports of the new combination of neprilysin inhibitor sacubitril and the angiotensin receptor blocker valsartan on MR.

There is substantial evidence that LV dys-synchrony is associated with adverse outcome in HF patients and that chronic resynchronization therapy (CRT) improves ventricular remodeling, HF symptoms, and survival [80]. Many patients with dys-synchrony have associated severe MR and CRT has been shown to improve MR grade in up to a third [81]. Improvement in MR grade with CRT has been shown to be associated with improved prognosis compared to non-responders [82]. Cessation of therapy has been associated with recurrence of MR [83]. Therefore following optimal medical therapy, persistent HF symptoms, LV dysfunction, and severe MR should be treated with resynchronization therapy. Guidelines for appropriate use of CRT have been published [84,85]. Since the release and update of these guidelines, the results of the Biventricular Pacing for Atrioventricular Block and Systolic Dysfunction in Heart Failure (BLOCK HF) trial were published showing benefit from CRT in patients with high-grade AV block, LVEF ≤50%, and NYHA class I, II, or II HF [86].

CRITICAL THINKING
Ischemic papillary muscle dysfunction MR from ischemia was once postulated to arise from papillary muscle dysfunction; however newer evidence indicates that MR occurs due to papillary muscle displacement and spherical LV dilation. Tethering of the papillary muscle and leaflets prevents adequate coaptation during systole and progressive annular dilation from maladaptive LV changes further exacerbates MR [84].

In some instances, MV function may improve with revascularization; however, retrospective analysis of the Surgical Treatment for Ischemic Heart Failure (STICH) trial did not show improvement in survival with coronary artery bypass grafting (CABG), but there may be survival improvement if a MV repair accompanies revascularization [59]. Prospective evaluation of CABG versus CABG + MVR has been performed but only to assess surrogate endpoints and was not powered to detect differences in survival [60]. MV surgery may be considered when patients are already undergoing concomitant cardiac surgery; however surgery for the sole purpose of correcting MR alone remains controversial, especially since there may be ongoing remodeling responsible for as high as a failure rate of 32.6% (Table 12.8) [87].

Correction of functional MR in dilated cardiomyopathy has mixed results as well. Although successful correction of MR in non-ischemic cardiomyopathy can result in ventricular remodeling and improvement in LV geometry, a significant amount of late failures have been observed for surgical repairs [56, 61]. A significant predictor of late repair failure includes the angle between the annular plane and a line that joins the anterior annulus and coaptation point (distal leaflet angle). This indicates that tethering of the distal anterior leaflet secondary to LV dilation is the mechanism of failure of mitral annuloplasty for dilated non-ischemic cardiomyopathy [56].

Surgery in functional mitral regurgitation

Until recently there were no randomized controlled trials comparing repair vs. replacement in functional MR. However, in a recent study for patients undergoing mitral-valve repair or replacement for severe ischemic MR, no significant between-group difference was observed in LV reverse remodeling or survival at 2 years. MR recurred more frequently in the repair group, resulting in more HF-related adverse events and cardiovascular admissions [88].

ACUTE MITRAL REGURGITATION

Background

Acute structural defect of the mitral apparatus results in immediate severe incompetence, sudden volume overload of an unprepared left atrium and loss in stroke volume [89]. Any initial presentation of acute pulmonary edema and/or cardiogenic shock should prompt consideration of acute MR. Possible etiologies include choral rupture, trauma, valvular destruction from endocarditis, or papillary muscle rupture secondary to myocardial infarction.

Challenges

Clinical detection of acute MR may be challenging. Tachycardia and tachypnea make auscultation difficult. The sudden equilibration in pressure between the LV and LA may cause the murmur to only appear early in systole and difficult to detect. ECG may only show sinus tachycardia and associated ST-T wave changes in the context of ischemia. Regurgitant volume may be selectively directed into only the left or right pulmonary veins yielding unilateral pulmonary edema on chest X-ray. TTE may show the structural abnormality and Doppler may assist in identifying a dense continuous wave MR signal with a 'V-wave cutoff'. Should visualization in a critically ill patient prevent high quality imaging, TEE should be considered to determine the etiology of valvular regurgitation. Of note, a percutaneous left ventricular assist device (LVAD) is sometimes rapidly deployed in the cardiac catheterization laboratories in the setting of cardiogenic shock and may mask detection of MR by TTE. Flow rate should be turned down during assessment to allow demonstration of MR by TTE. Meticulous quantification of the regurgitant jet should not be the top priority; it should rather be rapid diagnosis and triage for immediate correction of the valvular lesion in the face of possible respiratory or hemodynamic instability.

Strategic mapping

Priorities in treating patients with acute MR should revolve around relieving pulmonary edema, stabilizing hemodynamics, and triage to surgical repair. Diuretics are recommended for decreasing pulmonary congestion and intravenous sodium nitroprusside, should be considered for increasing forward flow and reducing filling pressures [90]. In the case of severe hemodynamic compromise, intra-aortic balloon counter-pulsation (IABP) should be initiated and reports of using a percutaneous LVAD to support a patient with acute ischemic MR have been reported [91, 92]. Should endocarditis be suspected, antibiotic administration should be considered immediately. Preoperative coronary angiography without left ventriculography should be considered if the patient is stable enough; however it should not delay surgery if hemodynamically unstable [22]. Finally, the ultimate goal remains expeditious MV repair or replacement. With rapid triage, the survival in the majority of patients with papillary muscle rupture depends on treatment of severe MR post-myocardial infarction [93].

The distinction between organic and functional causes is important. Organic causes frequently require surgical repair or valve replacement; conversely, functional causes may improve after the non-surgical treatment of underlying myocardial ischemia, infarction, or cardiomyopathy.

CLINICAL PEARLS
When to suspect acute mitral regurgitation
Clinicians typically encounter chronic, rather than acute, functional MR. However, processes that result in a rapid decline in ventricular function can present with acute functional MR as a manifestation of acute HF, such as in Takotsubo cardiomyopathy (left apical ballooning) and peripartum cardiomyopathy. In Takotsubo cardiomyopathy, functional MR can result from systolic anterior motion of the MV and obstruction of the LV outflow tract due to apical ballooning, with preserved basal ventricular function. The rapid onset of peripartum cardiomyopathy can include acute, severe MR. Leaflet inflammation and myocardial dysfunction from rheumatic carditis can cause acute MR, and some data suggest that the degree of valvular dysfunction influences outcomes [6]. Acute rheumatic carditis is more prevalent in developing countries than in industrialized nations.

Hemodynamically, the regurgitant volume in a normal-sized, non-compliant LA results in a marked increase in LA pressure – the mechanism by which acute pulmonary edema develops. In comparison, LA size and compliance are increased in chronic MR, but LA pressures remain normal despite the regurgitant volume. These findings parallel the changes in the LV in aortic regurgitation. Coexisting conditions may affect a patient's tolerance of acutely increased left atrial and LV volume. A patient with a history of chronic MR and preserved ventricular function might tolerate the marked increase in volume better than would a patient with impaired ventricular function. The LV of the latter would quickly decompensate upon acute worsening of MR causing acute volume overload into unprepared LA and LV and increasing their filling pressures. Increased filling pressures in LA with resultant increased pulmonary venous pressure can lead to pulmonary edema. Although, there is increased preload available to LV, in the absence of compensatory LV hypertrophy there is no increased forward flow.

CLINICAL PEARLS
Main symptoms and signs to be searched
Patients with acute MR are almost always symptomatic. Symptoms are due to pulmonary edema (dyspnea, respiratory distress) or due to poor cardiac output (altered mental status, weakness, fatigue).

Hypotension or even shock is usually present. Cardiac physical exam can be misleading. Physical signs present in chronic MR are usually absent. Apical impulse may not be displaced. There may be lack of holosystolic murmur. Signs of volume overload such as third heart sound or early diastolic flow rumble may be the only sign present. Auscultation of lungs will reveal rales if pulmonary edema is present.

Smart testing

All patients in whom acute valvular regurgitation is suspected should undergo electrocardiography and chest radiography. Electrocardiograms typically reveal sinus tachycardia with non-specific ST- and T-wave abnormalities. Ischemic ST changes can indicate regurgitation mediated by ischemia – CAD, or aortic dissection that affects the coronary ostia. Hemodynamic disturbances, such as very high LV end diastolic pressure (LVEDP), can exacerbate coronary insufficiency. Chest XR typically shows pulmonary edema and a left heart of normal size.

Transthoracic echocardiogram is the imaging modality utilized to detect presence of ruptured papillary muscle and diagnose MR. The estimation of EROA and regurgitant volume can be inaccurate in acute regurgitation (particularly in the presence of tachycardia) and depends upon dynamic loading conditions. In the presence of hyperdynamic LV with clinically suspected shock, acute MR should be suspected. The use of color-flow Doppler echocardiography can lead to an underestimation of the severity of regurgitation, particularly if the regurgitant jet is eccentric. If a transthoracic study is not conclusive, TEE can reveal the mechanism and severity of the regurgitation. In prosthetic valve dysfunction, TEE can also show artifacts. Interpreting the results of TEE is often crucial to the planning of operative repair, such as the identification of leaflet or annular involvement.

Left-heart catheterization is not routinely indicated in the preoperative evaluation of patients with acute MR. Catheterization can be considered when electrocardiographic changes suggest acute ischemia. Patients with acute MR from ischemia or papillary muscle rupture may benefit from revascularization along with MV repair or replacement. Conversely, patients whose mechanisms of regurgitation are non-ischemic (such as mitral regurgitation due to chordal rupture or aortic regurgitation) may poorly tolerate the contrast medium and the time needed for catheterization.

Management

Medical therapy   Medical therapy helps to stabilize hemodynamics before surgical correction. Nitroprusside has been shown to increase aortic flow by decreasing aortic impedance and, decrease MR by decreasing LV impedance, size and improving MV anatomy [31]. Hypotensive patients are treated with inotropic agents such as dobutamine and vasodilators such as nitroprusside. Inotropes likes dobutamine also have been found to be effective in reducing MR by increasing MV closing force. Similarly, nitrates and diuretics also help by decreasing LA pressure and thus increasing transmittal pressure with better MV closure.

Acute MR in the presence of acute cardiomyopathy or decompensated HF can respond to aggressive HF therapy. The use of IABP is effective in patients with acute functional MR of any cause, and IABPs are particularly useful in patients with underlying myocardial ischemia or cardiomyopathy. Although the role of LVAD has not been well studied in acute MR, these devices may be used in cases of decompensated HF that does not respond to medical therapy.

Decisions in regard to the treatment of acute MR are strongly influenced by the cause of the regurgitation. MV repair is almost always preferable to replacement. Therapeutic options, technical feasibility, and surgical priorities depend upon cause, acute pathophysiology, underlying pathology, and co-morbidities. If the initial repair is unsatisfactory, further cardiopulmonary bypass (CPB) and either repeat repair or valve replacement is necessary. Repair should therefore be undertaken when procedural success is likely, as a hemodynamically unstable patient may not be able to tolerate additional CPB time. Influential factors include papillary muscle rupture; chordal rupture; annular dilation; hibernating, stunned, or infarcted myocardium; and the severity of coronary artery disease. Repair techniques include ring annuloplasty, annular reconstruction with pericardium, leaflet resection, leaflet reconstruction with pericardium, chordal replacement, vegetation excision, and edge-to-edge (Alfieri) approximation. Valve repair is more useful when acute annular dilation is the cause, such as in ischemia, or when the pathology involves the posterior leaflet only, such as in myxomatous valve disease or endocarditis with or without annular dilation. In annular involvement with infection or in anterior leaflet involvement with degenerative disease, the ability to repair the MV dramatically decreases [94].

ACTION POINTS

1 Need to evaluate and stage the patient with MR for etiology and severity.

2 There is no medical treatment to delay the natural history of the disease process for patient with primary MR. Correction of conditions which dilate the left ventricle may delay the appearance or progression of secondary MR.

3 Need to look at the parameters such as LV size, volume, ejection fraction (EF) which serve as surrogates for judging appropriateness of surgical referral. Even so, LV dysfunction may still be observed despite timely referral to surgery indicating that the surrogates do not perfectly predict transition from compensated to decompensated phase of the LV.

4 Refer the appropriate patients for early surgery or percutaneous MR correction. The reason is because the myocardial damage often precedes the onset of symptoms.

REFERENCES

1. Enriquez-Sarano M, Tajik AJ, Schaff HV, et al. Echocardiographic Prediction of Left Ventricular Function After Correction of MR: Results and Clinical Implications. *J Am Coll Cardiol.* 1994;24:1534–1543.

2. Nishimura RA, Schaff HV. MR: Timing of surgery. In: Otto CM, Bonow RO, eds. *Valvular Heart Disease: A Companion to Braunwald's Heart Disease*, 3rd edn. Philadelphia: Elsevier, 2009:274–290.

3. Enriquez-Sarano M, Tajik AJ, Bailey KR, Seward JB. Color flow imaging compared with quantitative Doppler assessment of severity of MR: Influence of eccentricity and mechanism of regurgitation. *J Am Coll Cardiol.* 1993;21:1211–1219.

4. Baumgartner H, Schima H, Kuhn P. Value and limitations of proximal jett dimensions for the quantification of valvular regurgitation: an in vitro study using Doppler flow imaging. *J Am Soc Echocardiogr.*: official publication of the American Society of Echocardiography 1991;4:57–66.

5. Zoghbi W. Recommendations for evaluation of the severity of native valvular regurgitation with two-dimensional and doppler echocardiography. *J Am Soc Echocardiogr.* 2003;16:777–802.

6. Grayburn PA, Weissman NJ, Zamorano JL. Quantitation of MR. *Circulation.* 2012;126:2005–2017.

7. Enriquez-Sarano M, Avierinos JF, Messika-Zeitoun D, et al. Quantitative Determinants of the Outcome of Asymptomatic MR. *New Engl J Med.* 2005;352:875–883.

8. Enriquez-Sarano M, Seward JB, Bailey KR, Tajik AJ. Effective regurgitant orifice area: A noninvasive Doppler development of an old hemodynamic concept. *J Am Coll Cardiol.* 1994;23:443–451.

9. Topilsky Y, Michelena H, Bichara V, Maalouf J, Mahoney DW, Enriquez-Sarano M. Mitral valve prolapse with mid-late systolic MR: pitfalls of evaluation and clinical outcome compared with holosystolic regurgitation. *Circulation.* 2012;125:1643–1651.

10. Roberts BJ, Grayburn PA. Color flow imaging of the vena contracta in MR: technical considerations. *J Am Soc Echocardiogr.* 2003;16:1002–1006.

11. Buck T, Plicht B, Kahlert P, Schenk IM, Hunold P, Erbel R. Effect of dynamic flow rate and orifice area on mitral regurgitant stroke volume quantification using the proximal isovelocity surface area method. *J Am Coll Cardiol.* 2008;52:767–778.

12. Kizilbash AM, Willett DL, Brickner E, Heinle SK, Grayburn P. Effects of afterload reduction on vena contracta width in MR. *J Am Coll Cardiol.* 1998;32:427–431.

13. Ciarka A, Van de Veire N. Secondary MR: pathophysiology, diagnosis, and treatment. *Heart.* 2011;97:1012–1023.

14. Heinle SK, Hall SA, Brickner E, Willett DL, Grayburn P. Comparison of vena contracta width multiplane transesophageal echocardiography with quantitative Doppler assessment of MR. *Am J Cardiol.* 1998;81:175–179.

15. Ben Zekry S, Nagueh SF, Little SH, et al. Comparative accuracy of two- and three-dimensional transthoracic and transesophageal echocardiography in identifying mitral valve pathology in patients undergoing mitral valve repair: initial observations. *J Am Soc Echocardiogr*: official publication of the American Society of Echocardiography 2011;24:1079–1085.

16. Iwakura K, Ito H, Kawano S, et al. Comparison of orifice area by transthoracic three-dimensional Doppler echocardiography versus proximal isovelocity surface area (PISA) method for assessment of MR. *Am J Cardiol.* 2006;97:1630–1637.

17. Kahlert P, Plicht B, Schenk IM, Janosi RA, Erbel R, Buck T. Direct assessment of size and shape of noncircular vena contracta area in functional versus organic MR using real-time three-dimensional echocardiography. *J Am Soc Echocardiogr.*: official publication of the American Society of Echocardiography 2008;21:912–921.

18. Lang RM, Tsang W, Weinert L, Mor-Avi V, Chandra S. Valvular heart disease. The value of 3-dimensional echocardiography. *J Am Coll Cardiol.* 2011;58:1933–1944.

19. Dorosz JL, Lezotte DC, Weitzenkamp DA, Allen LA, Salcedo EE. Performance of 3-dimensional echocardiography in measuring left ventricular volumes and ejection fraction: a systematic review and meta-analysis. *J Am Coll Cardiol.* 2012;59:1799–1808.

20. Altiok E, Hamada S, van Hall S, et al. Comparison of direct planimetry of mitral valve regurgitation orifice area by three-dimensional transesophageal echocardiography to effective regurgitant orifice area obtained by proximal flow convergence method and vena contracta area determined by color Doppler echocardiography. *Am J Cardiol.* 2011;107:452–458.

21. Matsumura Y, Fukuda S, Tran H, et al. Geometry of the proximal isovelocity surface area in MR by 3-dimensional color Doppler echocardiography: difference between functional MR and prolapse regurgitation. *Am Heart J.* 2008;155:231–238.

22. Nishimura RA, Otto CM, Bonow RO, et al. 2014 AHA/ACC Guideline for the Management of Patients with Valvular Heart Disease: A Report of the American College of Cardiology/American *Heart.* Association Task Force on Practice Guidelines. *Circulation.* 2014;129.

23. Magne J, Lancellotti P, Pierard LA. Exercise-induced changes in degenerative MR. *J Am Coll Cardiol.* 2010;56:300–309.

24. Lancellotti P, Troisfontaines P, Toussaint AC, Pierard LA. Prognostic importance of exercise-induced changes in MR in patients with chronic ischemic left ventricular dysfunction. *Circulation.* 2003;108:1713–1717.

25. Magne J, Mahjoub H, Dulgheru R, Pibarot P, Pierard LA, Lancellotti P. Left ventricular contractile reserve in asymptomatic primary MR. *Eur Heart J.* 2014;35:1608–1616.

26. Magne J, Lancellotti P, Pierard LA. Exercise pulmonary hypertension in asymptomatic degenerative MR. *Circulation.* 2010;122:33–41.

27. Kizilbash AM, Hundley WG, Willett DL, Franco F, Peshock RM, Grayburn P. Comparison of quantitative Doppler with magnetic resonance imaging for assessment of the severity of MR. *Am J Cardiol.* 1998;81:792–794.

28. Thavendiranathan P, Liu S, Datta S, et al. Automated quantification of mitral inflow and aortic outflow stroke volumes by three-dimensional real-time volume color-flow Doppler transthoracic echocardiography: comparison with pulsed-wave Doppler and cardiac magnetic resonance imaging. *J Am Soc Echocardiogr.*: official publication of the American Society of Echocardiography 2012;25:56–65.

29. Shanks M, Siebelink HM, Delgado V, et al. Quantitative assessment of MR: comparison between three-dimensional transesophageal echocardiography and magnetic resonance imaging. *Circ Cardiovasc Imag.* 2010;3:694–700.

30. Ghoreishi M, Evans CF, DeFilippi CR, et al. Pulmonary hypertension adversely affects short- and long-term survival after mitral valve operation for MR:

implications for timing of surgery. *J Thoracic Cardiovasc Surg.* 2011;142:1439–1452.

31. Nishimura RA, Carabello BA. Hemodynamics in the cardiac catheterization laboratory of the 21st century. *Circulation.* 2012;125:2138–2150.

32. Nemoto S, Hamawaki M, De Freitas G, Carabello BA. Differential effects of the angiotensin-converting enzyme inhibitor lisinopril versus the beta-adrenergic receptor blocker atenolol on hemodynamics and left ventricular contractile function in experimental MR. *J Am Coll Cardiol.* 2002;40:149–154.

33. Harris KM, Aeppli DM, Carey CF. Effects of angiotensin-converting enzyme inhibition on MR severity, left ventricular size, and functional capacity. *Am Heart J.*2005;150:1106.

34. Rozich JD, Carabello BA, Usher BW, Kratz JM, Bell AE, Zile MR. Mitral valve replacement with and without chordal preservation in patients with chronic MR. Mechanisms for differences in postoperative ejection performance. *Circulation.* 1992;86:1718–1726.

35. Braunberger E, Deloche A, Berrebi A, et al. Very long-term results (more than 20 years) of valve repair with Carpentier's techniques in nonrheumatic mitral valve insufficiency. *Circulation.* 2001;104:I–8–I–11.

36. Gillinov AM, Blackstone EH, Nowicki ER, et al. Valve repair versus valve replacement for degenerative mitral valve disease. *J Thoracic Cardiovasc Surg.* 2008;135:885–93, 893 e1–2.

37. Tribouilloy CM, Enriquez-Sarano M, Schaff HV, et al. Impact of preoperative symptoms on survival after surgical correction of organic MR: Rationale for optimizing surgical indications. *Circulation.* 1999;99:400–405.

38. Enriquez-Sarano M, Tajik AJ, Schaff HV, Orszulak TA, Bailey KR, Frye RL. Echocardiographic prediction of survival after surgical correction of organic MR. *Circulation.* 1994;90:830–837.

39. Gillinov AM, Mihaljevic T, Blackstone EH, et al. Should patients with severe degenerative MR delay surgery until symptoms develop? *Ann Thorac Surg.* 2010;90:481–488.

40. Kang DH, Kim JH, Rim JH, et al. Comparison of early surgery versus conventional treatment in asymptomatic severe MR. *Circulation.* 2009;119:797–804.

41. Rosenhek R, Rader F, Klaar U, et al. Outcome of watchful waiting in asymptomatic severe MR. *Circulation.* 2006;113:2238–2244.

42. Sarris GE, Miller DC. Valvular–ventricular interaction: the importance of the mitral chordae tendinae in terms of global left ventricular systolic function. *J Card Surg.* 1988;3:215–234.

43. Hansen DE, Sarris GE, Niczyporuk MA, Derby GC, Cahill PD, Miller DC. Physiologic role of the mitral apparatus in left ventricular regional mechanics, contraction synergy, and global performance. *J Thoracic Cardiovasc Surg.* 1989;97:521–533.

44. Alfieri O, Maisano F, De Bonis M, et al. The double-orifice technique in mitral valve repair: a simple solution for complex problems. *J Thoracic Cardiovasc Surg.* 2001;122:674–681.

45. Feldman T, Young A. Percutaneous approaches to valve repair for MR. *J Am Coll Cardiol.* 2014;63:2057–2068.

46. Feldman T, Foster E, Glower D, et al. Percutaneous repair or surgery for MR. *New Engl J Med.* 2011;364:1395–1406.

47. Silbiger JJ. A novel mechanism by which MitraClip implantation may favorably alter the natural history of left ventricular remodeling in patients with MR: proposed role of the ventricular–valvular loop. *J Am Soc Echocardiogr.*: official publication of the American Society of Echocardiography 2013;26:217–219.

48. Lim DS, Reynolds MR, Feldman T, et al. Improved functional status and quality of life in prohibitive surgical risk patients with degenerative MR after transcatheter mitral valve repair. *J Am Coll Cardiol.* 2014;64:182–192.

49. Glower DD, Kar S, Trento A, et al. Percutaneous mitral valve repair for MR in high–risk patients: results of the EVEREST II study. *J Am Coll Cardiol.* 2014;64:172–181.

50. Nishimura RA, Otto CM, Bonow RO, et al. 2014 AHA/ACC Guideline for the Management of Patients with Valvular Heart. Disease: Executive Summary: A Report of the American College of Cardiology/American Heart Association Task Force on Practice Guidelines. *J Am Coll Cardiol.* 2014;63(22):2438–2488.

51. Wiebe J, Franke J, Lubos E, et al. for the German Transcatheter Mitral Valve Interventions (TRAMI) Investigators Percutaneous MV repair with the mitraclip system according to the predicted risk by the logistic EuroSCORE: Preliminary results from the German Transcatheter MV Interventions (TRAMI) registry. *Cathet Cardiovasc Intervent.* 84:591–8. doi: 10.1002/ccd.25493.

52. Siminiak T, Wu JC, Haude M, et al. Treatment of functional MR by percutaneous annuloplasty: results of the TITAN Trial. *Eur J HF.* 2012;14:931–938.

53. Hung J, Papakostas L, Tahta SA, et al. Mechanism of recurrent ischemic MR after annuloplasty: continued LV remodeling as a moving target. *Circulation.* 2004;110:II85–90.

54. Grigioni F, Enriquez-Sarano M, Zehr KJ, Bailey KR, Tajik AJ. Ischemic MR: Long-term outcome and prognostic implications with quantitative Doppler assessment. *Circulation.* 2001;103:1759–1764.

55. Enomoto Y, Gorman JH, 3rd, Moainie SL, et al. Surgical treatment of ischemic MR might not influence ventricular remodeling. *J Thoracic Cardiovasc Surg.* 2005;129:504–511.

56. Lee AP, Acker M, Kubo SH, et al. Mechanisms of recurrent functional MR after mitral valve repair in nonischemic dilated cardiomyopathy: importance of distal anterior leaflet tethering. *Circulation.* 2009;119:2606–2614.

57. Hunt SA, Abraham WT, Chin MH, et al. ACC/AHA 2005 Guideline Update for the Diagnosis and Management of Chronic HF in the Adult: a report of the American College of Cardiology/American Heart Association Task Force on Practice Guidelines (Writing Committee to Update the 2001 Guidelines for the Evaluation and Management of HF): developed in collaboration with the American College of Chest Physicians and the International Society for Heart and Lung Transplantation: endorsed by the Heart Rhythm Society. *Circulation.* 2005;112:e154–235.

58. van Bommel RJ, Marsan NA, Delgado V, et al. Cardiac resynchronization therapy as a therapeutic option in patients with moderate–severe functional MR and high operative risk. *Circulation.* 2011;124:912–919.

59. Deja MA, Grayburn PA, Sun B, et al. Influence of MR repair on survival in the surgical treatment for ischemic HF trial. *Circulation.* 2012;125:2639–2648.

60. Chan KM, Punjabi PP, Flather M, et al. Coronary artery bypass surgery with or without mitral valve annuloplasty in moderate functional ischemic MR: final results of the Randomized Ischemic Mitral Evaluation (RIME) trial. *Circulation.* 2012;126:2502–2510.

61. Bolling S, Deeb GM, Brunsting LA, Bach DS. Early outcome of mitral valve reconstruction in patients with end-stage cardiomyopathy. *J Thoracic Cardiovasc Surg.* 1995;109:676–683.

62. Kwan J. Geometric Differences of the mitral apparatus between ischemic and dilated cardiomyopathy with significant MR: Real-time three-dimensional echocardiography study. *Circulation.* 2003;107:1135–1140.

63. Trichon BH, Felker GM, Shaw LK, et al. Relation of frequency and severity of mitral regurgitation to survival among patients with left ventricular systolic dysfunction and heart failure. *Am J Cardiol.* 2003;91:538–543.

64. Tribouilloy CM, Enriquez-Sarano M, Schaff HV, et al. Impact of preoperative symptoms on survival after surgical correction of organic mitral regurgitation: rationale for optimizing surgical indications. *Circulation.* 1999;99:400–405.

65. Magne J, Mahjoub H, Pierard LA, et al. Prognostic importance of brain naturetic peptide and left ventricular longitudinal function in asymptomatic degenerative mitral regurgitation. *Heart.* 2012;98:584–591.

66. Wu AH, Aaronson KD, Bolling SF, et al. Impact of mitral valve annuloplasty on mortality risk in patients with mitral regurgitation and left ventricular systolic dysfunction. *J Am Coll Cardiol.* 2005; 129:860–868.

67. Dujardin KS, Enriquez-Sarano M, Bailey KR, Seward JB, Tajik AJ. Effect of Losartan on Degree of MR Quantified by Echocardiography. *Am J Cardiol.* 2001;87:570–576.

68. Neuberg GW, Miller AB, O'Connor CM, et al. Diuretic resistance predicts mortality in patients with advanced heart failure. *Am Heart J.* 2002;144:31–38.

69. Effect of enalapril on mortality and the development of heart failure in asymptomatic patients with reduced left ventricular ejection fractions. The SOLVD Investigators. *N Engl J Med.* 1992;327:685–691.

70. Granger CB, McMurray JJ, Yusuf S, et al. Effects of candesartan in patients with chronic heart failure and reduced left-ventricular systolic function intolerant to angiotensin-converting-enzyme inhibitors: the CHARM–Alternative trial. *Lancet.* 2003;362:772–776.

71. Eriksson SV, Eneroth P, Kjekshus J, et al. Neuroendocrine activation in relation to left ventricular function in chronic severe congestive heart failure: a subgroup analysis from the Cooperative North Scandinavian Enalapril Survival Study (CONSENSUS). *Clin Cardiol.* 1994;17:603–606.

72. Pitt B, Zannad F, Remme WJ, et al. The effect of spironolactone on morbidity and mortality in patients with severe heart failure. Randomized aldactone evaluation study investigators. *N Engl J Med.* 1999;341:709–717.

73. Krum H, Roecker EB, Mohacsi P, et al. Effects of initiating carvedilol in patients with severe chronic heart failure: results from the COPERNICUS Study. *JAMA*. 2003;289:712–718.

74. Cohn JN, Johnson G, Ziesche S, et al. A comparison or enalapril with hydralazine-isosorbide dinitrate in treatment of chronic congestive heart failure. *N Engl J Med*. 1991;325:303–310.

75. Lowes BD, Gill EA, Abraham WT, et al. Effects of carvedilol on left ventricular mass, chamber geometry, and mitral regurgitation in chronic heart failure. *Am J Cardiol*. 1999;83(8):1201.

76. Capomolla S, Febo O, Gnemmi M, et al. Beta-blockade therapy in chronic heart failure: diastolic function and mitral regurgitation improved by carvedilol. *Am Heart J*. 2000;139(4):596.

77. Keren G, Pardes A, Eschar Y, et al. One year clinical and echocardiographic follow up of patients with congestive cardiomyopathy treated with captopril compared to placebo. *Isr J Med Sci*. 1994;30(1):90.

78. Seneviratne B, Moore GA, West PD. Effect of captopril on functional mitral regurgitation in dilated heart failure: a randomized double blind placebo controlled trail. *Br Heart J*. 1994;72(1):63.

79. Dujardin KS, Enriquez-Sarano M, Bailey KR, et al. Effect of Lorsartan on degree of mitral regurgitation quantified by echocardiography. *Am J Cardiol*. 2001;87(5):570–576.

80. St. John Sutton MG, Plappert T, Abraham WT, et al. Multicenter In Synch Randomized Clinical Evaluation (MIRACLE) Study Group. Effect of cardiac resynchronization therapy on left ventricular size and function in chronic heart failure. *Circulation*. 2003;107:1985–1990.

81. Van Bommel RJ, Marsan NA, Delgado V, et al. Cardiac resynchronization therapy as a therapeutic option in patients with moderate–severe functional mitral regurgitation and high operative risk. *Circulation*. 2011;124(8):912.

82. Di Biase L, Auricchio A, Mohanty P, et al. Impact of cardiac resynchronization therapy on the severity of mitral regurgitation. *Europace*. 2011;13(6):829–838.

83. Brandt RR, Reiner C, Arnold R, et al. Contractile response and mitral regurgitation after temporary interruption of long term cardiac resynchronization therapy. *Eur Heart J*. 2006;27(2):187.

84. Tracy CM, Epstein AE, Darbar D, et al. 2012 ACCF/AHA/HRS focused update of the 2008 guidelines for device-based therapy of cardiac rhythm abnormalities: a report of the American College of Cardiology Foundation/American Heart Association Task Force on Practice Guidelines and the Heart Rhythm Society. *Circulation*. 2012;126(14):1784.

85. Yancy CW, Jessup M, Bozkurt B, et al. 2013 ACCF/AHA guideline for the management of heart failure: a report of the American College of Cardiology Foundation/American *Heart*. Association Task Force on practice guidelines. *Circulation*. 2013;128(16):e240.

86. Curtis AB, Worley SJ, Adamson PB, et al. Biventricular pacing for atrioventricular block and systolic dysfunction. *N Engl J Med*. 2013 Apr;368(17):1585–1593.

87. Acker MA, Parides MK, Perrault LP, et al. Mitral-valve repair versus replacement for severe ischemic MR. *New Engl J Med*. 2014;370:23–32.

88. D Goldstein, Moskowitz AJ, Gelijns AC, Ailawadi G. Two-year outcomes of surgical treatment of severe ischemic mitral regurgitation. *N Engl J Med.* 2015 Nov 09;[EPub Ahead of Print].

89. Yoran C, Yellin EL, Becker RM, Gabbay S, Frater RW, Sonnenblick EH. Dynamic aspects of acute MR: effects of ventricular volume, pressure and contractility on the effective regurgitant orifice area. *Circulation.* 1979;60:170–176.

90. Yoran C, Yellin EL, Becker M, Gabbay S, Frater RW, Sonnenblick EH. Mechanism of reduction of MR with vasodilator therapy. *Am J Cardiol.* 1979;43:773–777.

91. Harmon L, Boccalandro F. Cardiogenic shock secondary to severe acute ischemic MR managed with an Impella 2.5 percutaneous left ventricular assist device. *Catheterizat Cardiovasc Intervent:* official journal of the Society for Cardiac Angiography & Interventions. 2012;79:1129–1134.

92. Nishimura RA, Schaff HV, Shub C, Gersh BJ, Edwards WD, Tajik AJ. Papillary muscle rupture complicating acute myocardial infarction: Analysis of 17 patients. *Am J Cardiol.* 1983;51:373–377.

93. Nishimura RA, Schaff HV, Gersh BJ, Holmes DR, Tajik AJ. Early Repair of Mechanical Complications After Acute Myocardial Infarction. *JAMA: J Am Med Ass.* 1986;256:47–50.

94. Mokadam NA, Stout KK, Verrier ED. Management of acute regurgitation in left-sided cardiac valves. *Tex Heart Inst J.* 2011; 38(1): 9–19.

95. Thavendiranathan P, Phelan D, Collier P, Thomas JD, Flamm SD, Marwick TH. Quantitative assessment of mitral regurgitation: How best to do it. *J Am Coll Cardiol Img.* 2012;5:1161–1175 (figure 8).

CHAPTER 13

Cardiovascular Problems in Elderly Patients

Daniel E. Forman and Nanette K. Wenger

Management of Complex Cardiovascular Problems, Fourth Edition. Edited by
Thach N. Nguyen, Dayi Hu, Shao Liang Chen, Moo Hyun Kim and Cindy L. Grines.
© 2016 John Wiley & Sons, Ltd. Published 2016 by John Wiley & Sons, Ltd.

BACKGROUND

Longevity is increasing throughout the world, driven by widespread advances in infection control, nutrition, and medical management [1]. Ironically, these prevailing patterns of prolonged survival correlate with increased susceptibility to age-related cardiovascular disease (CVD). Coronary heart disease (CHD), heart failure (HF), valvular heart disease, peripheral arterial disease (PAD), arrhythmia and most cardiovascular (CV) pathophysiologic processes become endemic among older populations as a function of aging physiology, especially in relation to CV risk factors over a lifetime [2]. In most medical practices and hospitals the dominant patient demographic is the older adult. This pattern is expected to escalate as the vulnerable senior population continues to expand.

CHALLENGES

The **first challenge** is that health care providers for older CV patients must now address aging itself as a relevant parameter of CV management. In the past, CV providers had to expand their skill-sets regarding thrombogenesis and metabolism once their impact on CVD became apparent. Now the CV providers have to expand their skill-sets regarding geriatrics principles since they too fundamentally impact CVD and CV therapeutic outcomes (Table 13.1). In fact, all CV diagnosis, risk stratification, treatment, and even the metrics of quality care are affected by the pathological changes of advancing age.

The **second challenge** is that the occurrence of multiple cardiac and non-cardiac diseases in combination is a common feature in older adults with CVD [3]. Multiple cardiac pathologies can occur simultaneously (e.g. CAD, HF, atrial fibrillation [AF], PAD, and valvular disease), in simple or complex combination [4]. Then, CVD tends to occur at the same time with multiple non-CV pathophysiologies (e.g., renal insufficiency,

---

Table 13.1 New skill-sets required for care of older patients

1. Assess patient preferences.
2. Circumvent hazards of hospitalization.
3. Facilitate successful transitions from one care setting to the other.
4. Engage in useful risk-benefit discussions.
5. Provide care collaboratively within a care team responsive to the needs of the oldest patients.

diabetes mellitus, chronic obstructive pulmonary disease, and arthritis). Such multisystem disease combinations are more liable to overwhelm the diminished CV reserve capacity of aging, leading to adverse outcomes. So a new pivotal area of research regarding management of older CV patients is better understanding and assessment of non-CV parameters that affect CV management and outcomes. Therefore, the challenges for the CV providers are to separate the CV versus non-CV symptoms and signs, to differentiate the CV findings contaminated by non-CV pathologies.

The **third challenge** is that current CV guidelines are almost entirely based on data from predominantly younger adults and subsets of elderly patients free of most comorbidities [5]. While most current guidelines mention aging as distinct subsections, they only suggest that caregiving choices for elderly persons must be tailored to each patient's preferences and/or aggregate medical circumstances [6]. However, it is not reasonable to extrapolate from guidelines oriented to younger populations to older persons and to merely intuit strategies to determine patient-centered management choices. So an important contemporary challenge is to clarify which aspects of aging itself become the primary determinants of outcomes for older adults with valvular heart disease, CHD, HF, PAD and other types of CVD.

The **last challenge** is that while it is assumed that providers and patients can discern care that provides personalized value and efficacy, it often remains ambiguous how best to achieve this laudable goal. In reality, there are no standardized methods to guide this process reliably and efficiently. Specifically, there are no criteria by which to manage older CV patients which address the predictably confounding issues of multimorbidity, polypharmacy, frailty, falls, cognitive limits, chronic pain, and other intricacies of age that often overwhelm CV management and outcomes.

STRATEGIC MAPPING

Prioritize the goals of treatment

The average length of life is almost 80 years in the US and even longer in many other countries. Therefore, prolonging longevity remains an important clinical goal, even for someone who is very old. However, for many older adults, quality of life (QOL) is often as or more important than longevity and QOL consists of independence, self-efficacy, mobility and cognition, appetite, and contentment. Given these concerns, benefits of procedures, devices, medications, or other therapies may often seem less appealing than one might infer from their purported survival benefits. As many patients prioritize QOL, function, independence, and other clinical goals over longevity benefits, therapeutic strategies must shift and clinical trials relevant to older patients must address these outcome variables.

Holistic approach

In contrast to CVD in younger populations, management of CVD in older adults demands a relatively more holistic approach. Each medication, procedure, and transition of care must be regarded as a source of potential benefit as well as of potential instability. For older adults who are frail and/or have more complex health issues, their non-CV limitations may completely overshadow any perceived utility of CV therapy [7, 8].

Tiered management

As frailty emerges as one of the best predictors of outcome, a tiered medical approach based on frailty may help guide care more successfully for older adults. Frail adults may benefit from the same therapy as those who are not frail, but may require greater emphasis on pre-procedural rehabilitation, nutrition, and other supplemental treatments.

HIGH-RISK MARKERS

The assessment of older CV patients is an evolving science, especially in the quantification and integration of age-related parameters that affect CV diagnosis and management. Risk assessment is a related dimension of assessment that is particularly important in assessing eligibility of older adults for CV procedures. The goal is not to restrict treatment, but to better select those patients for therapy who are most likely to benefit. Assessments once seen as 'soft' or subjective (e.g., fatigue, weakness, gait speed) are now increasingly acknowledged as providing important prognostic information. Such innovative assessments have been reinforced by tools to increase their reliability and objectivity, which are important refinements to refute those who still see them as unreliable or inconsequential. Cognition (delirium risk), social support, and mood (depression) must be considered in assessing risk.

HIGH-RISK PREDICTORS

Frailty, multi-morbidities, polypharmacy and unstable social support are predictors of recurrent health problems, relapse and readmissions. They expand the concept of risk beyond traditional cardiovascular risk predictors (e.g., tobacco, diabetes).

INVESTIGATIONS

Symptoms to look for

In older patients, the symptoms can be subtle or even misleading because of the presence of multi-morbidity [9]. The classic manifestations of coronary heart disease (CAD), HF, and other CVD processes are less likely to be manifested in older adults. The so-called 'atypical symptoms' result from the overlap of multiple cardiac and non-cardiac morbidities, as well as the effects of age-related physiology. These often lead to notorious delays in initiating appropriate therapy. Even the prototypical CV symptoms such as chest pain or shortness of breath can be subtle as many older adults experience them as confusion, agitation, or malaise. Other older adults may complain of dyspnea instead of chest pain, so dyspnea becomes an extremely common presenting symptom for acute coronary syndromes (ACS) or chronic CHD.

Signs to look for

Clinical examinations may be less reliable amid age-related valvular changes (increased aortic sclerosis), pulmonary changes (increased atelectasis), changes in body habitus (increased kyphosis), or in vascular insufficiency and often obscure diagnostic signs. In the physical exam, there is a need to rule out significant aortic stenosis, to check for fluid retention or overload and especially frailty because as severe kyphosis often obscures the murmur, frailty emerges as one of the best predictors of outcome.

Frailty index

Frailty is a phenotypic characterization of features related to unsuccessful aging (weight loss, exhaustion, weakness, slowness, and low levels of activity). More than 20 tools have already been developed to measure frailty [11]. and the list is still growing. Many tools focus on 1 or more of 5 domains that are commonly used to define a frailty phenotype: slowness, weakness, low physical activity, exhaustion, and shrinking (Table 13.2). Tools entail assessments based on single domains as well as combined domains. Slowness is one of the most commonly applied domains; common indices include slow gait speed (measured during a comfortable-paced gait assessment). Weakness is also used frequently, typically by measuring handgrip strength using a dynamometer. More recently, cognition has been added as a sixth frailty domain.

Gait speed has advanced as one of most frequently used frailty indices, particularly because it is a relatively convenient and standardized procedure. A 5 meters gait assessment is usually used to assess gait speed;

Table 13.2 Factors related to frailty

1. Shrinking (unintentional weight loss).
2. Weakness.
3. Self-reported exhaustion.
4. Slowness.
5. Low activity.
6. Diminished cognition.

increased frailty-related risk is gauged by slow gait speed, >6 seconds for the 5 meter walk or <0.8 m/second is a common cut-point of risk [11,12]. This test also has strong inter-rater reliability (intra-class coefficient 0.88 to 0.96) and test–retest reliability (intra-class coefficient 0.86 to 0.91).

While frailty is often applied as a parameter that indicates poor prognosis, there is ongoing research to refine measures that can be used to enhance resiliency and tolerance to therapy, with better outcomes for patients identified as frail. Research efforts remain focused on identifying indices that can reliably gauge clinical improvements after therapeutic steps are taken to moderate frailty. For example, improved gait speed (estimated at 0.05 to 0.2 m/s) has been demonstrated to predict positive outcomes at a population level.

SMART TESTING

Biomarkers

As with younger patients, evaluation for acute coronary syndrome (ACS), HF and other instabilities in older patients includes serial assessment of biomarkers. More often than not, these biomarkers are assessed with a lower threshold given the subtlety and variability of these levels. Biomarkers are also often less reliable in older vs. younger populations due the confounding age-related effects of renal and hepatic metabolic changes, and/or concomitant disease states which can distort these levels. In general, the negative predictive value of most assessments is excellent, but the positive predictive value is often less certain. Clinicians must be thorough and watchful, and use multiple corroborating assessments to guide assessment and management.

Exercise stress testing

The baseline electrocardiography (ECG) in older adults is more likely to have baseline waveform abnormalities that may confound assessments of ischemia. Even so, exercise stress testing is still an important procedure to evaluate for chronic CHD as well as other CVD processes [13]. Exercise testing increases cardiac workload, and can provoke ischemic ECG changes and/or symptoms. Likewise, exercise testing provides a means to assess HF in terms of functional metrics and to clarify associated symptoms, heart rate responses, hemodynamics (pulmonary and systemic), arrhythmias, and other clinical parameters. Exercise testing for valvular heart disease and PAD help quantify how much these pathologies limit functional capacity. Therefore, exercise testing often has particular benefit for older adults, since the symptoms of CHD, HF, valvular disease or PAD are often obscured among elderly patients who claim to be asymptomatic, but only seem so owing to increasingly sedentary behaviors. Exercise testing exposes symptoms and signs masked by inactivity, clarifying utility for management (medications, revascularization, valvular replacement or repair, and/or cardiac rehabilitation) that can potentially restore physical function and improve quality of life and independence, as well as reduce morbidity and mortality. A more gradually progressive exercise test protocol may enable such testing even for a patient of advanced age.

Pharmacological stress test

While pharmacological stress testing with imaging is increasingly applied for older adults because it increases diagnostic sensitivity and specificity for CHD, it does not provide the same breadth of clinical perspective regarding physical function and exercise-associated symptoms/signs that help determine optimal clinical management choices for CHD and a wider spectrum of CV diseases [14]. Furthermore, assessments that rely exclusively on imaging increase the likelihood of an evaluation bias; i.e., CHD diagnosis that leads to revascularization and adjunctive medications, but without certainty that patients will benefit symptomatically from these management choices.

MANAGEMENT

As a result of aging and its associated risks, older adults with CV disease have the greatest conceptual potential for absolute risk reduction from revascularization, medications, and other aspects of care, but they also have the greatest potential for iatrogenesis and paradoxical detriment. Management choices entail a constant balance between rationale for aggressive therapy vs. rationale for reduced therapy. Multimorbidity, polypharmacology, and frailty, as well as geriatric conditions can affect cardiovascular care. Common geriatric conditions that are relevant include sensory limitations (vision, hearing), falls, delirium, cognitive decline, sarcopenia, fatigability, incontinence, and falls. They add to risks of therapy as well as to increased potential for poor compliance even when therapies are helpful [15].

Polypharmacy

The challenges of polypharmacy are typically linked to multimorbidity, as many older CV patients take numerous medications for concurrent pathologies [16]. Medications often compound problems, as age-related changes in absorption and metabolism alter the pharmacokinetics (PK) and pharmacodynamics (PD) of most drugs. As a result, medication dosing and effects, both beneficial and adverse, often differ from those in younger adults, and it cannot be assumed that the clinical utility of agents shown to be effective in younger individuals necessarily applies to the elderly. The problem is that concurrent medications and/or procedures often provoke uncertain responses, both because they have rarely been tested in a complex regimen (with efficacy of any one medication less clear in the context of many others), especially in the contexts of bed rest, hemodynamic lability, muscle weakness, confusion, and other risk-producing circumstances. These therapies are also often paradoxically associated with increased cumulative risks including falls, confusion, fatigue, loss of appetite, or other untoward effects [17].

While it is a common geriatric precept to treat iteratively, such as adding medications with small initial doses that are advanced only if tolerated, these principles contrast with more definitive treatment thresholds frequently required for CV management, e.g. device implantation, procedures (valve replacement, revascularization), and/or medications [18, 19], especially those oriented to non-hemodynamic benefits (e.g., neurohormonal, anti-inflammatory, and other therapeutic targets that commonly correspond to high dosing). It is challenging to divide standard medication regimens into a hierarchal organization such that one medication can be logically started before another. It is rarely clear which HF or CHD medication is more important than the other to evolve in an iterative fashion [20].

Specific disease management

Coronary heart disease   While aging predisposes to high incidence and prevalence of CHD, management of CHD for older adults is paradoxically ambiguous. Almost every aspect of care is transmuted by aging, confounding most traditional, guidelines-based standards of care.

So-called 'typical' CHD symptoms are less likely to be experienced by older patients, especially as ischemia is often associated with multiple co-morbid conditions that affect patients' complaints. Dyspnea is relatively more common than chest pressure or pain, in part because both heart failure with preserved ejection fraction (HFpEF) and heart failure with reduced ejection fraction (HFrEF) occur commonly in association with

CAD in older adults. Symptoms of confusion, agitation, or malaise may also be manifestations of acute or chronic CHD in older adults.

As in younger populations, evidence-based therapies for CHD in older adults include medical therapy and revascularization, but amidst the aggregate complexities of older adults, there is less clarity how these therapies should be applied. High vulnerability to CHD-related mortality and morbidity risks that are theoretically modifiable with aggressive care are counterbalanced by treatment-related risks (e.g., bleeding, renal failure, confusion/delirium). These risks are compounded by the predictable problems of frailty, polypharmacy, and geriatric conditions [21, 22].

Acute coronary syndrome   Just as in younger adults, the initial management for acute coronary syndrome (ACS) patients (both ST segment elevation myocardial infarction (STEMI) and non-ST segment elevation myocardial infarction (NSTEMI) focuses on options of acute revascularization. Landmark trials such as the Treat Angina With Aggrastat and Determine the Cost of Therapy With an Invasive or Conservative Strategy (TACTICS-TIMI 18) trial show relatively greater mortality reduction with revascularization (and associated anti-thrombin and antiplatelet adjunctive therapy) vs. medical therapy for ACS patients aged ≥75 and over. Nonetheless, only a minority of eligible older ACS patients receive reperfusion therapy. While advanced age is cited as the most common reason for its omission, care is omitted for many older candidates without a comprehensive assessment or rationale.

ST segment elevation myocardial infarction   Mechanical revascularization with percutaneous coronary intervention (PCI) within 90 minutes remains standard of care, especially given the increased bleeding risk associated with thrombolysis at elderly age. However, misinterpretation of STEMI symptoms in very old adults often contributes to delay in transporting patients to appropriate PCI capable hospitals. Furthermore, high prevalence of baseline ECG abnormalities often hinder time-sensitive ECG diagnostic assessments. High prevalence of co-morbidity and/or polypharmacy also contributes to uncertainty regarding the benefit: risk ratio when considering revascularization (and adjunctive therapy) vs. risks (e.g., bleeding, renal failure, delirium).

Clinical tools to help gauge composite health and vigor of older adults are potentially helpful to guide therapy. Frailty helps gauge the potential efficacy of aggressive therapy and provides an opportunity to consider reinforcements of therapy. Theoretically, a tiered medical approach based on frailty may help guide care more successfully for older adults. However, as compared to gait speed, assessments of frailty in the context of an ACS are relatively less clear cut. Moreover, even if when identified, it remains uncertain how frailty should be integrated into acute or chronic CHD management. Frail ACS adults may, for example, benefit from the same therapy as those who are not frail, but may require greater emphasis on rehabilitation, nutrition, and other supplemental treatments to ensure good outcomes [23]. More research in this area is needed to sort out these relationships.

Older CHD patients can benefit from evolving techniques to mitigate age-related risks. Radial artery catheterization may provide superior outcomes to femoral artery access by facilitating more rapid mobilization and less bleeding risk. Precise hydration can help mitigate heart failure and/or pre-renal failure. Specific anti-thrombin choices (e.g. bivalrudin vs enoxaparin) and antiplatelet agents (e.g., clopidogrel vs. prasugrel) as well as renal- and weight-adjusted dosing help reduce bleeding complications. Measures to hasten mobilization, reduce sedation, and avoid polypharmacy are also useful in their capacity to reduce delerium.

A related issue is consideration of drug eluting stents (DES) vs. bare metal stents (BMS) for older CAD patients. Whereas revascularization is usually more complete and durable with DES vs BMS at all ages, the medicated stent technology requires prolonged use of multiple antiplatelet agents, usually aspirin and clopidogrel for at least a year, and ideally even longer. This is complicated by increased age-related bleeding risks (e.g., GI bleeding, cystitis, epistaxis). Bleeding risks are compounded by polypharmacy especially among the many elderly who have concurrent atrial fibrillation, deep vein thrombosis, pulmonary emboli, or other diseases for which antithrombin therapy is indicated to reduce stroke and other morbidity (e.g., warfarin or a newer oral antithrombin agents [dabigatran, rivaroxaban, or apixaban] [24]). Since BMS require shorter courses of antiplatelet therapy, they may be better suited for older adults, but at the expense of the relatively better outcomes attributed to DES technology. The WOEST Trial is pertinent as it showed that treatment with double therapy (warfarin as well as clopidogrel) as compared to triple therapy (warfarin, clopidogrel, and aspirin) for PCI patients requiring anticoagulation (mostly for atrial fibrillation) was associated with significantly reduced episodes of bleeding, and even significantly reduced mortality, but without associated increases in thromboembolic events. Many other trials are exploring similar relationships with novel oral anticoagulation agents in combination with different thienopyridines as double agent adjunctive therapy for atrial fibrillation patients undergoing PCI [25].

Non-ST segment elevation myocardial infarction   Given the relatively greater leeway between guidelines recommendations for revascularization and medical management for NSTEMI as compared to STEMI, the management of NSTEMI in older adults is particularly ambiguous. While higher risk NSTEMI patients tend to derive the greatest benefit from revascularization and most older NSTEMI patients are at high risk, revascularization decisions in older NSTEMI patients still tend to be complicated. Management is often tailored relative to each patient's frailty, physical function, cognition, aggregate morbidity, prognosis and other dimensions of health status.

Chronic coronary heart disease   Just as in younger adults, older adults may be treated with medical therapy or revascularization; however decisions are compounded by the complexities of age. Optimal medical therapy is usually an initial strategy with revascularization particularly oriented to those with persistent symptoms and/or goals to reduce reliance on multiple anti-ischemic medications.

Older patients with severe coronary artery disease (left main or multivessel disease), left ventricular systolic dysfunction, and/or concomitant valvular disease are frequently referred for coronary artery bypass surgery. Comparing older vs. younger coronary artery bypass surgery (CABG) candidates, co-morbid conditions are more common (including diabetes mellitus, hypertension, chronic obstructive pulmonary disease, peripheral arterial disease and chronic kidney disease) in older adults and contribute to increased perioperative morbidity and mortality, including longer lengths of intensive care unit and hospital stay and prolonged post-hospital recovery.

A key consideration for CHD management in older adults is referral to cardiac rehabilitation. Older CHD patients benefit significantly from cardiac rehabilitation with reduced mortality, and improved quality of life, reduced symptoms, and increased functional capacity, independence, and self-efficacy. Cardiac rehabilitation addresses many issues associated with CHD management, from the emotional trauma associated with an AMI and/or revascularization to the complexities of polypharmacy, multimorbidity, and frailty, and to the critical value of increasing exercise and risk factor modification. Older patients both frail and robust, benefit. Cardiac rehabilitation provides care that can be tailored to address each older patient's circumstances [26, 27].

It is beyond this chapter to assess every aspect of management pertinent to older CV patients, as it would essentially entail the entire field of cardiology. Other resources are available with this kind of information such as the American College of Cardiology's Essentials in Cardiovascular Care for Older Adults (www.cardiosource.org/ECCOA).

For heart failure, valvular heart disease, arrhythmia, peripheral arterial disease, hypertension, and even for CV risk factors such as diabetes and hypercholesterolemia, complexities of aging fundamentally modify management choices. Currently most standards of care are extrapolated from younger adults, but with limited efficacy in the context of age-related vulnerabilities to polypharmacy, iatrogensesis and paradoxical detriments (fatigue, anorexia, dizziness). Furthermore, many CV diseases are particularly precipitated by mechanisms of aging (e.g., HF with preserved ejection fraction, aortic stenosis), such that research is increasingly focused on aging itself rather than disease as a theoretical way to forestall disease in the future.

General points regarding aging and management decisions

Given the multiple uncertainties and value-based judgements regarding caregiving choices, patients must be engaged in the selection of the management choices bearing on their health. To facilitate this, it is incumbent on the medical system (and cardiologists in particular, but also hospitalists, nurses, and other members of the caregiving team) to achieve processes, organization, and standards that ensure that seniors receive lucid, relevant, and consistent information in a straightforward and comprehensible manner.

Life circumstances of bereavement, diminished access to care, and/or chronic pain are also more common among the elderly, and impact on patients' priorities regarding their CV management. Relative differences in psychology (e.g., interpersonal capacities, self-efficacy, coping skills), social structure (e.g., class, community, access, spouse, family support), economic resources (personal, governmental), and culture (religion, ethnicity, transcendent sense of meaning and purpose) also impact the aging process.

Idiosyncratic effects of age must be anticipated. Complexities are exacerbated by cognitive decline, confusion, mood changes, and loss of appetite, especially in the context of the stress of hospitalization, loss of independence, functional decline, polypharmacy and sensory impairments (vision, hearing, taste).

Access to caregivers is often more limited (hindering assessments and monitoring); vision, hearing, and cognitive limitations can complicate comprehension and compliance; arthritis impedes exercise goals; financial constraints and altered taste may frustrate dietary recommendations; finances may also prohibit use of vital ancillary services; even the ability to stand on a scale can become difficult for someone challenged by dizziness, stroke, or Parkinsonism.

ACTION POINTS

1 The efficacy of mainstream cardiology is now very much affected by the advanced age of most CV patients. There is no systematic approach that incorporates age-related complexities into routine clinical decision making. It is incumbent on the cardiologist to embrace a broader paradigm that links CV care to the multisystem effects of aging, including co-morbidities, polypharmacy, psychosocial factors, and personal preferences into an individualized approach to care.

2 More research is essential to establish reliable diagnostic criteria despite often nebulous symptoms and often non-specific biomarkers.

3 Medication reconciliation is an essential part of comprehensive care, and should be repeated at every transition (at home, admission into the hospital, transfer within the hospital, and at discharge).

4 Provocative testing is often useful to clarify symptoms and signs of CVD.

5 Most standard therapies entail relative trade-offs between traditional standards of benefit (usually assessed in terms of increased longevity) and the risks associated with treatment burden, iatrogenesis, and the uncertain effects of multiple medications in combination. While therapeutic strategies vary from one older patient to another, stringent monitoring is usually necessary in every case as effects of therapy vary substantially, particularly because of the unpredictable impacts of multimorbidity and polypharmacy. Undesirable effects of CV therapy may be subtle, including changes in appetite, cognition, or mood, so thorough evaluations are useful. It also is necessary to consider the challenges commonly associated with access and logistics for monitoring to be successful.

REFERENCES

1. http://transgenerational.org/aging/demographics.htm
2. Forman DE, Rich MW, Alexander KP, Zieman S, Maurer MS, Najjar SS, Cleveland JC Jr, Krumholz HM, Wenger NK. Cardiac care for older adults. Time for a new paradigm. *J Am Coll Cardiol.* 2011;57:1801–1810.
3. Boyd CM, Wolff JL, Giovannetti E, Reider L, Weiss C, Xue QL, Leff B, Boult C, Hughes T, Rand C. Healthcare task difficulty among older adults with multimorbidity. *Med Care.* 2014;52:S118–125.

4. Lakatta EG, Levy D. Arterial and cardiac aging: major shareholders in cardiovascular disease enterprises: Part I: Aging arteries: a 'set up' for vascular disease. *Circulation.* 2003;107:139–146.

5. Alexander KP, Newby, LK, Cannon, CP, et al. Acute coronary care in the elderly. Part I: Non-ST-segment-elevation acute coronary syndromes: a scientific statement for healthcare professionals from the American Heart Association Council on Clinical Cardiology: in collaboration with the Society of Geriatric Cardiology. *Circulation.* 2007;115:2549–2569.

6. Forman DE, Wenger NK. What do the recent American Heart Association/American College of Cardiology Foundation Clinical Practice Guidelines tell us about the evolving management of coronary heart disease in older adults? *J Geriatr Cardiol.* 2013;10:123–128.

7. Abley C. Responding to vulnerability in old age: patient-centred care. *Nurs Stand.* 2012;27:42–46.

8. Reynolds MR1, Magnuson EA, Lei Y, Leon MB, Smith CR, Svensson LG, Webb JG, Babaliaros VC, Bowers BS, Fearon WF, Herrmann HC, Kapadia S, Kodali SK, Makkar RR, Pichard AD, Cohen DJ; Health-related quality of life after transcatheter aortic valve replacement in inoperable patients with severe aortic stenosis. *Circulation.* 2011;124:1964–1972.

9. Milner KA, Vaccarino V, Arnold AL, Funk M, Goldberg RJ. Gender and age differences in chief complaints of acute myocardial infarction (Worcester Heart Attack Study). *Am J Cardiol.* 2004;93:606–608.

10. Fried LP, Tangen CM, Walston J, et al. on behalf of the Cardiovascular Health Study Collaborative Research Group. Frailty in older adults: evidence for a phenotype. *J Gerontol A Biol Sci Med Sci.* 2001;56:M146–57.

11. Afilalo J, Alexander KP, Mack MJ, Maurer MS, Green P, Allen LA, Popma JJ, Ferrucci L, Forman DE. Frailty Assessment in the Cardiovascular Care of Older Adults. *J Am Coll Cardiol.* 2014;63:747–62.

12. Yano Y, Inokuchi T, Kario K. Walking speed is a useful marker of frailty in older persons. *JAMA Intern Med.* 2013;173:325–326.

13. Fletcher GF, Ades PA, Kligfield P, Arena R, Balady GJ, Bittner VA, Coke LA, Fleg JL, Forman DE, Gerber TC, Gulati M, Madan K, Rhodes J, Thompson PD, Williams MA. Exercise standards for testing and training: a scientific statement from the American Heart Association. American Heart Association Exercise, Cardiac Rehabilitation, and Prevention Committee of the Council on Clinical Cardiology, Council on Nutrition, Physical Activity and Metabolism, Council on Cardiovascular and Stroke Nursing, and Council on Epidemiology and Prevention. *Circulation.* 2013;128:873–934.

14. Mehta N, Chokshi NP, Kirkpatrick JN. Cardiac imaging in the geriatric population: What do we think we know, and what do we need to learn? *Prog Cardiovasc Dis.* 2014 Sep–Oct;57(2):204–214.

15. Knafl GJ, Riegel B. Patient prefer adherence. What puts heart failure patients at risk for poor medication adherence? *Patient Prefer Adherence.* 2014;8:1007–1018.

16. Tinetti ME, Bogardus ST Jr, Agostini JV. Potential pitfalls of disease-specific guidelines for patients with multiple conditions. *N Engl J Med.* 2004 Dec 30;351:2870–2874.

17. Murphy TE, Agostini JV, Van Ness PH, Peduzzi P, Tinetti ME, Allore HG. Assessing multiple medication use with probabilities of benefits and harms. *J Aging Health*. 2008;20:694–709.

18. Forman DE, Ahmed A, Fleg JL. Heart failure in very old adults. *Curr Heart Fail Rep*. 2013;10:387–400.

19. Inampudi C, Parvataneni S, Morgan CJ, Deedwania P, Fonarow GC, Sanders PW, Prabhu SD, Butler J, Forman DE, Aronow WS, Allman RM, Ahmed A. Spironolactone use and higher hospital readmission for Medicare beneficiaries with heart failure, left ventricular ejection fraction <45%, and estimated glomerular filtration rate <45 ml/min/1.73 m^2. *Am J Cardiol*. 2014;114:79–82.

20. Tinetti ME, Han L, Lee DSH, et al. Antihypertensive medications and serious fall injuries in a nationally representative sample of older adults. *JAMA Intern Med*. Apr 2014; 174(4): 588–595.

21. Fleg JL1, Aronow WS, Frishman WH. Cardiovascular drug therapy in the elderly: benefits and challenges. *Nat Rev Cardiol*. 2011;8:13–28.

22. Verbrugge FH, Dupont M, De Vusser P, Rivero-Ayerza M, Van Herendael H, Vercammen J, Jacobs L, Verhaert D, Vandervoort P, Tang WH, Mullens W. Response to cardiac resynchronization therapy in elderly patients (≥70 years) and octogenarians. *Eur J Heart Fail*. 2013;15:203–210.

23. Forman DE, Goyette RE. Oral anticoagulation therapy for elderly patients with atrial fibrillation: Utility of bleeding risk covariates to better understand and moderate risks. *Clin Appl Thromb Hemost*. 2014 Jan;20(1):5–15.

24. Barreto-Filho JA, Wang Y, et al. Transfer Rates From Nonprocedure Hospitals After Initial Admission and Outcomes Among Elderly Patients With Acute Myocardial Infarction *JAMA Intern Med*. 2014;174(2):213–222.

25. Dewilde WJ, Oirbans T, Verheugt FW, et al. Use of clopidogrel with or without aspirin in patients taking oral anticoagulant therapy and undergoing percutaneous coronary intervention: an open-label, randomised, controlled trial. *Lancet*. 2013;381:1107–1115.

26. Fleg JL, Forman DE, Berra K, Bittner V, Blumenthal JA, Chen MA, Cheng S, Kitzman DW, Maurer MS, Rich MW, Shen WK, Williams MA, Zieman S. Secondary prevention of atherosclerotic cardiovascular disease in older adults: a scientific statement from the American Heart Association; American Heart Association Committees on Older Populations and Exercise Cardiac Rehabilitation and Prevention of the Council on Clinical Cardiology, Council on Cardiovascular and Stroke Nursing, Council on Lifestyle and Cardiometabolic Health. *Circulation*. 2013;128:2422–2446.

27. Daniels KM, Arena R, Lavie CJ, Forman DE. Cardiac rehabilitation for women across the lifespan. *Am J Med*. 2012;125:937.e1–7.

CHAPTER 14

Cardiovascular Problems in Women

Kahroba Jahan, Ainol Shareha Sarar, Nisa Arshad, Nguyen Phuc Nguyen, Amsa Arshad, Sajaj Agarwal, Thach Nguyen and Kwan Lee

Management of Complex Cardiovascular Problems, Fourth Edition. Edited by Thach N. Nguyen, Dayi Hu, Shao Liang Chen, Moo Hyun Kim and Cindy L. Grines.
© 2016 John Wiley & Sons, Ltd. Published 2016 by John Wiley & Sons, Ltd.

BACKGROUND

Ischemic heart disease (IHD) continues to be the leading cause of death in women throughout the United States and other western countries. The term IHD encompasses a new concept of multifactorial pathophysiology for coronary atherosclerosis. It includes obstructive coronary artery disease (CAD) and dysfunction of the coronary microvasculature and endothelium resulting in arterial expansive remodeling and non-obstructive plaque [1]. A lot of information in this chapter was updated after the release of the 2014 American Heart Association (AHA) Consensus Statement on the Role of Non-invasive Testing in the Clinical Evaluation of Women with Suspected IHD [1].

CHALLENGES

The first challenge is the overall awareness of the prevalence of IHD in women. The misconception that IHD occurs mainly in men is now being disputed by the estimate that 1 out of 2 women in the U.S. will die of heart disease or stroke, while it is only estimated that 1 out of 25 women will die from breast cancer (the second leading cause of death from cancer in women). Of particular concern is the observation of the ever-increasing and growing prominence of coronary related death among young women in recent years. In a study by Ford et al. who examined age-specific mortality rates from IHD in younger adults, the mortality rate among women aged 35 to 44 years has increased on average 1.3% per year since 1980. These findings closely correlate with an array of emerging coronary risk factors such as increasing obesity in young adults as well as diabetes mellitus (DM), hypertension (HTN), and metabolic syndrome [2].

The second challenge is the misinterpretation of symptoms by both female patients and their physicians during clinical evaluation, leading to delays in diagnosis and therapy. The Euro Heart Survey of Stable Angina found that women with angina less often undergo exercise ECG stress testing and coronary angiography [3].

Lastly, the third challenge is the discrepancy in outcome, which is partially driven by a tendency for more conservative treatment when compared to male patients – especially in acute coronary syndrome (ACS). Underrepresentation of women in clinical trials and scant attention for differences between genders with the current sex-neutral guidelines form a significant barrier towards effective diagnosis and treatment of women with IHD [4].

HIGH-RISK MARKERS

In general, frail older women who have engaged in smoking and have had heart failure (HF) are at high risk. When associated with any of the high-risk factors listed in Table 14.1, a female patient, regardless of age and status, is considered high risk – except in the case of diabetes mellitus (DM) [1].

STRATEGIC MAPPING

The first step in the assessment of cardiovascular (CV) disease in women is to obtain a comprehensive history and physical examination (looking specifically for high-risk markers). In the investigation of IHD,

---

Table 14.1 High-risk markers for women regardless of age

1. Presence of significant atherosclerotic disease
   a Peripheral arterial disease
   b Diabetes mellitus: 10-year history or poorly controlled in a woman >40 years of age
   c Transient ischemic attacks or cerebrovascular accident
2. Severe co-morbidities
   a Chronic obstructive lung disease
   b Chronic kidney disease
3. Severe functional disability
   a Inability to perform activities of daily living or <5 estimated Duke Activity Status Index metabolic equivalents.

associated symptoms such as dyspnea, nausea, vomiting, fatigue, dizziness, etc. should be investigated further because women may not report chest pain as the predominant symptom. The second step is to calculate the pretest probability (PTP) in order to classify the patient on the basis of risk. Further non-invasive and invasive tests can be ordered according to the patient's risk. The tactic is to avoid the use of expensive non-invasive and invasive imaging procedures, except when the evidence clearly supports their benefit in improved diagnostic and prognostic accuracy. When qualified evidence is available that highlights a particular lower-cost procedure, this lower cost procedure should be selected. Once a diagnosis is made, patient management based on women-specific results from randomized clinical trials (RCT) should be applied judiciously.

INVESTIGATIONS

Symptoms to look for

Chest pain is the most common presenting symptom of IHD, although its characteristics and associated symptomatology differ significantly between men and women. Women may not report chest pain as the predominant symptom and tend to report more associated symptoms including—epigastric discomfort; nausea; the radiation of discomfort to the neck, arms and the interscapular area; dyspnea; and fatigue [5]. Compared with men, women's ischemic symptoms are more often precipitated by mental or emotional stress and less frequently by physical exertion. Also, symptoms in women are often less associated with the level of physical activity [6]. Women who are older, diabetic, and have a prior history of HF are more likely to have little or no chest discomfort [7].

Signs to look for

As there are no specific physical findings for IHD, the goal of a physical examination is often to detect possible precipitating factors or identify clues of alternative diagnoses. Several of these related physical findings could rank the patients in a higher risk category especially patients with acute coronary syndrome (ACS), pulmonary edema, a worsening mitral regurgitation murmur, a third or fourth heart sound, hypotension, bradycardia, or tachycardia.

Pretest probability calculations

The second step in the evaluation of stable IHD is to calculate the pretest probability (PTP). The first method of calculation is based on risk factors in the asymptomatic population such as the Framingham risk scores.

The second method of calculation is used by Diamond and Forrester to estimate the pretest likelihood of IHD, defined by age, sex, and symptoms, along with the sensitivity and specificity of four diagnostic tests. The results would then be based upon Bayes' theorem of conditional probability [7]. The third method of calculation classifies the symptomatic patient according to age by decade and the presence or absence of high risk factors and co-morbidities.

The Framingham Risk Score   These were derived from a predominantly male and asymptomatic patient population, and therefore present inherent difficulties in predicting risk in asymptomatic women. For example, application of the 10-year Framingham Risk Score in a clinical population revealed that three quarters of all women, even up to the age of 80, would have a risk score <10% [8]. In order to improve the predictive power of the Framingham Risk Score, the Reynolds Risk Score was designed to include other risk factors such as: age, systolic blood pressure, hemoglobin Alc, smoking status, total high density lipoprotein cholesterol (HDL-C), high-sensitivity C-reactive protein (hsCRP), and family history of myocardial infarction (MI) <60 years of age. With more data, the Reynolds Risk Score calculation was able to reclassify 15% of women who were initially at an intermediate risk group into a high-risk group. However, this represented only a small incremental shift in diagnostic accuracy over the Framingham Risk Scores [9].

The updated calculation based on conditional probability   The second method is to calculate the PTP according to Diamond and Forrester's method (conditional probability), but based on contemporary data. In this calculation, chest pain is divided into three types: (a) typical angina which is substernal chest discomfort provoked by physical or emotional stress and relieved by rest or nitroglycerin; (b) atypical chest pain which is chest discomfort with only one of the two aforementioned characteristics; and (c) non-cardiac chest pain which has neither of the two aforementioned characteristics. Based on age, type of pain, and presence of risk factors, the PTP can be calculated and confirmed by the prevalence of significant CAD (>70% significant stenosis) on a coronary angiogram. The patient is considered at high risk if the PTP is >90%. The patient has intermediate risk if the PTP is between 10 to 90%. Low PTP is from 5 to 10% and very low PTP is <5% (Table 14.2) [10, 11].

The newest and latest calculation   The third and latest method to calculate the PTP is to classify the symptomatic patients according to age, daily activities (ADL), risk factors, and co-morbidities as suggested in the

Table 14.2 Pretest probability of significant ischemic heart disease in women according to age, symptoms and risk factors

	Non angina chest pain	Atypical angina	Typical angina	Non-angina chest pain	Atypical angina	Typical angina
Age bracket	Low-risk	Low-risk	Low-risk	High-risk	High-risk	High-risk
35–44	1%	2%	10%	19%	39%	30%
45–54	2%	5%	20%	22%	43%	51%
55–64	4%	10%	38%	21%	47%	80%
>65	9%	20%	56%	29%	51%	93%

Note: % = percentage of significant CAD on angiogram.

2014 AHA Consensus Statement on the role of non-invasive testing in the clinical evaluation of women with suspected IHD [1]. The two main high-risk factors are peripheral arterial disease and longstanding poorly controlled DM. The two main co-morbidities are chronic obstructive lung disease and chronic kidney disease (CKD). In this calculation, a reasonable level of functional capability is defined as the patient is able to achieve the maximal heart rate and peak exercise greater than stage I of Bruce protocol (i.e., >5 metabolic equivalents [METs]). The level of functional capability can be calculated by the Duke Activity Status Index (DASI), which is a self-administered 12-question form designed to provide an estimate of physical exercise capacity (Table 14.3). If performance of routine ADL is compromised, then a woman is considered to be functionally limited.

In this new and latest method of PTP calculation, female patients can be classified as low-, intermediate-, or high-risk according to her age, ADL, and risk factors by following the three steps in Table 14.4.

Differential diagnoses

The common differential diagnoses of chest discomfort for symptomatic women with the possibility of IHD are listed in Table 14.5. Once a significant CAD is ruled out, other specific diagnoses (which occur more frequently in women presented with chest pain) are listed in Table 14.6.

Table 14.3 How to calculate the Duke Activity Status Index

1. Can you take care of yourself by eating, dressing, bathing, toileting? (2.75 METS)
2. Can you walk indoors such as around the house? (1.75 METS)
3. Can you walk a block on level ground? (2.75 METS)
4. Can you climb a flight of stairs or walk up hill? (5.50 METS)
5. Can you run a short distance? (8.00 METS)
6. Can you do light housework such as dusting or washing dishes? (2.70 METS)
7. Can you do moderate housework: vacuuming, sweeping, or carrying groceries? (3.50 METS)
8. Can you do heavy housework such as scrubbing floors or moving furniture? (8.0 METS)
9. Can you do yard work such as raking, weeding, or pushing a mower? (4.5 METS)
10. Can you have sexual relations? (5.25 METS)
11. Can you exercise such as golf, bowl, dance, doubles tennis, throw a ball? (6 METS)
12. Can you perform strenuous exercise such as swim, ski, singles tennis, football, basketball? (7.5 METS)

Duke Activity Status Index (DASI) = sum of 'Yes' replies _____
VO_2 peak = $(0.43 \times DASI) + 9.6$
VO_2 peak = _____ ml/kg/min ÷ 3.5 ml/kg/min = _____ METS

Table 14.4 Risk stratification of female patients

Step 1 Stratify the female patients by age

50 or less	Low-risk (premenopausal)
60	Intermediate-risk
70	High-risk

Step 2 The patient would be advanced to a higher level if there is one extra risk

1. Multiple cardiac risk factors (smoking, early menopause, hypertension), etc
2. Functional disability (activities of daily living <5 METS)
3. Extensive co-morbidities (chronic obstructive pulmonary disease, chronic kidney disease)

Step 3 The patient at any age could be advanced to the high-risk category if there is high-risk equivalent

1. Peripheral arterial disease (including stroke or transient ischemic attack)
2. Longstanding poorly controlled diabetes mellitus

Table 14.5 Common differential diagnoses of acute chest pain in women

1. Acute myocardial infarction
2. Pulmonary embolism
3. Pneumonia
4. Esophageal disease
5. Acute pericarditis
6. Hypertensive crisis
7. Hypertrophic cardiomyopathy
8. Aortic stenosis
9. Costochondritis
10. Herpes zoster
11. Pneumothorax
12. Acute aortic dissection

Table 14.6 Cardiac conditions presenting as chest pain with higher frequency in women

1. Takotsubo cardiomyopathy
2. Spontaneous coronary dissection
3. Syndrome X
4. Coronary vasospasm
5. Amniotic embolism

SMART TESTING

In the comprehensive investigation of IHD, a sequence of testing modalities (electrocardiogram, biomarkers, non-invasive imaging, stress test) are suggested.

Electrocardiogram (EKG)

In healthy men, the amplitude of the ST junction in V2 and V3 is greater than those in women. As a consequence, the threshold value for abnormal J-point elevation should be 0.15 mV (1.5 mm) in leads V2 and V3, and greater than 0.1 mV (1 mm) in all other leads, as opposed to the J-point elevation of 0.2 mV (2 mm) in leads V2 and V3 in men 40 years of age and older, and 0.25 mV (2.5 mm) in men younger than 40 [12].

Biomarkers

In patients presenting with symptoms suggestive of acute coronary syndrome (ACS), cardiac troponins (cTnI) are the most sensitive and specific biomarkers for myocardial injury. In 2009, the Chest Pain Evaluation by Creatine Kinase-MB, Myoglobin, and Troponin I (CHECKMATE) study assessed the accuracy and gender variability of the cTnI assay and creatine phosphate kinase (CK-MB) enzyme in the diagnosis of non-STEMI [13]. The results showed no differences in accuracy of cTnI among men and women, while the CK-MB markers showed more true positive results in men. So for patients suspected of MI, the troponin marker may improve the diagnosis of MI in women.

The biomarker hs-CRP was studied in the Justification for the Use of Statins in Primary Prevention. The Intervention Trial Evaluating Rosuvastatin (JUPITER) showed that hs-CRP levels may be used to tailor the dose of statins after an ACS event [14]. However, the question of correlation between hs-CRP and CV outcomes in women has not been specifically studied.

The biomarkers natriuretic peptides (biologically active B-type NP [BNP] and the inactive N-terminal prohormone BNP [Nt-proBNP]) are produced in the myocardium in response to wall stress and are used widely in the diagnosis and prognostication of patients with HF. Although women seem to have a higher baseline concentration of natriuretic peptides, whether BNP or NT-proBNP can be used to improve CV risk stratification has not yet been studied.

Exercise stress test

In the 2014 AHA consensus statement on the Role of Non-invasive Testing in the Clinical Evaluation of Women with Suspected IHD, the recommendations for exercise treadmill testing (ETT) are summarized below [1].

- **Low-risk women** are generally not candidates for further diagnostic testing. In patients deemed to be low-risk (young age, negative cardiac enzymes, and no electrocardiogram changes) adverse events, such as death and non-fatal MI, are rare and occur with similar frequency in those who undergo ETT as those who do not. Even when stress test results were abnormal, follow-up angiography frequently did not demonstrate any significant signs of IHD. Further, in a recent meta-analysis of studies using diagnostic testing in low risk populations, ETT did not reduce patient symptoms or anxiety and only a small decrease in office visits was observed. Based on this data, ETT in patients with a low pretest probability of IHD should generally be avoided [15].
- **The low intermediate-risk or the intermediate-risk women** are candidates for an ETT if they are functionally capable and have a

normal, or interpretable, resting ECG. Women with an intermediate–high IHD risk and with an abnormal 12-lead resting ECG (i.e. with resting ST-segment abnormalities) may be referred for stress imaging (myocardial perfusion imaging [MPI], echocardiography, or cardiac magnetic resonance imaging [CMR] or coronary computed tomographic angiography [CCTA]) [1].

- **Women with a high IHD risk** and with stable symptoms may be referred for a stress imaging modality for functional assessment of their ischemic burden and also to guide post-test, anti-ischemic therapeutic decision-making [1].

ST-T segment changes

In an ETT, the ST segment changes are the standard criteria for ischemia. The STT changes are the differences in ST segment (at 60 ms after the J point) between peak exercise (or recovery) and rest ECG. They include:

1 ST-segment depression ≥ 2 mm.
2 ST-segment depression ≥ 1 mm at <5 METs or >5 min into recovery.
3 ST-segment elevation ≥ 2 mm (not in q-wave lead or aVR).

In a study by Barolsky et al. looking at exercise ECG in both symptomatic men and women who later underwent coronary angiography, the positive predictive value of ST-segment depression with exercise ECG in women was only 47% versus 77% in men ($P < 0.05$) [16]. This significant difference has been attributed to multiple factors. Women have been known to have non-specific baseline ST-segment changes and more depression with exercise testing [17]. Moreover, it has been suggested that the hormone estrogen may have a 'digoxin-like effect' on ST segments, which also change according to menstrual cycle [18]. As women get older, they have more functional disabilities and thus decreased exercise tolerance, which leads to an overall inaccurate study. To make the problem worse, the Bruce protocol is commonly used in the US ETT laboratories and requires an initial workload of 4.7 METs (stage 1). Then the workload increases quickly 2 to 3 METs per stage, which may precipitate early fatigue in women with less muscle mass—particularly for less physically-fit women [1].

In these studies, which compared the exercise ECG with angiography, only a minority of female patients underwent invasive angiography. Therefore, post-test referral bias contributed to the artificial elevation of diagnostic sensitivity and reduced specificity. This statistical bias is operational for all diagnostic test modalities [1].

Beyond the STT changes on the ECG, the diagnostic and prognostic accuracy of ETT in women can be improved by incorporating parameters such as exercise capacity, chronotropic response, heart rate recovery, blood pressure response, and the Duke Treadmill Score (DTS).

The first parameter is the exercise capacity (or cardiorespiratory fitness), which is one of the strongest predictors of outcomes for women. Women who achieve <5 METs during ETT are at an increased risk of death and other related IHD events, independent of traditional cardiac risk factors. The age-predicted maximal fitness is calculated using the formula below:

$$100\% \text{ Age predicted METS} = 14.7 - (0.13 \times age)$$

The second parameter is that the patient can achieve at least 85% of maximum age-predicted heart rate (MPHR) with exercise. The inability to achieve at least 85% of the MPHR results in an increased risk of obstructive CAD. Recently, the calculation of a woman's age-predicted heart rate has been revised as shown in the following formul [1]:

$$\text{Age-predicted heart rate for women} = 206 - (0.88 \times age)$$

The third parameter is heart rate recovery. An abnormal heart rate recovery can be defined as a decrease in the heart rate less than 12 beats per minute at 1 minute of recovery from the peak heart rate.

The fourth parameter is blood pressure (BP) increase with exercise. The failure to raise BP with exercise is a strong negative prognostic factor that is suggestive of left main disease or 3-vessel disease.

The last parameter is the Duke Treadmill Score (DTS) which is a weighted index combining treadmill exercise time using the standard Bruce protocol, maximum net ST segment deviation (depression or elevation), and exercise-induced angina. It was developed to provide accurate diagnostic and prognostic information for the evaluation of patients with suspected IHD [28]. The typical observed range of DTS is from –25 (highest risk) to +15 (lowest risk). A low DTS is a better indicator to exclude ischemic heart disease in women when compared to men. The calculation of DTS is shown in Table 14.7 [19].

Table 14.7 How to calculate the Duke Treadmill Scores

DTS = Exercise Time – (5 × Max ST) – (4 × Angina Index)		
Results	≥5	Low-risk
	+4 to –10	Moderate-risk
	≤ –11	High-risk
Max ST = Maximum net ST deviation (except aVR)		
Angina Index 0 for no angina during exercise		
1 for non-limiting angina		
2 for exercise limited angina		

CLINICAL PEARLS
How to perform and interpret exercise stress test in women Adaptive protocols that use small increases or start at lower workloads are preferable for most symptomatic women, such as the Asymptomatic Cardiac Ischemia Pilot [20] or the modified Bruce [21]. (or Balke [22]) protocols [23]. Regardless of whether imaging is used, important prognostic and diagnostic parameters (exercise capacity, heart rate increase and recovery, blood pressure increase, and DTS) should be assessed and reported. Nevertheless, despite the common notion that exercise ECG leads to more 'false-positive' results in women, a negative exercise stress test is an effective way to rule out IHD. Once a conclusion is made, the stress test abnormalities are no longer defined as having a false-positive test, but rather the patient's test is classified as abnormal, and the patient is noted as being at an elevated IHD risk [1].

Myocardial perfusion imaging

In women with an abnormal baseline ECG, the addition of imaging to exercise with either single-photon emission computed tomography (SPECT) or echocardiography is strongly recommended in the AHA Consensus Statement [1].

Stress echocardiography

Stress echocardiography is recommended for identification of obstructive IHD and for an estimation of prognosis for symptomatic women who are at intermediate–high IHD risk and have any of the following: (a) resting ST-segment abnormalities; (b) functional disability; or (c) indeterminate or intermediate-risk stress ECG *(Class I: Level of Evidence B)*. At the same time, diastolic function and pulmonary artery pressures can be assessed in women presenting with dyspnea *(Class IIb: Level of Evidence C)*. Other important information such as left ventricular (LV) global and regional systolic function, as well as the extent of scarred myocardium and stress-induced myocardial ischemia can be obtained and used as a basis for diagnosis, selection of treatment options, and follow-up [24]. When exercise stress echocardiography images are suboptimal due to a poor acoustic window with associated difficulty obtaining accurate images during maximal stress, or in patients with functional disability, pharmacological stress echocardiography is recommended. The markers of high IHD risks in women with stress echocardiography are listed in Table 14.8.

Table 14.8 Markers of high risk in stress echocardiography

1. Rest left ventricular ejection fraction ≤40%.
2. Extensive rest wall-motion abnormalities.
3. Extensive ischemia (≥4–5 left ventricular segments).
4. Right ventricular ischemia.
5. Increase in end-systolic size with stress (dilation of left ventricle).
6. Left ventricular ejection fraction decrease with stress.

SPECT myocardial perfusion imaging (MPI)

For symptomatic women at intermediate-high IHD risk and with (a) resting ST-segment abnormalities; (b) functional disability; or (c) indeterminate or intermediate-risk stress ECG; stress myocardial perfusion imaging (MPI) with single-photon emission computed tomography (SPECT), or positron emission tomography (PET) is recommended to identify obstructive IHD and estimate prognosis *(Class I: Level of Evidence B)*. In younger women, the choice of a test should be based on concerns about radiation exposure and increased projected cancer risk and not higher reported accuracy *(Class II: Level of Evidence C)*. Radiation dose-reduction techniques should be used whenever possible when radiation exposure levels are ≥3 mSv. It should be noted that soft tissue attenuation due to either breast tissue or large body habitus can yield false-positive results in exercise SPECT imaging [1]. The markers of high IHD risk in women with SPECT imaging are listed in Table 14.9.

Radiation

Patients should undergo testing which involves the lowest dose of radiation. The levels of radiation by different modalities of imaging are listed in Table 14.10.

Nonetheless, despite the above limitations, the addition of either imaging method to ETT increases both diagnostic accuracy and prognostic

Table 14.9 Markers of high risk in women with SPECT imaging

1. Summed stress score >8.
2. ≥10% of the abnormal myocardium at stress.
3. ≥10% of the ischemic myocardium.
4. Left ventricular dilation.
5. Peak stress or post-stress left ventricular ejection fraction ≤45%.

Table 14.10 Levels of radiation in different modalities of imaging (units?)

Annual background exposure	≈3
Invasive coronary angiography	≈7
Rest-stress MPI SPECT	
Technetium Tc 99m	≈11
Stress-only MPI SPECT	≈3
Dual-isotope MPI SPECT	22
Rest-stress MPI PET	
Rubidium Rb 82	≈3
Nitrogen N 13	≈2
CCTA	
Overall	≈10
With dose-reduction techniques	<2–5
Coronary artery calcium scoring	2

CCTA = coronary computed tomographic angiography; MPI = myocardial perfusion imaging; PET = positron emission tomography; and SPECT = single-photon emission computed tomography.

value. In the case of exercise stress echocardiography, specificity increases from 81% to 86% and sensitivity increases from 80% to 88% in symptomatic women with an intermediate risk [25]. Similarly, the diagnostic accuracy of exercise SPECT is much greater than that of exercise ECG alone, with improved sensitivity and specificity to approximately 88% in symptomatic postmenopausal women, which is equivalent in diagnostic accuracy as is in men [25]. Exercise stress echocardiography and SPECT are also have prognostic value in predicting overall CV mortality in women [26].

Cardiac computed tomography angiography (CCTA)

By measuring the coronary artery calcium (CAC) score, cardiac computed tomography angiography (CCTA) provides a unique and non-invasive strategy in the evaluation and diagnosis of IHD in women. The prevalence and prognostic significance of subclinical coronary calcium in asymptomatic, 'low-risk' women, who were classified based on the Framingham Risk Score (estimated risk <10% in 10 years), was analyzed in The Multi-Ethnic Study of Atherosclerosis (MESA) trial. This study revealed that the prevalence of coronary artery calcification (CAC score >0) in the low-risk subset (which was ~90% of all MESA women excluding diabetics) was 32%. The results showed that these women were at increased risk for

IHD disease, and so the presence of CAC provided incremental predictive power for CV events [27]. The use of coronary CTA for the detection of IHD in symptomatic women was studied in the ACCURACY (Assessment by Coronary Computed Tomographic Angiography of Individuals Undergoing Invasive Coronary Angiography) trial which showed a sensitivity and specificity for detection of >50% stenosis to be 95% and 83%, and for >70% stenosis to be 94% and 83%, respectively [28]. However, CCTA is not the first choice or the preferred method in detecting IHD (indication class of 2b) if other modalities are available and/or are more affordable.

INVASIVE TESTING

Coronary angiography

Coronary angiography helps to confirm the diagnosis and guide the treatment of IHD. Not infrequently, women with clinical symptoms of cardiac ischemia are found to have no obstructive CAD on angiography suggesting the presence of coronary microvascular dysfunction ('microvascular angina' or 'syndrome X') or in the setting of appropriate accompanying diagnostic criteria—Tako-tsubo cardiomyopathy. A systematic review, of 47 studies on microvascular angina with a total patient population of 1934 patients, found a relative frequency of 56% with cardiac Syndrome X^{32} – clearly posing a challenge to physicians taking care of this type of patient. While earlier studies suggested fewer cardiac events and overall better prognosis in such patients [33, 34], more recent studies indicate that patients with symptomatic cardiac ischemia and non-obstructive IHD on angiography may not have such a benign prognosis [35]. The Women's Ischemia Syndrome Evaluation (WISE) study followed women with clinical signs and symptoms of ischemia with no angiographic evidence of IHD for a mean 5.2 years and showed that WISE women with clinical signs and symptoms of ischemia without obstructive IHD were at elevated risk for CV events compared with asymptomatic community-based women [35].

MANAGEMENT

Primary prevention

Overall, most primary prevention interventions are similar for women and men, but there are some notable exceptions. In a 20-year long study of 88,940 female participants, in which the mean age was 37.1 years, the adoption of six healthy lifestyle behaviors averted up to 72.7% of IHD cases, 92.9% of DM cases, 57.0% of HTN cases, and 40% of cases of hypercholesterolemia in women over 20 years of age. Optimal healthy lifestyle behaviors included not smoking, engaging in at least 2.5 hours of physical activity a week, watching television no more than 7 hours per week, maintaining a lower BMI, consuming 0.1–14.9 g of alcohol daily, and eating a healthy diet [33].

Aspirin (ASA) is routinely recommended for the primary prevention of MI in men, but is not recommended in healthy women <65 years of age [34]. Low-dose ASA is recommended for women with a 10-year risk of a first coronary event that exceeds 20%, and can be considered for women with a 10-year risk of 10% to 20% [34]. The potential benefit of ASA should be individualized and balanced against the increased risk of gastrointestinal bleeding by ASA [35]. Hormone therapy and selective estrogen-receptor modulators (SERMs) are currently a Class III intervention and should not be used for primary or secondary prevention of IHD [36].

Secondary prevention

A daily dose of 75–162 mg of ASA is recommended in all patients with IHD unless contraindicated. Cardiac rehabilitation is recommended as a Class I guideline in all eligible patients – after an ACS presentation, post-coronary artery bypass grafting (CABG), or post-percutaneous coronary intervention (PCI) and also in patients with chronic angina or with peripheral vascular disease. In a community-based cohort study, disparities in the participation of cardiac rehabilitation after myocardial infarction (MI) mainly included women and the elderly. This was associated independently with a decreased mortality rate and a lower risk of recurrent MI [37]. Further effort to encourage women to participate in a cardiac rehabilitation program is needed.

Acute coronary syndrome (ACS)

Female representation in large RCTs of IHD was low and resulted in lack of data on the difference in the effects of anti-ischemic drugs between genders. Therefore, the current guidelines for treatment of STEMI and unstable angina/non-ST segment elevation myocardial infarction (UA/NSTEMI), which are sex-neutral, remain the standard of care for both sexes regardless of their innate differences [38, 39]. It is important to be aware of differences in the underlying etiology of women presenting with ACS. There is a significantly higher incidence of spontaneous coronary dissection in women during the third trimester and post-partum period, accounting for up to 43% of women presenting in this time frame [40]. Overall, women also account for a disproportionate 89,8% of all cases of takotsubo cardiomyopathy, although the initial diagnostic management should not change as the diagnosis can only be made after excluding significant CAD [41]. The acute pharmacological management of women should take into account sex-based differences in body size and creatinine clearance, and should avoid fixed dosed medication regimens. Dosages should be administered according to body weight.

Another mechanism to explain inter-gender differences in response to therapy among patients with ACS is the increase in platelet function in women, which may suggest that women may benefit more from treatment with antiplatelet therapy than men. With respect to gender outcomes with clopidogrel, a meta-analysis of all blinded, randomized placebo controlled trials was performed. It involved 79,613 patients of which 30% were women. Overall, no significant difference was noted between men and women with the same therapeutic effect. In women, the risk reduction was greatest for MI rather than stroke or total death while in men, a reduction for all endpoints was shown [42]. No significant gender differences have been noted thus far regarding the use of the new oral antiplatelet agents, such as prasugrel or ticagrelor.

Invasive treatment

It has been hypothesized that a higher mortality rate exists among women undergoing coronary revascularization. The many mechanisms explaining the high mortality include: the delay in diagnosis; atypical presentation of women with ACS; an increased number of co-morbidities such as DM, HTN, hypercholesterolemia, peripheral vascular disease; and a smaller caliber of female coronary vessels. Taking into account the different characteristics of women with IHD, several studies have examined the response of women with ACS to contemporary medical methods, invasive therapies, and the patient's overall outcome.

The results of these studies confirmed the benefits of direct invasive strategy over initial conservative strategy for men, but not for women. The Thrombolysis in Myocardial Infarction (TIMI), IIIB, and the FRagmin and Fast Revascularisation during InStability in Coronary artery disease (FRISC) II trial, demonstrated either an improved outcome in men only, or similar outcome between both sexes (adjusted for co-morbidities) and showed no differences between invasive and conservative therapy [43]. In the RITA-3 (randomized intervention trial of unstable angina-3) trial, early invasive treatment provided no benefit for women and was in fact associated with worse outcomes. At one year, death or MI occurred in 5.1% of men, compared to 8.6% of women. In the conservative and invasive groups, it was 10.1% in women compared to 7.0% in men [44]. The Treat Angina With Aggrastat and Determine the Cost of Therapy With an Invasive or Conservative Strategy (TACTICS-TIMI 18) trial assessed the outcome of early invasive strategy (within 48 hours of presentation) in patients with ACS and treated them with a combination of glycoprotein IIb/IIIa inhibitor and stenting. The results showed that early PCI was equally beneficial in both men and women in reducing the rate of death, MI, and re-hospitalization and also showed an enhanced benefit in high-risk women showing dynamic ST changes and elevated cardiac enzymes [45, 46].

In general, the results of the published literature show that low-risk women had worse outcomes (including higher risk of major bleeding) with early PCI, whereas low-risk men were neither harmed nor benefited by early PCI [47]. However, the above trials were conducted prior to the evolution of drug-eluting stents (DES).

In the new recommendations, women presenting with UA/NSTEMI and high-risk features should proceed with an early invasive strategy. In contrast to men, low-risk women proceeding with an early invasive strategy may result in harm and an initial conservative approach should be adopted. An invasive strategy should be reserved only for patients who fail medical therapy or show objective evidence of significant ischemia [48].

Drug-eluting stents (DES)

DES have led to significant improvement in PCI outcomes. None of the individual major RCTs have been powered to evaluate an assessment of the safety and efficacy of DES in women. A recent patient level meta-analysis of 26 RCTs showed continued improvements in rates of death, or MI, at 3 years in the transition from BMS to early-generation and newer generation DES [49]. Promisingly, newer generation DES were found to result in improvements in the rates of stent thrombosis when compared to early generation DES. Dramatic reductions in the rates of target lesion revascularization were also found [49].

In conclusion, the most important implication is that the use of DES in women is more effective and safer than the use of bare-metal stents during long-term follow-up. Newer-generation DES are associated with an improved safety profile compared with early-generation DES.

Complications of percutaneous coronary interventions (PCI)

Women were known to be of higher risk for vascular complication with higher access site and non-access site bleeding, possibly due to: a smaller vessel size, hormonal influences on vessel fragility, and/or hemostasis. Notably, the use of interventional devices such as rotablation, laser therapy, and directional coronary atherectomy appear to correlate with higher complication rates in women [50, 51]. Despite early observational studies suggesting reduced bleeding in women who utilized a radial approach, a recent registry-based randomized trial failed to show a reduction in bleeding in women undergoing PCI through the radial approach; however, it did show less bleeding in women undergoing either cardiac catheterization or PCI [52].

ST segment elevation myocardial infarction (STEMI)

Despite the overall benefit of appropriate invasive management of women presenting with ACS, women still have a higher rate of complications, notably cardiogenic shock, stroke, and bleeding. In a large retrospective study involving 833 patients who had undergone PCI, the rate of short- and long-term cardiac events in men and women were similar. Nonetheless, in the subgroup of STEMI, the rates of death were significantly greater for women than for men (20% vs. 8.1%) and women were significantly less likely to have received effective treatment, including the use of DES [53]. However, the results of the Optical Coherence Tomography Assessment of Gender Diversity In Primary Angioplasty (OCTAVIA) trial showed no differences in the pathophysiology of STEMI in response to primary PCI between women and men such as differences in age other than biological factors [54].

Coronary artery bypass graft surgery (CABG)

In general, women undergoing coronary artery bypass graft surgery (CABG) are at a higher perioperative risk and postoperative mortality compared to men due to smaller stature and smaller vessel diameters [55]. Despite having a lower overall graft patency rate than men, the overall survival rate at 5 and 10 years was not significantly different [55].

Acute coronary syndrome (ACS) in pregnancy

Ischemic heart disease during childbearing age is rare, with an incidence of 1 acute MI in about 16,000 deliveries [57]. During pregnancy, there is a 3–4 times increase in risk of ACS, likely due to an increase in blood volume and cardiac output which in turn may lead to exacerbated shear force within blood vessels, as well as an overall hypercoaguable state. Additionally, elevated female hormone levels during pregnancy are well-known to be a major cause of spontaneous coronary artery dissection because of biochemical and structural changes in the coronary vessel wall [57]. With advances in reproductive technology and the increasing maternal age in women, the number of incidents is expected to rise. Due to the vulnerable physiological state of pregnancy, maternal mortality is 11%, while fetal mortality is 9% [58]. Rather, the underlying etiology of acute MI in pregnancy is 40% due to atherosclerosis, 50% due to coronary dissection, 13% due to transient coronary spasm, and 8% due to thrombosis without atherosclerosis. Primary PCI for acute MI in pregnant women is similar to that of non-pregnant women, but extra care should be taken in order to minimize radiation exposure to the fetus. Echocardiography is the imaging modality of choice for the detection of wall motion abnormalities. Non-invasive risk stratification is generally favored and especially if stress testing is performed – certain modifications should be adopted in response to the physiology of pregnancy, risk of radiation to the fetus, and potentially harmful pharmacological effects to the fetus.

Exercise stress testing should be performed with use of submaximal protocol (<70% of max predicted HR) and with simultaneous fetal monitoring. Dobutamine stress echocardiography is presumably safe with no fetal risk and dobutamine (pregnancy category B) is favored over adenosine (category C) for stress testing [58]. Nuclear perfusion imaging with tech-99 or thallium, yields <1 rad of radiation exposure to the fetus. Cardiac catheterization and PCI have been shown to result in <1 rad fetal exposure. Measures such as the use of radial access for catheterization should be considered to minimize direct fetal radiation. External shielding of the maternal pelvis is of limited value and the radiation dose absorbed by the fetus without shielding was found to be only 3% higher than without any external shield [59]. Complex PCI results and longer exposure could yield up to 5–10 rad fetal exposure. Termination of pregnancy is not necessary for fetal doses <5 rads, but may be considered for >10 rads [58]. Iodinated contrast used during PCI crosses the blood-placental barrier. Although it cannot be proven as teratogenic, it can cause fetal hypothyroidism if directly administered into amniotic fluid [58]. The safety of DES is still unknown and should be avoided. Thrombolytic therapy is a relative contraindication. Based on anecdotal information, however, if alternative therapy is not available, thrombolytic therapy should not be withheld [56, 57]. Care and expert pharmacological consultation should be sought when choosing therapeutic options. Additional awareness should be placed on which drugs may cross the placenta. There is also a possibility of breast milk excretion should not be forgotten.

ACTION POINT [60]

1 IHD develops at a later age for women compared to men; however, rates of IHD have been increasing among younger women. Although rates of HTN and dyslipidemia are lower in men than premenopausal women, with older age, these gender differences disappear. Diabetes appears to be a stronger risk for IHD in women compared to men. Rates of impaired glucose are higher among women than men. Mechanistic studies are needed to understand these differences.

2 Additional risk factors for IHD include depression and other forms of mental stress (anxiety, anger, work, and marital stress).

Coronary heart disease risk related to mental stress is similar for men and women; however, the prevalence of these factors is higher among women.

3 Women with symptoms of cardiac ischemia have a higher frequency of no obstructive epicardial CAD. Women with NSTEMI are more likely to demonstrate myocardial ischemia independent of coronary stenosis. Microvascular disease, coronary artery spasm, and spontaneous coronary artery dissection are more often seen in women than men.

4 The pretest probability of IHD is different in women compared to men under the age of 60 and can be stratified by the nature of the chest pain, age, high risk factors and co-morbidities. This pretest probability should specify if the use for further testing is appropriate.

5 Diagnostic testing of coronary microvascular disease includes measurement of coronary blood flow reserve by echocardiography or positron emission tomography-computed tomography (PET-CT). Calculation of microcirculatory resistance index can be performed during coronary catheterization (i.e., coronary flow reserve). Women with chest pain and non-obstructive CAD have an increased risk for obstructive CAD; thus, diagnosis of microvascular disease is warranted.

6 Several unique ACSs occur more commonly in women, such as Tako-tsubo cardiomyopathy, vasospastic angina, cardiovascular 'Syndrome X', and spontaneous coronary dissection.

7 In ACS a conservative invasive strategy is preferable for low-risk women while an invasive therapy is preferable for high-risk women.

8 DES has been demonstrated to be efficacious in women with clear improvements in the transition from BMS to newer generation DES.

9 Despite an early promise, a radial approach for PCI in women has not been shown to clearly reduce bleeding.

10 Acute CV events in pregnancy, although rare, can be catastrophic for mother and child. Special considerations in management should include efforts to minimize fetal radiation exposure and raising awareness about the increased risks of bleeding, fetal distress, and teratogenic potential with routinely used cardiovascular drugs.

11 The prevalence of heart failure with preserved ejection fraction (HFpEF) is greater in women than men; while rates of heart failure with reduced ejection fraction (HFrEF) and dilated cardiomyopathies in general are higher in men. Rates of Takotsubo cardiomyopathy are higher among women than men. Understanding differences related to inflammation, sex hormones, hyperglycemia, and ventricular remodeling is warranted.

12 Although rates of HTN are lower among young women compared to young men, rates are higher in women and the elderly. Sex-related differences have been observed related to the renin-angiotensin system; however, no differences related to efficacy of antihypertensive medications have been consistently noted. Polycystic ovarian syndrome and postmenopausal status have been associated with increased incidence of HTN among women. Left ventricular hypertrophy (LVH) related to HTN is more difficult to treat among women than men, with less regression of hypertrophy with antihypertensive treatment. Increases in LVH and myocardial stiffness predispose women to HFpEF and stroke at older ages.

13 Aortic stenosis is one of the most common valvular abnormalities among both men and women. Perioperative complications are higher among women than men with aortic valve replacement. Transcatheter aortic valve replacement (TAVR) appears to have similar success rates for men and women with greater short- and mid-term survival for women, and similar stroke rates among women and men. Mitral valve prolapse (MVP) is more common among women than men; however, the need for MV surgery is higher among men. Underdiagnosis of symptomatic MV among women may be present given women often have higher LVEFs and smaller LV dimensions compared to men.

14 Sex and gender differences exist related to the pharmacokinetics of many cardiac drugs. Oral bioavailability, clearance, body fat distribution, plasma protein binding, and metabolism all can differ by sex. Furthermore, women have a longer repolarization phase (longer QT duration on electrocardiogram), which may increase a woman's risk for ventricular arrhythmias in the setting of certain drugs including antidepressants. It is also important to consider teratogenicity in women of child-bearing age and the degree of breast milk excretion in breast-feeding women.

REFERENCES

1. Mieres JH, Gulati M, Merz NB; Berman DS, Gerber TC, Hayes SN, Kramer CM, Min JK, Newby LK, Nixon JV, Srichai MB, Pellikka PA, Redberg RF, Wenger NK, Shaw LJ; on behalf of the American Heart Association Cardiac Imaging Committee of the Council on Clinical Cardiology and the Cardiovascular Imaging and Intervention Committee of the Council on Cardiovascular Radiology and Intervention. Role of noninvasive testing in the clinical evaluation of women with suspected ischemic heart disease: a consensus statement from the American Heart Association. *Circulation.* 2014;130:350–379.

2. Ford ES, Capewell S. Coronary heart disease mortality among young adults in the U.S. from 1980 through 2002: concealed leveling of mortality rates. *J Am Coll Cardiol.* 2007;50:2128–2132.

3. Daly C, Clemens F, Lopez Sendon JL, et al. Gender differences in the management and clinical outcome of stable angina. *Circulation* 2006;113:490-8.

4. Kim ES, Menon V. Status of women in cardiovascular clinical trials. *Arterioscler Thromb Vasc Biol.* 2009;29:279–283.

5. Patel H, Rosengren A, Ekman I. Symptoms in acute coronary syndromes: does sex make a difference? *Am Heart J.* 2004;148:27–33.

6. Kimble LP, McGuire DB, Dunbar SB, et al. Gender differences in pain characteristics of chronic stable angina and perceived physical limitation in patients with coronary artery disease. *Pain.* 2003;101:45–53.

7. Diamond GA, Forrester JS. Analysis of probability as an aid in the clinical diagnosis of coronary-artery disease. *N Engl J Med.* 1979;300:1350–1358.

8. Pasternak RC, Abrams J, Greenland P, Smaha LA, Wilson PWF, Houston-Miller N. Task force #1—identification of coronary heart disease risk: is there a detection gap? *J Am Coll Cardiol.* 2003;41:1863–1874.

9. Ridker PM, Buring JE, Rifai N, Cook NR. Development and validation of improved algorithms for the assessment of global cardiovascular risk in women: the Reynolds Risk Score. *JAMA.: the Journal of the American Medical Association* 2007;297:611–619.

10. Stone NJ, Robinson J, Lichtenstein AH, et al. 2013 ACC/AHA guideline on the treatment of blood cholesterol to reduce atherosclerotic cardiovascular risk in adults: a report of the American College of Cardiology/American Heart Association Task Force on Practice Guidelines. *J Am Coll Cardiol.* 2014;63:2889–2934.

11. Fihn SD, Gardin JM, Abrams J, Berra K, Blankenship JC, Dallas AP, Douglas PS, Foody JM, Gerber TC, Hinderliter AL, King SB 3rd, Kligfield PD, Krumholz HM, Kwong RY, Lim MJ, Linderbaum JA, Mack MJ, Munger MA, Prager RL, Sabik JF, Shaw LJ, Sikkema JD, Smith CR Jr, Smith SC Jr, Spertus JA, Williams SV. 2012 ACCF/AHA/ACP/AATS/ PCNA/SCAI/STS guideline for the diagnosis and management of patients with stable ischemic heart disease: a report of the American College of Cardiology Foundation/American Heart Association Task Force on Practice Guidelines, and the American College of Physicians, American Association for Thoracic Surgery, Preventive Cardiovascular Nurses Association, Society for Cardiovascular Angiography and Interventions, and Society of Thoracic Surgeons. *Circulation.* 2012;126:e354–e471.

12. Wagner GS, Macfarlane P, Wellens H, et al. AHA/ACCF/HRS recommendations for the standardization and interpretation of the electrocardiogram: part VI: acute ischemia/infarction: a scientific statement from the American Heart Association Electrocardiography and Arrhythmias Committee, Council on Clinical Cardiology; the American College of Cardiology Foundation; and the Heart Rhythm Society. Endorsed by the International Society for Computerized Electrocardiology. *J Am Coll Cardiol.* 2009;53:1003–1011.

13. Shoaibi A, Tavris DR, McNulty S. Gender differences in correlates of troponin assay in diagnosis of myocardial infarction. *Transl Res.* 2009;154:250–256.

14. Ridker PM, Danielson E, Francisco AH, Fonseca FAH, et al. for the JUPITER Study Group Rosuvastatin to Prevent Vascular Events in Men and Women with Elevated C-Reactive Protein *N Engl J Med.* 2008; 359:2195–2207.

15. www.cardiosource.org/en/News-Media/Special-Features/ACC14-Meeting-Coverage/Perspectives-Testing-in-Low-Pretest-Probability-Women-With-Exercise-Treadmill-vs-Stress-Echo.aspx

16. Barolsky SM, Gilbert CA, Faruqui A, Nutter DO, Schlant RC. Differences in electrocardiographic response to exercise of women and men: a non-Bayesian factor. *Circulation.* 1979;60:1021–1027.

17. Weiner DA, Ryan TJ, McCabe CH, et al. Exercise stress testing. Correlations among history of angina, ST-segment response and prevalence of coronary-artery disease in the Coronary Artery Surgery Study (CASS). *N Engl J Med.* 1979;301:230–235.

18. Grzybowski A, Puchalski W, Zieba B, et al. How to improve noninvasive coronary artery disease diagnostics in premenopausal women? The influence of menstrual cycle on ST depression, left ventricle contractility, and chest pain observed during exercise echocardiography in women with angina and normal coronary angiogram. *Am Heart J.* 2008;156:964.e1–e5.

19. Shaw LJ, Peterson E, Shaw LK, et al. Use of a prognostic treadmill score in identifying diagnostic coronary disease subgroups. *Circulation.* 1998; 98: 1622–1630.

20. Chaitman BR, Stone PH, Knatterud GL, Forman SA, Sopko G, Bourassa MG, Pratt C, Rogers WJ, Pepine CJ, Conti CR; ACIP Investigators. Asymptomatic Cardiac Ischemia Pilot (ACIP) study: Impact of anti-ischemia therapy on 12-week rest electrocardiogram and exercise test outcomes. *J Am Coll Cardiol.* 1995;26:585–593.

21. Bruce RA. Evaluation of functional capacity and exercise tolerance of cardiac patients. *Mod Concepts Cardiovasc Dis.* 1956;25:321–326.

22. Froelicher VF Jr, Thompson AJ Jr, Davis G, Stewart AJ, Triebwasser JH. Prediction of maximal oxygen consumption: comparison of the Bruce and Balke treadmill protocols. *Chest.* 1975;68:331–336.

23. Gulati M, Shaw LJ, Thisted RA, Black HR, Bairey Merz CN, Arnsdorf MF. Heart rate response to exercise stress testing in asymptomatic women: the St. *James Women Take Heart Project. Circulation.* 2010;122:130–137.

24. Pellikka P, Nagueh S, Elhendy A, Kuehl C, Sawada S. American Society of Echocardiography recommendations for performance, interpretation, and

application of stress echocardiography. *J Am Soc Echocardiogr*. 2007;20:1021–1041.

25. Kohli P, Gulati M. Exercise stress testing in women: going back to the basics. *Circulation* 2010;122:2570–80.

26. Lakoski SG, Greenland P, Wong ND, et al. Coronary artery calcium scores and risk for cardiovascular events in women classified as 'low risk' based on Framingham risk score: the multi-ethnic study of atherosclerosis (MESA). *Arch Intern Med*. 2007;167:2437–2442.

27. Lewis JF, Lin L, McGorray S, et al. Dobutamine stress echocardiography in women with chest painPilot phase data from the National Heart, Lung and Blood Institute Women's Ischemia Syndrome Evaluation (WISE). *J Am Coll Cardiol*. 1999;33:1462–1468.

28. Budoff MJ, Dowe D, Jollis JG, et al. Diagnostic performance of 64-multidetector row coronary computed tomographic angiography for evaluation of coronary artery stenosis in individuals without known coronary artery disease: results from the prospective multicenter ACCURACY (Assessment by Coronary Computed Tomographic Angiography of Individuals Undergoing Invasive Coronary Angiography) trial. *J Am Coll Cardiol*. 2008;52:1724–1732.

29. Vermeltfoort IA, Raijmakers PG, Riphagen, II, et al. Definitions and incidence of cardiac syndrome X: review and analysis of clinical data. *Clin Res Cardiol*.: official journal of the German Cardiac Society 2010;99:475–481.

30. Lichtlen PR, Bargheer K, Wenzlaff P. Long-term prognosis of patients with anginalike chest pain and normal coronary angiographic findings. *J Am Coll Cardiol*. 1995;25:1013–1018.

31. Radice M, Giudici V, Marinelli G. Long-term follow-up in patients with positive exercise test and angiographically normal coronary arteries (syndrome X). *Am J Cardiol*. 1995;75:620–621.

32. Gulati M, Cooper-DeHoff RM, McClure C, et al. Adverse cardiovascular outcomes in women with nonobstructive coronary artery disease: a report from the Women's Ischemia Syndrome Evaluation Study and the St James Women Take Heart Project. *Arch Intern Med*. 2009;169:843–850.

33. Busko M, Zawahir N, Vaga CP, Bernard A. Healthy life style play vital role in preventing CHD in women. Medscape.<to be completed>

34. Mosca L, Benjamin EJ, Berra K, et al. Effectiveness-based guidelines for the prevention of cardiovascular disease in women—2011 update: a guideline from the American Heart Association. *Circulation*. 2011;123:1243–1262.

35. Berger JS, Brown DL, Becker RC. Low-dose aspirin in patients with stable cardiovascular disease: a meta-analysis. *Am J Med*. 2008 Jan;121(1):43–9.

36. Howard BV, Rossouw JE. Estrogens and cardiovascular disease risk revisited: the Women's Health Initiative. *Curr Opin Lipidol*. 2013;24:493–499.

37. Witt BJ, Jacobsen SJ, Weston SA, et al. Cardiac rehabilitation after myocardial infarction in the community. *J Am Coll Cardiol*. 2004;44:988–996.

38. O'Gara PT, Kushner FG, Ascheim DD, et al. 2013 ACCF/AHA guidelines for the management of ST-elevation myocardial infarction: executive summary: a report of the American College of Cardiology Foundation/American Heart Association Task Force on Practice Guidelines: developed in collaboration with

the American College of Emergency Physicians and Society for Cardiovascular Angiography and Interventions. *Catheter Cardiovasc Interv.* 2013;82:E1–27.

39. Blomkalns AL, Chen AY, Hochman JS, et al. Gender disparities in the diagnosis and treatment of non–ST-segment elevation acute coronary syndromes: Large-scale observations from the CRUSADE (Can Rapid Risk Stratification of Unstable Angina Patients Suppress Adverse Outcomes With Early Implementation of the American College of Cardiology/American Heart Association Guidelines) National Quality Improvement Initiative. *J Am Coll Cardiol.* 2005;45:832–837.

40. Elkayam et al. *Circulation.* 2014;129:1695–1702.

41. Templin et al. *N Eng J Med.* 2015;373:929–938.

42. Berger JS, Bhatt DL, Cannon CP, et al. The relative efficacy and safety of clopidogrel in women and men a sex-specific collaborative meta-analysis. *J Am Coll Cardiol.* 2009;54:1935–1945.

43. Hochman JS, McCabe CH, Stone PH, et al. Outcome and Profile of Women and Men Presenting With Acute Coronary Syndromes: A Report From TIMI IIIB. *J Am Coll Cardiol.* 1997;30:141–148.

44. Clayton TC, Pocock SJ, Henderson RA, et al. Do men benefit more than women from an interventional strategy in patients with unstable angina or non-ST-elevation myocardial infarction? The impact of gender in the RITA 3 trial. *Eur Heart J.* 2004;25:1641–1650.

45. Cannon CP, Weintraub WS, Demopoulos LA, et al. Comparison of early invasive and conservative strategies in patients with unstable coronary syndromes treated with the glycoprotein IIb/IIIa inhibitor tirofiban. *N Engl J Med.* 2001;344:1879–1887.

46. Glaser R, Herrmann HC, Murphy SA, et al. Benefit of an early invasive management strategy in women with acute coronary syndromes. *JAMA.* 2002;288:3124–3129.

47. O'Donoghue M, Boden WE, Braunwald E, et al. Early invasive vs conservative treatment strategies in women and men with unstable angina and non-ST-segment elevation myocardial infarction: a meta-analysis. *JAMA.* 2008;300:71–80.

48. Anderson JL, Adams CD, Antman EM, et al. 2011 ACCF/AHA Focused Update Incorporated Into the ACC/AHA 2007 Guidelines for the Management of Patients With Unstable Angina/Non-ST-Elevation Myocardial Infarction: a report of the American College of Cardiology Foundation/American Heart Association Task Force on Practice Guidelines. *Circulation.* 2011;123:e426–579.

49. Stefanini GG, Baber U, Windecker S, et al. Safety and efficacy of drug-eluting stents in women: a patient-level pooled analysis of randomised trials. *Lancet.* 2013;382:1879–1888.

50. Bell MR, Garratt KN, Bresnahan JF, Holmes DR, Jr. Immediate and long-term outcome after directional coronary atherectomy: analysis of gender differences. *Mayo Clin Proc.* 1994;69:723–729.

51. Casale PN, Whitlow PL, Franco I, Grigera F, Pashkow FJ, Topol EJ. Comparison of major complication rates with new atherectomy devices for percutaneous coronary intervention in women versus men. *Am J Cardiol.* 1993;71:1221–1223.

52. Rao S, Vora A. Transfusion in ischemic heart disease correlation, confounding, and confusion. *J Am Coll Cardiol.* 2015;66(22):2519–2521. doi:10.1016/j.jacc.2015.09.058.

53. Mehta LS, Beckie TM, DeVon H, et al. Acute myocardial infarction in women a scientific statement from the american heart association. *Circulation.* 2016;133:00–00. DOI: 10.1161/.

54. Guagliumi G, Capodanno D, Saia F, et al. Mechanisms of Atherothrombosis and Vascular Response to Primary Percutaneous Coronary Intervention in Women Versus Men With Acute Myocardial Infarction Results of the OCTAVIA Study. *J Am Coll Cardiol Intervent.* 2014;7(9):958–968.

55. Fisher LD, Kennedy JW, Davis KB, et al. Association of sex, physical size, and operative mortality after coronary artery bypass in the Coronary Artery Surgery Study (CASS). *J Thorac Cardiovasc Surg.* 1982;84:334–341.

56. James AH, Jamison MG, Biswas MS, Brancazio LR, Swamy GK, Myers ER. Acute myocardial infarction in pregnancy: a United States population-based study. *Circulation.* 2006;113:1564–1571.

57. Roth A, Elkayam U. Acute myocardial infarction associated with pregnancy. *J Am Coll Cardiol.* 2008;52:171–1780.

58. Colletti PM, Lee KH, Elkayam U. Cardiovascular imaging of the pregnant patient. *AJR, Am J Roentgenol.* 2013;200:515–521.

59. National High Blood Pressure Education Program Working Group Report on High Blood Pressure in Pregnancy. *Am J Obstet Gynecol.* 1990;163:1691–1712.

60. Regitz-Zagrosek V, Oertelt-Prigione S, Prescott E, et al. on behalf of the EUGenMed, Cardiovascular Clinical Study Group. Gender in Cardiovascular Diseases: Impact on Clinical Manifestations, Management, and Outcomes. *Eur Heart J.* 2015;Nov 3:[Epub ahead of print]. See more at: www.acc.org/latest-in-cardiology/ten-points-to-remember/2015/11/19/23/53/gender-in-cardiovascular-diseases?WT.mc_ev=EmailOpen&w_pub=JScan151203&w_nav=JScan#sthash.9SrSs2FQ.dpuf

Index

Note: Page numbers ending in an f refers to a figure; page numbers ending in a t refers to a table.

Management of Complex Cardiovascular Problems, Fourth Edition. Edited by Thach N. Nguyen, Dayi Hu, Shao Liang Chen, Moo Hyun Kim and Cindy L. Grines.
© 2016 John Wiley & Sons, Ltd. Published 2016 by John Wiley & Sons, Ltd.